ALIEN LANDSCAPES?

ALIEN LANDSCAPES?

Interpreting Disordered Minds

Jonathan Glover

The Belknap Press of Harvard University Press
Cambridge, Massachusetts and London, England
2014

Printed in Canada

First printing

Pages 419–422 constitute an extension of the copyright page.

Library of Congress Cataloging-in-Publication Data

Glover, Jonathan.
Alien landscapes? : interpreting disordered minds / Jonathan Glover.
pages cm
Includes bibliographical references and index.
ISBN 978-0-674-36836-1 (alk. paper)
1. Psychiatry—Decision making. 2. Mental illness—Diagnosis. I. Title.
RC455.2.D42G56 2014
616.89'17—dc23 2014005635

To Sam

alienist: former term for psychiatrist. Origin: mid 19th century: from French *aliéniste,* based on Latin *alienus* "of another"

—Oxford Dictionaries Online

Homo sum, humani nihil a me alienum puto.
I am human; I think nothing human alien to me.

—Terence

CONTENTS

PREFACE

This book is about mental disorders: how to think about them and how well those of us outside can get a feel for what they are like from inside.

Some dispute the boundaries of mental disorder. Is autism a disorder, or should it be seen as "neurodiversity"? Is antisocial personality disorder rightly named, or is it just ruthless amorality? Is addiction mental illness or just moral weakness? Is either medication or psychotherapy appropriate to ease the devastating grief of bereavement, or should we avoid medicalizing this normal human experience?

When and how much do mental disorders impair agency and responsibility? When should acting under the influence of severe depression excuse someone from responsibility for what she does? What do some disorders do to a person's identity? When someone with schizophrenia shows unprovoked hostility and aggression, does that reflect him, or is it his illness? How should we draw boundaries here? How much is the original person still present in severe dementia?

This book is about the human interpretation of disordered states. Are mental disorders impenetrably alien? The genetics and brain chemistry of some of these states are starting to be understood, but do the inner landscapes of these states defy empathy at the psychological level? The question of human interpretation is important, not only for psychiatrists, psychotherapists, psychoanalysts, and psychiatric nurses. It is important for, above all, people who have these disorders, and for their families and friends, and for others who are simply interested in this area of human experience. This book is written for anyone who hopes it may be possible to interpret and understand disordered states—and for anyone who hopes, despite a disorder, to be interpreted, to be understood.

It may be presumptuous for someone who is neither a psychiatrist nor any other kind of mental health professional to write a book about these questions. Inevitably the limits of my knowledge will sometimes show through, although I hope these limits may be outweighed by the ideas and the reasons behind them. Mental disorder straddles the boundary between the sciences and the humanities. The subject I teach—philosophy—is in the humanities, and this book has a humanities approach. Many mental health professionals are notably open to viewing mental disorder through the lenses of art, philosophy, poetry, novels, and the humanities in general. Some of them may feel the book presumes too much in this regard. Again, I hope there may be justifying benefits.

The book has several different origins.

In Broadmoor, a secure psychiatric hospital, I interviewed a group of men who had been diagnosed as having "antisocial personality disorder." The aim was to explore the claim sometimes made that they "lack a conscience." This was part of a larger project carried out with the psychiatrist Dr. Gwen Adshead. The other part of the project, under the stimulus of an invitation from the neurologist Martin Rossor, involved asking similar questions of a group of people diagnosed with frontotemporal dementia.

In 2003 I gave the Tanner Lectures on Human Values at Princeton. I chose the title "Towards Humanism in Psychiatry" and lectured on psychiatric interpretation and on the relations between psychiatric disorder and a person's identity. The part on identity developed thoughts I had first aired in the 2002 Aubrey Lewis Lecture at the Institute of Psychiatry at King's College London.

I have a long-standing interest in the intersection of psychiatry and philosophy. My first book, *Responsibility,* published more than forty years ago, included chapters on the concept of mental illness and on mental illness and responsibility. I was drawn then to the depth and difficulty of the philosophical questions raised by psychiatry. Rereading those chapters after writing this book, I was pleased that, although my ideas have developed since, there was little I wanted to repudiate in that earlier effort. I was less pleased to notice how very little I then knew about psychiatry. I admit, however, to being now a bit envious of the youthful effrontery.

The interest remained. Fifteen years ago, on coming to the Centre of Medical Law and Ethics at King's College London, I cooperated with colleagues in the Institute of Psychiatry and the Department of Philosophy to set up and teach a master's course in the philosophy of mental disorder. In the Centre's master's course in medical ethics and law, I also set up and taught a module on psychiatric ethics.

This book did not originate purely in intellectual curiosity. Although I have not been hit by psychiatric disorder, its shadow has touched my family. A minor consequence of that has lasted for nearly a quarter of a century. Without their permission, and without their realizing it, I have been watching many psychiatrists and psychiatric teams at work. They have provided stimulus to reflect on their different approaches—their assumptions, their patterns of thought, and their ways of interpreting other people. I have also noticed how important are both the strengths and the limitations of the different kinds and degrees of perceptiveness and sensitivity they bring to their work. They have provided stimulus to reflect on their different approaches, on their assumptions, their patterns of thought, and their ways of interpreting other people. Although this is not on the surface of the book, I hope it has given it an extra dimension.

ALIEN LANDSCAPES?

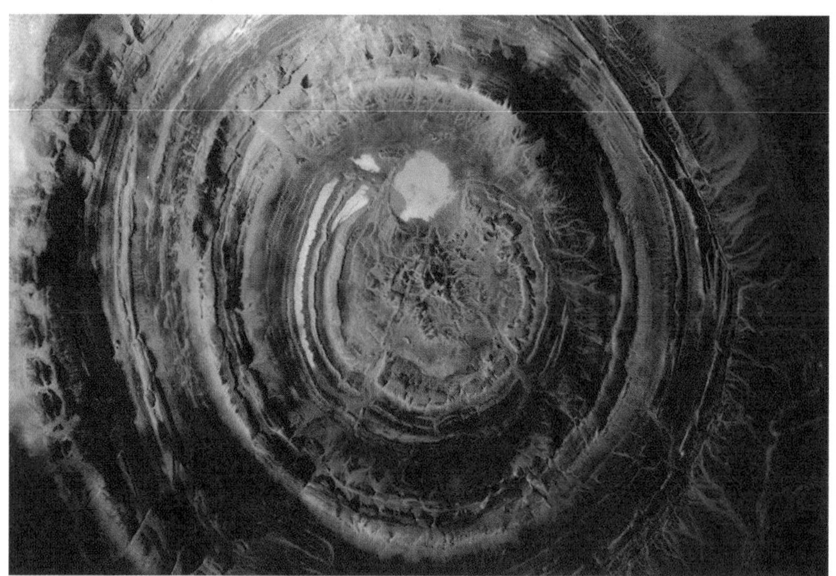

Figure I.1: Richat Structure, NASA.

PROLOGUE

Alien Landscapes?

An alien landscape? One of the landmarks when Earth is seen from space is the thirty-mile-wide Richat Structure, or Eye of the Sahara, found in Mauritania (Figure I.1). Some thought the Richat Structure was the work of extraterrestrials. Current evidence suggests it is a dome-shaped rock, first pushed to the surface and then eroded over hundreds of millions of years. The process of understanding is not yet over. We still do not know why the Eye of the Sahara is circular. But a dramatic "alien" landscape can yield to undramatic incremental interpretation.

A century ago Karl Jaspers published a great philosophical book on psychiatry, his *General Psychopathology*. It included some classic pessimism about the limits of psychiatric interpretation. Jaspers said it was possible to have empathy for people with mood disorders, but not for those with schizophrenia: "These personalities have something baffling about them, which baffles our understanding in a peculiar way. There is something queer, cold, inaccessible, rigid and petrified there, even when the patients are quite sensible and can be addressed and even when they are eager to talk about themselves. We may think we understand dispositions furthest from our own, but when faced with such people, we feel a gulf which defies description."[1] Anyone familiar with schizophrenia will recognize the bafflement Jaspers describes. But the discussion here will challenge the pessimism and oppose giving up too soon.

People often see the inner lives of those with a major mental disorder like schizophrenia as impenetrably alien. This assumption should be challenged. *Homo sum, humani nihil a me alienum puto.* We long ago moved beyond "possessed by devils," the equivalent of the "extraterrestrials" account of the Richat Structure. We are starting—still patchily—to decipher the genetic, neurobiological, and environmental causes of mental disorders. Is it really impossible at the *psychological* level to get deeper inside people with such disorders? Can we hope for interpretations that make the alien inner landscapes more intelligible to us?

Psychiatry is both humanist and scientific. Here, as elsewhere, humanism and science are not opposed. But the compatibility is not always obvious. In psychiatry it is sometimes necessary to resolve what seem to be tensions between the two.

Human activities take place at many different levels, which need to be understood in different ways. Here is one basic contrast. We are vastly complex physical and chemical systems: genetic, epigenetic, neurochemical, and other mechanisms interact to produce what we do—whether in its "normal" undisturbed versions or in psychiatrically disturbed ones. But we are also human beings: people with thoughts, emotions, hopes, beliefs, decisions, intentions, relationships, and interpretations of each other. Out of this human side also comes what we do—whether in its "normal" undisturbed versions or in psychiatrically disturbed ones. How these two "levels" or "sides" can be integrated into a single coherent whole is a deep problem for all the human sciences, including psychiatry.

At a practical level psychiatrists need to excel on the scientific side and on the human side. The scientific side requires a decent understanding of the outlines of the relevant sciences, including current developments. It needs a scientific cast of mind: basing treatment on evidence, not being more confident than the evidence warrants, being willing to change beliefs as new evidence emerges. In research it means coming up with new questions and ideas, competently testing them, and not overinterpreting the results. This is an ideal to which even the best probably only approximate.

On the scientific side we have a reasonably clear idea of what to aim for. On the human side things are much less clear. Here too psychiatrists, psychotherapists, and others vary in quality. There is the whole range from the humanly obtuse to the wonderfully perceptive, from the arrogant or bored to the supportive, intuitive, and imaginative. Psychiatrists who excel at connecting with patients sometimes express concern that they are being guided by impressions of a person rather than by strictly applying diagnostic categories. "Am I being unscientific?" "When I do this, am I only pretending to exercise professional skills as a psychiatrist?"

The disciplines dealing with mental disorder are both human and scientific, although we will look mainly at the human issues here. One reason for addressing them is that it is so much less clear what it is to be good on that side. When this is explored, it turns out that psychiatry is bound up both with deep conceptual issues and with questions about human values. This book has two central themes: psychiatric interpretation and the role of values. These themes are analyzed separately at first but come together in mutual support at the end.

Interpretation

While I will take for granted the great value of biological psychiatry, I will make a case for placing much more emphasis than is common on human interpretation.

Part 1 of this book presents an interpretation of interviews I conducted at Broadmoor Hospital with people who have a diagnosis of antisocial personality disorder. Such people are sometimes said to "lack a conscience." Those interviewed were asked about right and wrong and other questions about how they thought about moral issues. The aim was to sketch a map of their moral worlds. How far do theirs differ from, or overlap with, the moral worlds of other people? Are there gaps that might fit the view that people with this diagnosis lack a conscience? The interviewees also talked a lot, unbidden but appreciated, about their lives. This suggested some tentative interpretations of how they may have come to be as they are.

These interviews offer a first glimpse of the theme of human interpretation. I will argue that bland, abstract accounts of antisocial personality disorder obscure much about the condition. The voices of people with psychiatric diagnoses should be listened to attentively. Efforts should be made to interpret what they say as clues to their inner worlds.

Part 2 makes a case for relying on human interpretation. It draws on neuroscience, psychology, philosophy, literature, and art to show how our experience is saturated with interpretation, and I outline some of the main ways we interpret the world, especially people. These chapters aim to show the scientific basis for broad reliance on human interpretation of people. Our interpretations are obviously fallible, but there are good reasons for expecting them to be reliable enough to be valuable.

Part 3 is about the role of human interpretation in psychiatry. I identify lines of inquiry worth pursuing and discuss the interpretation of autism and of delusions in schizophrenia and other disorders. Part of interpreting people with these conditions is trying to piece together how they in turn interpret other people and the world, and seeing how their interpretation may be going wrong. The account of delusions draws on, and aims to extend, psychologists' work on what may be going on. My focus here is on how normal mechanisms of interpretation may be distorted in delusions. There is also a chapter seeking clues about the inner world of people with psychiatric problems by looking at their art.

Values, the Good Life, and the Boundaries of Mental Disorder

The history of psychiatry has a dark side. Part 4 links this dark side with questions about the boundaries of disorder. One lesson learned is that not everything a culture considers deviant should be medically treated. The boundaries of psychiatry matter. Where should they be? Is psychiatry simply a medical discipline? Should problems such as "personality disorders" really be seen as illnesses? If psychiatry's boundaries are wider than the boundaries of psychiatric medicine, can they be drawn without psychiatry becoming a general social service for dealing with *all* the problems people have?

Answers to these questions bring out the relevance to psychiatry of human values, especially ideas of what a good human life is. When these values are invoked in drawing the disputed boundaries of the field, they also shape both the justification and the content of psychiatric treatment.

Human flourishing can be impaired in ways that make psychiatric help appropriate. Psychiatrists try to restore human beings, not Martians, to how they should be. Ideas of what human beings need, if they are to think, feel, and function well, are linked to ideas of human nature. Two of the currently important ways of thinking about human nature involve very different approaches, with different implications for psychiatry. One set of ideas comes from evolutionary psychology. The other comes from thinking about values. The picture of human nature coming from evolutionary psychology is relevant to psychiatry, but it needs to be supplemented with ideas rooted in human values.

Values and Interpretation

Parts 5 and 6 bring together these central themes of interpretation and values by investigating the interaction between psychiatric disorders and aspects of a good human life. In particular I argue that the interpretation of some psychiatric conditions can be deepened by a framework of thought explicitly linked to the values that shape our conception of a flourishing life.

What are the relevant contours of human flourishing? Here are two. We think of ourselves as responsible agents, able to make decisions and act on them. And we think of ourselves as having our own identity and, to some extent, being able to shape the kind of person we are. Psychiatric disorders can undermine these contours in ways that present serious intellectual challenges.

I approach the topic of individual flourishing from the human end, with the unscientific categories of agency, responsibility, values, and identity. Starting here presents many problems. In everyday life people take these concepts for granted and do not spell them out. We need to sharpen our focus and define our terms if we are to enlist such concepts in approaching problems raised by psychiatry. Philosophers, aiming for greater precision, have done much analytical work on these concepts. As elsewhere, philosophical analysis can be "applied" to psychiatry. But in the often paradoxical world of psychiatric disorder, the concepts themselves may need to be changed and extended to fit the human phenomena.

Part 5 draws on philosophy in discussing some psychiatric conditions that obstruct agency. What is the contrast between normal and impaired agency? What is going on at the human, psychological level in addictions? Are people with antisocial personality disorder victims of a disability or should they be blamed for their antisocial acts? Is there a coherent account of when someone with a psychiatric disorder should or should not be held responsible for an action? Part 6, about identity, continues to ask philosophical questions. In what ways can individuals' sense of their own identity can be impaired? Can we make a clear distinction between what comes from the person and what comes from his or her psychiatric illness?

In these last parts of the book philosophy is not the main focus. First-person accounts figure prominently throughout the book—as surely they should, in any attempt to understand the inner landscapes of these conditions?—but in these last two parts, they occupy most of the foreground.

The voices in Broadmoor were ones I heard. I was lucky to be able to ask follow-up questions designed to help in the interpretation. In these last parts of the book, I have drawn on many published first-person accounts. Whether interpreting the interviews or the published accounts, I have been searching for patterns in the hope of sketching maps of inner landscapes going beyond a single person. Obviously not all people with a particular psychiatric diagnosis are the same. Where a general map is sketched, it is likely that later, finer-grained investigation will bring out variations between different individuals and different groups.

This method is a first stage. Generalizations about people diagnosed as having some psychiatric disorder are not established by a few anecdotes or by the quoted responses of a few people. The focus here is on the close—often intuitive—interpretation of what people say. The hope is to see things that get lost in large-scale studies. But of course, one hope is that these intuitive sketches will stimulate proper scientific testing of their suggestions.

We now have many first-person reports, a rich resource that was not available in the time of Karl Jaspers. They start to reveal the contours of impaired agency. They show something of impaired, diminished or distorted identity from the inside. Because they do not have the limiting abstractness of textbook lists of symptoms or neurochemical accounts, they offer a deeper understanding of the inner landscape that those accounts too often flatten.

PART ONE

"Antisocial Personality," Values, Psychiatry

That girls are raped, that two boys knife a third,
Were axioms to him, who'd never heard
Of any world where promises were kept,
Or one could weep because another wept.

—W. H. Auden, "The Shield of Achilles"

I and the public know
What all schoolchildren learn,
Those to whom evil is done
Do evil in return.

—W. H. Auden, "September 1, 1939"

1

Socratic Questions in Broadmoor

"Psychopaths" are at the extreme. The tool most used to diagnose "antisocial personality disorder" is the Hare Psychopathy Checklist, a scale devised by the Canadian psychologist Robert D. Hare. There is a cutoff score above which the test taker is given the diagnosis of antisocial personality disorder. Being a "psychopath" is widely considered to be an extreme version of this. Something often said about those called psychopaths, and by extension about the others within the broader category, is that they lack a conscience.

This claim is intriguing. Are there really people who completely lack a conscience? If so, how does this come about? Are they born with something missing? Or does something happen to them that destroys their conscience? Most fundamentally, what does it mean to say that they lack a conscience?

I have spent a lot of my life teaching ethics, which is still taught by the method invented by Socrates. This starts by asking people what they think is right or wrong, pressing them to state their views with maximum clarity and explicitness. Then they are challenged to defend their beliefs in the face of counterexamples and opposing argument. The student is pushed into a journey of self-exploration, rather than being given "the answers" by the teacher. Some students, those who think being taught is being given information or conclusions to take away, are baffled by this and doubt that they are being taught properly. Be that as it may, the teacher learns a lot about the students and about the very different structures and styles of moral belief and thinking that people have. There are very different views about what conscience is.

To say that people with antisocial personality disorder lack a conscience could mean one or more of several things. It could mean that they lack any empathy for other people: that they cannot imagine how other people feel. Or it could mean that they lack sympathy: that they can imagine the feelings of, for instance, those they hurt, but do not care about them. It might mean that they do not feel guilt. It could be that they lack certain moral concepts, such as "cruel," "unfair," "dishonest," "right," or "selfish." Or it might mean that they lack a sense of moral identity: a conception of the sort of person they are, or of the sort of person they hope to be, together with a set of values guiding those hopes. The conscience or lack of conscience of people with this diagnosis seemed a promising field to investigate.

Dr. Gwen Adshead, a psychiatrist at Broadmoor Hospital, has many patients with the diagnosis of antisocial personality disorder. She and I found that we shared an interest in their morality or lack of it, and we jointly devised a project to investigate these questions in some of those patients in Broadmoor.

My part of the project used a series of interviews with men who had a diagnosis of antisocial personality disorder. The aim was to probe their morality and values by asking questions about ethics. Partly in homage to the inventor of the approach, but perhaps with a touch of pretentiousness, I called this series "the Socratic interviews." The following account reports on these "Socratic" interviews. To introduce them, I will say a bit about antisocial personality disorder and then outline briefly the content of the interviews and the guiding questions behind them.

Antisocial Personality Disorder

There are many questions, to be raised later, about the general category "personality disorders." The particular diagnosis of antisocial personality disorder—including psychopathy at the severe end—is heir to a tangled history of moral, legal, and psychiatric concepts. They include those marked out by the nineteenth-century term "moral insanity" and the early twentieth-century terms "constitutional psychopathic inferiority" and "sociopath."[1] The modern conception of a psychopath has been greatly influenced by Hervey Cleckley, who in the mid-twentieth century was a professor of psychiatry at the University of Georgia Medical School. He reported on the psychopaths among his patients in *The Mask of Sanity*.[2]

Cleckley's hunch (though he knew he lacked evidence to support it) was that psychopaths were born that way: "Increasingly I have come to believe that some subtle and profound defect in the human organism, probably inborn but not hereditary, plays the chief role in the psychopath's puzzling and spectacular failure to experience life normally and to carry on a career acceptable to society."[3] His book has two sides, one influencing popular stereotypes and legends about psychopaths and the other influencing psychiatric thinking.

Cleckley had many of the prejudices of his time and place. His book attacks modern "permissiveness," and "intellectuals and esthetes" for their liking of "what is generally regarded as perverse, dispirited or distastefully unintelligible." What they liked included the writings of Gide (who "openly insists that pederasty is the superior and preferable way of life for adolescent boys") and Joyce ("a collection of erudite gibberish indistinguishable to most people from the familiar word salad produced by hebephrenic patients on the back wards of any state hospital").[4] In his description of one male patient who had had oral sex with four black men, Cleckley's disapproval focuses, not on whether the men's consent was genuine, but mainly on the choice of partners. The man "hit upon the notion of picking up four Negro men who worked in the fields not far from his residence. In a locality where the Ku Klux Klan (and its well-known attitudes) at the time enjoyed a good deal of popularity, this intelligent and in some respects distinguished young man showed no compunction about taking from the field these unwashed laborers whom he concealed in the back of a pickup truck, with him into a well-known place of amorous rendezvous . . . Although he expressed regret and said his prank was quite a mistake, he seemed totally devoid of any deep embarrassment."[5]

Cleckley helped create the popular stereotype of the psychopath as not really human, a satanic monster hiding behind the mask of sanity—"the exquisitely deceptive mask of the psychopath," who uses extraordinary facility and charm to pose as a normal person.

> We are dealing here not with a complete man at all but with something that suggests a subtly constructed reflex machine which can mimic the human personality perfectly. This smoothly operating psychic apparatus reproduces consistently not only specimens of good human reasoning but also appropriate simulations of normal human emotion in response to nearly all the varied stimuli of life. So perfect is the reproduction of a whole and normal man that no-one who examines him in a clinical setting can point out in scientific or objective terms why, or how, he is not real. . . . The psychopath, however perfectly he mimics man theoretically, that is to say, when

> he speaks for himself in words, fails altogether when he is put into the practice of actual living.[6]

Cleckley's influence on psychiatrists lay not in his image of the monster behind the mask but in his powerful descriptions of the behavior of some of his psychopathic patients.

One memorable case was "Milt," who was 19 when he arrived at the hospital. He had done a lot of antisocial things. When criticized for them, he made charming apologies, but he never seemed really to appreciate the seriousness of what he had done, and he continued to carry on in the same way. Here is one example: Once he was driving his mother back from the hospital after she had major surgery. The car broke down in the middle of a very long bridge. With darkness falling, Milt set out to walk to a garage half a mile away to get a fuse. He said he would get a ride and be back in less than fifteen minutes. After an hour his distraught mother managed to get a ride home. She called hospitals to see if Milt had had an accident.

On the way to the garage, Milt had stopped at a cigar store for ten to fifteen minutes to check football results. Then he called on a girl living nearby and chatted casually for an hour. All this time he remembered his mother was waiting. When he finally collected the car and came home, he was cross with his mother for not having waited. He showed "a bland immunity to any recognition that he had behaved irresponsibly or inconsiderately."[7]

Cleckley used this and other case descriptions to draw up a list of the distinguishing characteristics of psychopaths. These included superficial charm, unreliability, insincerity, lack of remorse, egocentricity, emotional poverty, and a failure to follow any life plan. This "Cleckley psychopath" is the origin of current diagnosis, including the Hare Psychopathy Checklist.[8]

In the Psychopathy Checklist, Robert Hare distinguishes two factors that are highly correlated with each other but have different patterns of intercorrelations with other variables. Factor One represents personality traits typical of the syndrome: "selfish, callous and remorseless use of others." Factor Two reflects socially deviant behavior: "chronically unstable, antisocial and socially deviant lifestyle." If the diagnosis of being a psychopath is supposed to explain antisocial behavior, Factor One does the work, as Factor Two hardly gets beyond listing the behavior to be explained. And Factor One is more relevant to questions about conscience. It includes glibness and superficial charm, a grandiose sense of self-worth, pathological lying, being conning and manipulative, lack of remorse or guilt, shallow emotions, being callous and lacking empathy, and failure to accept responsibility for one's own actions.

Hare himself sees psychopathy in terms of Factor One, and sees the diagnosis of antisocial personality disorder (based on both factors) as being of limited use. He claims that the personality traits of Factor One have predictive value, whereas a diagnosis of antisocial personality disorder catches a mixed bag and predicts little.[9]

There are questions about how people end up with a diagnosis of antisocial personality disorder. The people I interviewed in Broadmoor were there because they had committed a major crime and because they were assessed as having a psychiatric problem. The latter distinguished them from "ordinary" criminals needing punishment. There are also questions about whether a medical diagnosis is appropriate. How different are they from ruthless people in ordinary life who manage to get their way either without committing crimes or else without getting caught? How do they compare with some of the politicians, businesspeople, media magnates, heads of academic institutions, captains of industry, and others who may also sometimes be lying, callous, manipulative charmers with a grandiose sense of self-worth and little remorse? And how do they compare with people who have committed similar crimes but who are sent to prison rather than to see psychiatrists?

Amoralists?

One obvious question is how far someone with the antisocial record of Factor Two, combined with the glib, conning, callous personality of Factor One, should qualify as having a disorder rather than just as being morally bad. Could the person with antisocial personality disorder turn out to be the "rational amoralist" who haunts philosophical books on ethics?

At least as far back as Plato, philosophers have tried to meet the challenge of explaining why anyone should bother about the claims of morality. One form of the challenge is the demand for arguments that will defeat the amoralist. But this theoretical construct, the "amoralist," turns out to be a slippery character.

The simple version of the amoralist is someone utterly self-interested and prepared to trample ruthlessly on anyone else. But because society is set up to deter people from acting like this, a rational amoralist will have to operate in heavy disguise. To avoid legal punishment or social ostracism, a self-interested person must try to "pass" as someone who respects the interests of others. Whatever the underlying attitude, at least the behavior is less of a threat. A second change results if the amoralist has ordinary human desires for relationships. The deepest relationships are incompatible with being approached in a spirit of self-interested calculation. Emotional involvement with others may make some cracks in the barrier against altruism.

As a result of these changes, there is a paring down to the conceptual core of amoralism. The pure "conceptual" amoralist might not be selfish. He might often care about other people and act toward them with benevolence and even generosity. But he does this because he wants to, not because of thoughts that he ought to do so or about moral obligations. To "moral" uses of words like "ought," "right," "wrong," "duty," and "obligation," he will react as Oscar Wilde did when asked if he was patriotic: "Patriotism is not one of my words." One aim of these interviews was to see how far people diagnosed with antisocial personality disorder are like either the original or the modified amoralist.

The Moral Restraints

The people being interviewed had all done some terrible things. (All their names and initials have been changed.) The interview plan started from a framework I used for previous work on the psychology of twentieth-century atrocities. Thinking about Auschwitz, the Gulag, Hiroshima, or the Rwandan genocide, there is an obvious question: How can people do such things? I approached this by asking about the restraints in everyday life that prevent people from torturing or killing each other. I proposed a set of restraints and then asked what had happened to them in Nazi Germany, Rwanda, and other places. In these interviews I used a similar strategy. When the people I was interviewing committed their terrible crimes, were the normal restraints overwhelmed by other things? If so, how were they overwhelmed, and by what? Or did they lack the normal restraints? Either way, what went on inside them? How did they think about what they did?

What are the factors that, most of the time, restrain people from cruelty, violence, and killing? One obvious factor is self-interest. The death of a competitor might be profitable. Assaulting an enemy might give psychological satisfaction. But society is usually organized in ways intended to make the cost too high. For rational self-interested people, such temptations usually are outweighed by the risks of social disgrace and long-term imprisonment.

Of course, self-interested calculation is not the whole story for most people. Plato's brilliantly simple "ring of Gyges" thought experiment is designed to bring this out. If you had a ring that made you invisible, so that you could commit crimes without suffering punishment and disgrace, would you have any reason not to steal, not to rape, or not to attack people who antagonize you? The ring of Gyges is a challenge to spell out the moral resources we have: the restraining motives that are not just self-interested.

These moral restraints are rooted in our psychology. Central are what can be called "the human responses." We are capable of feeling sympathy for other people. Although the response can be deadened or overridden, we can be delighted by others' joy or distressed by their suffering. And we have a tendency to show other people respect. Again the response can be deadened or overridden, but most of us avoid behavior that humiliates others. We are appalled to see someone being spat on. These human responses of sympathy and respect are linked to empathy: to our imagining what it is like for someone else to experience suffering or indignity.

Another key moral restraint is our sense of our own moral identity. Most of us have an idea of the sort of person we are. We sometimes have a picture of the sort of person we would like to be, together with values that shape that picture. Even if the picture is not well worked out or is partly unconscious, it may function as a moral restraint. We may at least know the kind of person we do *not* want to be, and this may hold us back from working in the arms trade or becoming a television evangelist.

The questions were designed mainly to see how far these moral restraints were present in the men I interviewed. Hoping to make the questions unthreatening, I avoided asking "Do you have a sense of right and wrong?" Instead I asked about what they would teach children about right and wrong.

I also asked whether, if they drove a car, they would park in a disabled space, and what their reasons were for doing or not doing so. If they said they would not park there, the follow-up question about reasons could tap into self-interest: "I would not want to get wheel-clamped" or "It might be awkward if people noticed." There was also the hope of exploring some of the moral resources: sympathy for disabled people, respect for their rights, or even the sense of moral identity: "I would not want to be the kind of person who was so mean as to do that." Some questions were intended to explore their sense of moral identity: "How would you describe the sort of person you think you are? Do you have an idea of the sort of person you would like to be?" Others explored their understanding of moral concepts such as fairness, or whether there were things that made them feel guilty.

I knew that the men I would interview not only had been diagnosed with antisocial personality disorder but had also been convicted of at least one serious crime, such as murder or rape, but before the interviews I avoided finding out what crimes they had committed, as I did not want to be biased by this knowledge. In the interviews I did not ask what their crimes had been. (Sometimes they volunteered this information without being asked.) But in order to explore their capacity for empathy and sympathy, I did ask questions along the lines of "When you did whatever it was, did you imagine how the people you harmed felt? *Could* you imagine how they felt? Did you care about how they felt?"

The Interviews as Conversational and Intuitive

The interviews were "semistructured." That is, a standard set of questions was in place, but I did not rigidly adhere to it. I felt free sometimes to ask "leading questions," where it seemed this might trigger something interesting or clarify an obscure comment. The aim was something conversational rather than a strictly scientific interview. My hope was to encourage the sort of informality and ease that conversations can have in a more ordinary context. The flexibility of semistructured interviews gave scope to intuitive hunches about what might be interesting or revealing. When a person said something of that kind, I felt free to follow it up regardless of the original plan.

The interviews were intended to be qualitative rather than quantitative, employing open-ended questions rather than those requiring yes-or-no answers. The aim has been an intuitive understanding of how members of the group think about right and wrong, about themselves, and about their values. The intuitive understanding can perhaps be compared to that of a historian trying to get an idea of what H. H. Asquith was like from his letters, or trying to get a feel for the mind of Hitler from the records of his table talk or of the books he read. While not lending themselves to numerical analysis, these sources may still give a useful feel for the person.

A piece of qualitative research will often raise questions that require quantitative research. In this study, for instance, these interviews were not also given to a control group. Gwen Adshead and I considered doing this but decided against it. The control group could have been students, people in a psychiatric hospital with a different diagnosis, soldiers, nurses, or people in regular prisons. Different control groups would generate very different sets of similarities and contrasts. Each possible control group would have tilted the emphasis of the study in a different direction. Having a control group would have allowed measurement, but we thought the advantages of this would have been outweighed by the tilting effect. We wanted a broad picture of this group, not a picture mainly of the particular contrasts between them and, say, students.

But the picture based on the intuitive and conversational interviews needs further testing. The conclusions to be outlined here are suggestions. They need to be placed on firmer foundations by studies using comparative and quantitative methods. Our interviewees were psychiatric patients. They were convicted violent criminals. They had the diagnosis of antisocial personality disorder. To establish how far their distinctive personality contributed to what they said would of course require quantitative comparisons with those in the other categories. A first step would be to test some of the suggestions by a study with a control group of people without a psychiatric diagnosis but convicted of similar crimes. The picture here is a sketch. It aims partly to give an intuitive feel for a group of people whose own way of seeing things is not much understood and partly to suggest hypotheses that can be tested in future studies.

2

The Contours of a Moral Landscape

One of the questions was, What sorts of things are wrong, and what makes them so? (This question was usually put in terms of what children should be taught, in an attempt to make it less threatening or accusing.) The question tapped into the continuum between what can be called moral "depth" and "shallowness."

Moral Depth and Shallowness

The question about what things are wrong sometimes elicited answers of striking shallowness.

> CQ: They shouldn't swear, you know, do what your mother tells you to do, you know, do well at school, when you grow up, you know. Be careful who you mix with. Don't talk to strangers, you know. Things like that.
> *Which is more wrong—bullying or swearing?*
> Hmm, swearing and bullying is wrong, both wrong in my eyes.
> *Both the same?*
> Yeah, both the same.

> IQ: But they said I've set myself a pretty high moralistic standard.
> *What can you say about your very high moralistic standards?*
> Well, I don't swear in front of females. I'm respectful. I mean I believe in opening doors, and if a female is walking along, be it a patient, or a member of staff, I let them go through the door first, and things like that.

Some were inarticulate when asked to go beyond listing specific things they thought wrong and to give reasons for items being on the list. But sometimes a more general view (such as "things you would not like if they were done to you" or "things that in the long run will not make you happy") did emerge.

QA: One day I bought my wife a dozen red roses and put them on top of the television for when she come in and when my son see them he cut them off with a pair of scissors. Well, I didn't chastise him. My wife chastised him.

If you had been talking to him, what would you have liked to put across? What do you think children should be taught about right and wrong?

Not to go out stealing. Not to go out fighting and just walk away. It takes a better man to walk away than just standing and fight. Not to go out and call people names and all that. Not to get in trouble, really.

But if you were bringing up your children, you'd think of telling them these things . . . They mustn't cut roses off, they mustn't shout after other people. Supposing the children said, "What makes all these things wrong?" What is it they have in common that makes them wrong?

Well, it's just abusive, that's all. It's just abusive . . . being abusive all the time.

Supposing you were bringing up a child and he says, "You tell me all these things are wrong, but what makes them wrong?" What makes all these things—stealing and lying and abusing people—what makes them all wrong?

Well, it makes them wrong—it isn't their property. It belongs to someone else. Someone else has bought it, or built it or had it given, or something like that, and it's not your property. It's their possession. It's theirs.

What about shouting after old people? What makes that wrong?

Shouting after old people? Well, I find that's mickey-taking [making fun of them] more than anything. That's wrong, abusing old people . . . I used to chastise my two little girls when they used to shout at Mrs. Hopkins who used to live next door. She had two sticks and they used to take the mickey out of her . . . One day they could be the same and somebody could start shouting at you and how would you like it?

What is the distinction between depth and shallowness here? Depth can come from serious reflection on why things matter. This reflection might be about oneself. What sort of life do I want to lead and why? What sort of person do I want to be? It might be about religion or society. None of this necessarily involves much concern for other people. On the other hand, depth can come, not from reflection, but from an intuitive feel for other people and for what matters to them. The question about how you would like it if someone started shouting at you has at least some depth. But the emphasis on letting women go through the door first and on not swearing are shallow because conventional. They show no signs either of reflection on reasons or of a feel for what really affects people. This applies most clearly to the view that swearing and bullying are equally bad.

Self-Interest, Amoralism, and the Ring of Gyges

What principles of selection, if any, were they using? Why would they teach children to do some things but not others? Some interviewees oscillated between reasons that appealed to ideas of right and wrong or to concern for other people and reasons appealing to self-interest. The emphasis was strongly on self-interest.

> *When you're talking about younger children, say children aged about 6 or 7, what would you teach them about right and wrong?*
>
> ZC: Well, I would teach them . . . not to misbehave, not to steal. I would tell them the reasons, though. I would not just say to them—don't steal because it's wrong. I would tell them the reason. Because if you steal, the police would catch you eventually, they would lock you up and you would suffer. I would tell them that way.
>
> *Do you know any other reasons?*
>
> Well, that it's wrong. I would explain to them—how would you like someone to steal your property? You wouldn't like. So don't steal other people's property. And also because it's important—you'll be locked up, locked in prison and well—you suffer. You lose your freedom.

Others gave reasons that appealed simply to self-interest.

> *What would you teach them is right and wrong? What have you got in mind?*
>
> NB: Um, teach them not to talk to strangers, um, not to get on the wrong side of the law, break the law, um, teach them things that I've been through, teach them not to do what I did, type of thing, so teach them different. Get a good education, get a good job.
>
> *Suppose you were teaching your children not to talk to strangers, get a good education, not to break the law. They turn 'round at the age of 13 and say, "Well, OK, you're telling us all this, but why? What's the reason behind it all?" What would you say?*
>
> Um. [long silence] Because you need a job in life and a good education in life to get anywhere. If you don't, then you're just going to be um, on the dole, living in hostels and bedsits for ages, no money, hardly any clothes, can't get yourself a good meal. And that's why you need a good education and a job, and when you're on the dole and living in a bedsit, and you've got nothing to your name, then you start stealing from shops, food from shops. You get caught, you get in trouble with the law.

When the results of getting caught are so prominent in the replies, it is natural to wonder what the question about the ring of Gyges will elicit. Some, understandably, were a bit thrown by it. Sometimes it was hard to be sure how much their responses reflected a real attitude and how much they reflected the need to say *something* as an answer to questions they found hard and perhaps stressful.

> *In general you think people should do the right thing?*
>
> LF: Yeah.
>
> *Even if they could get away with doing the wrong thing? What's the reason for doing the right thing if you can get away with not doing it?*
>
> Say again?
>
> *Well, suppose you could get away with not getting caught, what's the point of bothering about doing the right thing?*

Well, I don't know [he laughs] to be honest. Um, depends, I don't know, I don't know.

There was once a philosopher who said that if we had a ring that made us invisible, there would be a question about whether we need bother about morality at all . . . What would you think about somebody who said, "Well, we don't need to bother about right and wrong, if we can get away with it because of being invisible"?

I dunno.

Would you feel you had any reason to do the right thing?

No, not really.

You could steal but you were invisible so nobody would see it's you. You'd do it?

Well, I suppose so, yeah.

Others were not so thrown by the question. Often the first response is to doubt the plausibility of what such fairytale thought experiments assume. Would invisibility really be a reliable protection against being caught?

The Greek philosopher Plato had the idea that if we had a ring that made us invisible, there would be a question that we had any reason not to steal. If we had a ring that made us invisible, we'd never be caught. Would there be any reasons for not stealing then?

ZC: Say you're invisible, you may get away with it maybe one hundred times. But eventually they will suss [figure] you out—somebody who is invisible is doing this and they will probably be more . . . look out for.

So you will get caught in the end?

Yeah . . . They suss out that some invisible person is doing this. There's some films where they show invisible people and eventually they caught them.

But the next response was often to think that an effective version would remove any problems about stealing, though the detail of this line of thought was sometimes bizarre.

But if I could get away with it—if I could really get away with it forever—supposing I just knew I could get away with something, would there be any problem in doing it then?

ZC: There wouldn't. No, you're right. There wouldn't be a problem. If you were invisible and, say, kept killing people and you couldn't be caught, then eventually, and you'd be the only person on the planet, and you would be lonely by yourself if you killed everybody.

One view was that wearing the ring of Gyges would not stop acts from being wrong, but that the lack of consequences would mean the wrongness did not matter.

If a child had that ring, what would you teach them? Would there be anything they . . .
JF: Be above the law, one step above the law.
Would those things that would still be wrong, even if you could always get away with them . . .
It would be wrong, yeah, but if you could get away with it, you'd be one step above the law.
Then, that's all right?
That's all right, yeah.

For some, the ring would have results that were better than "all right." It would be a wonderful opportunity.

If we had a ring that made us invisible, would there be a reason to bother about right and wrong? Because you could still have a good life, because you'd never get caught?
NB: That would be my perfect dream, which would.
That would be your perfect dream.
It would, yeah. If you just did anything, could have anything.
And would you do that?
I would, yes.
If you could get a good life by doing things that are wrong, because you couldn't get caught, then there would be no problem?
I do think, because I knew that I could get away with it, but can you use the ring in a way where you could not just do wrong things, but get a good life out of using the ring as well?
OK, how would you use the ring for a good life?
Um, houses, cars, boats, holidays.

However, not everyone shared the general enthusiasm for the ring. One thought conscience would still function.

> *If we could be made invisible . . . we wouldn't have any reason to bother about respecting other people's rights because no one would know it was us. What do you think of that?*
>
> BF: Er, I think if you had the ultimate psychopath with no conscience, then you may get away with it, yes. But I don't think there is anybody here who . . . I can't imagine, perhaps there is, that there is anybody whose conscience would allow them to get away with it. Or, I don't know, it sounds, if you were in the sort of position where you want to do that, um, I could guess that you wouldn't just be happy with doing that.

The widespread enthusiasm for the liberating effects of the ring of Gyges suggests the ruthless self-interest of simple amoralism. This fitted with my expectations, based on the stereotype about "lacking a conscience." Against that stereotype, their outlook did not fit the conceptual core of amoralism: the rejection of the vocabulary of moral concepts. For the most part they did have a moral vocabulary of right and wrong, good and bad, fair and unfair. And for many of them, certain moral concepts and thoughts in particular were deeply embedded in their outlook.

Fairness and Respecting Rights

Two of the moral concepts that had a strong hold on many interviewees were fairness and respect for people's rights. Sometimes respecting rights was linked to letting people live their own lives, and fairness was seen as equal treatment. These combined in the idea that different groups, such as men and women, should be equally free to live their own lives.

> ZC: In my sister's case, I wish she did give birth to the baby, because I like to have plenty of nephews and nieces. But it's not up to me. I mean, I can't go and tell my sister—oh, go on, you have the baby, whether you like it or not. I can't do that. It's up to my sister. It's up to the individual.

So one of your values is respecting individuals? What other values do you think you have?

Who, me?

Yes.

Values, eh? [long pause] Well I spoke to a psychologist a long time ago. I do believe in—I do believe that women should be as equal as men are. I believe women should be allowed to do whatever job the men do—they should be allowed to do it as well. If they are good at it, they should be allowed to do it. I also believe that the woman—I mean, if the woman goes out and has plenty of sex with men, some men would call her a slut. But I don't agree with that. Men like to go and have plenty of sex with women, so a woman should be allowed to have plenty of sex with men.

Is this a matter of fairness?

It is, yes.

What is fairness? What does it mean to be fair or unfair?

Equality to everybody. Whatever they're allowed to be, the others should be allowed to live.

Sometimes concern for fairness and for rights was linked to imaginative awareness of how others might feel when treated unfairly or when their rights are ignored. The man whose conscience wouldn't let him get away with using the ring of Gyges appealed to imagination here.

Taking your car to get the groceries, what would you do if there was a shortage of space and there was a disabled space, would you park in the disabled space sometimes or not?

BF: No.

Not at all?

Not at all, no.

Why not?

Er, because there's a specific reason. Disabled have trouble with mobility, and you know there would be nothing stopping me parking a long way away and walking with the shopping . . . but some people have a . . . need wheelchairs, whatever, to get around . . . or walking frames, so I wouldn't, it'd be very unfair, um . . .

Unfair?

Yes, on any potential disabled person who wanted to use it. Yes.

How do you decide what's fair and what's unfair?

Um, I suppose part of that is down to, would it cause distress, create trouble for somebody?

Yes.

And, er, you know, it's looking at pros and cons of any decision I suppose, er, yes it would save me time and effort if I parked there but the amount of effort and time a disabled person would lose would massively outweigh that.

So it's partly a kind of greatest happiness for greatest number sort of issue (or least misery)?

Um, partly, but it's not solely just that.

No. What else is it?

Um, I suppose it's partly how I feel about it anyway.

When you say "how you feel," what do you have in mind?

Um, well I suppose anybody has experienced at some point disabled people being ignored, their rights being ignored, and the way that can make them feel. And if you're quite happy to just put up with that, then, er, you probably won't have so much of a problem with using their parking space, but, er, if you're not, then . . .

But this appeal to imagination was rare. Most thought respect for people's rights was important, but it was not particularly linked to any empathy or sympathy for people whose rights are overridden.

Do you think it is wrong to park in a disabled space?

OA: Yeah, I do.

Why is it wrong?

Because there might be somebody who comes in to use the space who is disabled and can't park there. It's not what I would do.

Is that because you feel sorry for the disabled person?

No, it's because disabled people have got rights just like normal people.

Yes, it's just respecting their rights?
Yeah, I respect their basic rights.

It is worth exploring this strong commitment to fairness and respecting rights that does not stem from imaginative sympathy with people who are unfairly treated. It is a dominant feature of this moral landscape. Where does it come from?

Sources of Morality without Sympathy

The philosopher David Hume argued that we should follow the conventions for respecting others' property because this would result in stability and other social benefits. One interview brought out a motive for respecting people's rights that echoed Hume.

QA: I have never heard of a patient stealing from another patient in this hospital.
Why do you think that is?
Well, I suppose they respect each. I've got a telly, I've got a budgie, a Walkman—all that kind of stuff. And I leave my door open. Every patient has already got the same kind of things. They do a bit of swapping, wheeling and dealing between each other, but they don't go stealing from each other.
You mentioned about respecting each other. Do you respect people much?
I respect people if they talk to me and treat me OK. If they don't, I just ignore them. I won't have nothing to do with them. I don't want nothing to do with any troublemakers or anything like that now.

In the hospital the set of tacit conventions went beyond respect for property.

In the hospital here, is there a kind of moral code that people obey about what you do with each other, how you treat each other and so on? Or not? Are there things that most patients would agree were wrong when some person does it to another patient?

JQ: Yeah, I think so. There is nothing actually said, or written down, but it's sort of generally accepted that, without anything ever being said, of what is and what isn't done.

What would you say are the things in that moral code?

Um, I mean, like, homosexuality, in private OK, in public, no. Things like that, you know . . . It's a sort of accepted rule that you don't ask people about their history or anything like that.

The growth of such an agreement needs some idea of what others are likely to want and how they are likely to respond to the understanding being broken. But having empathy for, or caring about, the feelings of others is not essential. This strategy is at best a minimal step away from self-interested amoralism.

Sympathy is not the only route away from amoralism. Most people's moral outlook comes from a variety of sources. Some are linked to sympathy and some are not. In the interviews, three elements not linked to sympathy played a large part. One is what can be called "command morality." The other two are versions of fairness, one based on what can be called "primitive equality" and the other based on what people deserve.

Command Morality

One example of command morality is found in authoritarian versions of religion: "This is wrong because God has said so, and there is no room for further discussion." Another version is the attitude many people have to the law of the land: "It is not for me to judge whether the reasons for a law are good or bad; this is illegal, and so it should not be done." Immanuel Kant's phrase "the moral law" brings out parallels between his secular morality and both divine and governmental laws. Some have complained that his approach has a hidden dependence on the idea of a divine lawmaker still lurking behind the supposedly secular moral law. And Freud famously saw, lurking in turn behind the divine lawmaker, the commands and rebukes of a child's actual father. The divinely inspired "voice of conscience" was in his view the internalized echo of the guilt-inducing parental voice.

None of the interviewees mentioned God or gave religious reasons in support of their moral beliefs, and there was only one of them who even might have heard of Kant. Whatever truths or illusions underlie its various theoretical versions, command morality was a presence in the interviews. Unsurprisingly, parental commands were the important ones, as in the case of the man quoted above who thought bullying and swearing were equally wrong:

> *Why is swearing wrong?*
> CQ: Well it's just the way that I was brought up, not swearing at people. It's the way my Mum and Dad brought me up, you know. We were brought up as to what was wrong and what was right and that, you know.

Others hinted at parental authority as the reason for holding beliefs. In one case this was combined with the Queen being central to some of their content. Possibly being brought up with a command morality encourages a general willingness to defer to those seen as having authority.

> LN: I think capital punishment for certain crimes should be mandatory.
> *For which crimes?*
> Murder of children, murdering people under the age of 16, er, arson with intent to danger, arson of Her Majesty's property, arson, like arson in any place where the Crown's at threat . . . If I was to [be in] Portsmouth and try to set fire to one of her majesty's frigates I should be hung for it. Because it's arson of her Majesty's docks.
> *I suppose the thing you said that surprises me the most is the thing about "people ought to be executed for arson of her Majesty's property." That makes it sound as though, if somebody's in prison and they set fire to one of the waste paper baskets, it's Her Majesty's prison . . .*

That's not arson. I mean like set fire to, like try to set fire to, say, Kensington Palace, set fire to Buckingham Palace, Clarence House, Glamis Castle.

Why does it make a difference if it is one of those palaces rather than just a block of flats?

Because it's the Queen's property, Queen's property.

What's special about the Queen?

It's the way I was brought up, respect the Crown, respect the uniform, respect the royal family.

If I say I'm not so interested in respecting the royal family, can you give me a good reason why I should?

Where would you be without them? . . . I'd say to you, you got to look at it, without the Queen you ain't going to have a decent way of living . . . I look at it, I mean, the way I've been brought up, the Queen, how can I put it, the Queen is the number one person, you know what I mean, after yourself. You know what I mean, you've got yourself, and then you should respect the monarchy because the monarchy respects you . . . [A] prime example is Prince Charles. He's involved in conservation, he's involved in art . . . He's not like, even though he is royal, he will take time to sit, talk to you, and probably understands you better than yourself, probably.

I'm not sure I believe he understands me better than I do myself, but . . .

But he's got more experience . . . I don't know, it's just the way I been brought up.

This deference to authority sometimes combined with ideas about loyalty to your own country. The result was a "my country right or wrong" belief in unconditional obedience to the demands of patriotism.

Some people say that one problem with the army is that you have to obey orders, sometimes you kill people if there's a war, and it may not be right to do that always.

OA: To defend your country, yeah, too right it is.

In war, is it right?

Yeah, of course it is. You're not just defending your homeland, you're defending the women, the children, people in it. You're defending their right to be free.

It takes two sides to make a war, and one side is defending and the other side is attacking. Can you always rely on our side to be the ones who are defending?

If you're British, you stand for Britain, whether it's right or wrong. You're part of that country. If Britain says, "Right, I'm at war with this bunch," you don't argue. You just say, "Fair enough" and "Let's go to do what we've got to do."

Fairness as Primitive Equality

Another source of moral beliefs independent of sympathy is the sense of fairness. One version is concern is for equal treatment. Most parents know the deep passion for this. This "primitive equality" seems deeply entrenched in children at a very young age. Anyone with three children and three pieces of cake, who distributes them in any way other than the obvious one, comes across this passion.

The strong support for equal treatment was often linked to primitive equality. One reference harked back to childhood, when one child was given pocket money and one was not.

NB: My Mum gave me pocket money but not my sister. That's unfairness as well.

So fairness is treating people the same?

Yeah, to be treated equally to the other person . . . So I'd give you £1.50 and I'd give the other person £1.50 so it's equal so it's fair. He's not getting more than you.

Fairness as What People Deserve, and Retribution

One version of fairness is about what people deserve: that people should be rewarded or punished, blamed or praised, according to what they have done. The deep unfairness of undeserved punishment was a recurring theme.

What is fairness and what is unfairness?

NB: Unfairness is like when someone is blamed for something they haven't actually done. I've been blamed for things that I haven't actually done and that's unfairness.

There was also a strong sense of unfairness when others had not given them the support and loyalty they thought they deserved.

Do you think you'll see anything of your family, or are they really out of the picture?

QA: I was in touch with my wife last year because my son died. I think the last time I hear from my wife was sixteen years ago, and it took my son to die for her to be in touch with me. I went home to see her for the day after the funeral. A couple of months later we went home. The staff took me out to visit my wife for the day, and me and my wife went up to the grave. Then we went back to the flat and she said, "I've all the paint and the wallpaper and all that indoors ready for when you come home." I said, "I'm not coming home." After sixteen years, she's not been in touch with me and because my son died and she's on her own now, she wanted me back. After sixteen years when I've been locked away. That's not fair.

The importance of what people deserve was not just something that cropped up about undeserved blame or abandonment in their own lives. It shaped their thinking about more public matters. For instance, one suggested that although the killings by the Kray twins were not justified, the twins' guilt was at least mitigated by the thought that their victims might have got what they deserved.

JF: The Krays only killed their own. They didn't kill innocent people.

I see. Who did they kill?

They killed Jack "The Hat" McVitie and George Cornell. George Cornell was with the Richardsons. The Richardsons used to torture people and George Cornell was always shouting his mouth off about Ronnie Kray, calling him a fat poof and that and this business, saying how he wasn't scared of the Krays and that they're ponces and shouting his mouth off. And he worked with the Richardsons and he was a gangster himself. So Ronnie Kray shot him in the head. He was just killing another gangster. And Jack "The Hat" McVitie—he was supposed to be with the Krays but he was always shouting his mouth off that he was going to get the Krays . . . He pushed a woman out the car and she had her spine broke and she couldn't walk again and the Krays had to look after her. They gave money so that she could be all right financially, and this Jack "The Hat" McVitie was causing nothing but trouble. He was doing the Krays out of money and he was shouting his mouth off. So Reggie killed him. He stabbed him to death.

Does that make it all right to kill him?

It doesn't make it right, no, but he only killed wrong people. He didn't kill innocent people.

What about people who do kill innocent people? What do you think should happen?

That's bad. I reckon they should be hung.

There was a lot of support for capital punishment.

Why should we think it is all right to kill somebody because they've committed these crimes?

LN: Because it's inhumane to do certain things like that. I look at it like, this is one of my opinions, anybody who can harm a child . . . doesn't deserve to live . . . I mean if you hurt a child,—boom—you know what I mean, there's punishing a child and then there's just going out of your way to hurt a child. That's out of order.

Some people say two wrongs don't make a right. That it's terrible to kill a child, but it's also terrible to kill the person who killed the child? You don't agree with that?

It's just the way I've brought myself up, really, you know what I mean. Even though I'm a devout Catholic, I still think pedophilia is the worst crime in the world, and there is only one sentence for it—death.

Some supporting reasons were strikingly shallow, but this could be combined with a strong sense of the unfairness of innocent people being executed.

> NB: I think serious offenders should be executed.
> *Why do you think that?*
> Um, I just look at England. There's no spaces, there's prisoners everywhere, there's criminals hanging around and that, and I reckon that if there was execution then, more execution than normal, I think it'd be a more quieter world to live in.
> *Some people say that one of the problems with executing people is that people who are innocent sometimes wrongly get convicted.*
> Yeah, I think that, OK yeah, I think then the law should make sure you've got 100 percent proof before execution.
> *Yes, but you can't always get 100 percent proof.*
> No, you can't.
> *Some people would say, "Well, if it would hugely reduce the murder rate, never mind if a few people get executed because fewer people die overall." Would you say that's right or do you think that's wrong?*
> I think that's wrong.
> *Why?*
> Because they're just killing innocent people. So they end up being murderers themselves.

Sometimes ideas of what made someone deserve execution were bound up with a network of other distinctive moral views.

> OA: If a man murders a man, then, as far as I am concerned, that's acceptable, because a man can defend himself. If somebody attacks a man from the front, or two men have a fight and one of them dies, someone hits him and he falls down and dies, that's acceptable because they've had a fight and accidentally somebody's died. If you go out with the intent of killing somebody, then you should lose your life. If you kill a child you should lose your life.

Sometimes, though rarely, support for capital punishment was linked to remorse about the person's own past and to sympathy for his victims.

Some people think it's wrong to have capital punishment. What do you think?

QA: In some cases—yes, and in some cases—no.

Which cases would be "yes"?

There's been innocent people electric-chaired and the guilty one's been found later. In rape there should be the birch—give them the birch, or cat-of-nine-tails—in the case of raping. In the case of sexual assault on children, the same and they should be castrated. In the case of actually murder, I would agree with hanging. I have killed twice—two people, and I never forget it. I didn't only hurt them. I hurt their family mentally, not physically but mentally, and their loved ones.

A strong commitment to retribution and desert could lead people in different directions. The concern about the execution of innocent people led one interviewee to reject capital punishment, although he also thought that, where someone *did* deserve punishing, a private violent response could be justified.

LF: Say you got someone that's . . . beating up and burgling, beating up old women and taking all their money. The police haven't got enough evidence for conviction and they're sitting there driving these nice motors and throwing all this money around and stuff like that, and then, I'd no compun . . . no guilt about, er, taking money off him or stealing off him, or what, lying to him or, do you know what I mean, or attacking him . . .

Do you think there should be capital punishment?

No.

Why not?

Well, it depends. If you admit it and it's definitely right that they did do it, then maybe, but you always have these cases where innocent people . . .

Patterns in the Landscape

Three themes stand out in interview responses: moral shallowness, the dominance of self-interest over imaginative concern for others, and a morality emphasizing fairness and rights, but again with its roots not in empathy for others. (These are the dominant impressions, but I have quoted comments by particular people that go against each of these generalizations.)

The shallowness is obvious in the triviality of some of the proposed moral teaching about letting women through the door first, or swearing being as bad as bullying. The few reasons that were given showed little thoughtfulness or any sense of what mattered to other people. The dominance of self-interest is obvious in the welcome given to the ring of Gyges, provided it works. These two factors taken together might suggest a group of amoralists who have no real conception of what morality is about.

But this picture of the flat amoral landscape is at most a half-truth. What goes against it is the highly visible outcrop of moral concepts clustered around ideas of fairness and what people deserve. It is a *moral* landscape, but a narrow and hard one. In a few of the men interviewed, beliefs about rights and equality grew out of a concern for other people being able to live their own lives, or out of imagining how disabled people feel when their rights are trampled on. But for most, imaginative concern for others was not central. The focus on primitive equality and on what people deserve seemed to come from gut reactions, without much thought about them. The ideas of what people deserve were often linked to their own feelings of being unfairly treated. In most of the group, these ideas seemed largely independent of empathy or sympathy.

Again, the shallowness is striking. This comes out in the importance attached to the Queen's property and in belief in the acceptability of "attacking a man from the front." It comes out in the view that if a victim has been causing trouble and "shouting his mouth off," then it is less wrong to murder him. It comes out in giving as a reason for supporting capital punishment that "I just look at England. There's no spaces, there's prisoners everywhere, there's criminals hanging around . . ." All this has the same triviality as letting women through the door first and believing that swearing is seriously wrong. Some of the shallowness may come from being brought up with a command morality, which is not about imagining how people feel. Nor does it develop thoughtful reflection. Instead, it encourages immediate and uncritical obedience: "If Britain says, 'I'm at war with this bunch,' you don't argue. You just say, 'Fair enough.'"

3

Childhood and After

In the interviews I did not initiate discussion of either the interviewees' crimes or their childhoods. But they often raised these topics. Many saw a strong connection between the two. It started to seem important to look more closely into their sense that their violent actions were linked to a disastrous childhood.

Childhood Rejection

> LF: Well, I knew it was wrong, um, but there was a lot of, I'm not sort of mitigating but, I was getting married the next day and . . . it's a long story really. Whenever things are going well, I sort of always, muck 'em up, mess 'em up.
>
> *Do you want to tell me how it happened, or not?*
>
> Well, I had to go and get my suit, and there was different things we had to pay for. Girlfriend was going on about this that and the other and what we, what needed to be paid for, money, bills, and not just bills but like for this wedding and that. And I went out and I done a burglary and when I was in there I saw all these pictures, all these happy families you know, and um, smashed the place up and set fire to it.
>
> *Was that because you felt you hadn't had a happy family?*
>
> Well I know I haven't had a happy family. But it's just all my life everything's always gone wrong, it just feels, well this is just how it is. But when things are going right, I just know that things are just going to go . . .

The project continued to be about their morality and values, but it took on an extra dimension. How had their childhoods shaped what they cared about, and how in turn did this shaping contribute to their antisocial violence? Many described childhoods in which they were shown little love.

Why didn't you want to be at home?

OA: Because I wasn't loved. There was nine of us in the family and there was just my mum. My mum couldn't give love to all of us and I was left out. Not on purpose but I felt I was and I felt unwanted but I always wanted to be with my mum because that's where a child should be. So I was always wanting to be with her but when I was with her I wasn't loved. So I didn't want to be with her when I was, and when I wasn't I did.

Sometimes their families were violent. Some of them were brought up by parents who punished them severely. Many were physically or emotionally abused. The common theme was emotional rejection.

IQ: I was brought up till I was 7 in a very violent family. Yes, where weapons were used and stuff like that . . . [My mother] was indifferent really, you know, it was a very volatile relationship . . . I remember many a time the police were called to stop her I suppose what you'd call now domestic disputes and such like that, but there was some quite extreme violence from time to time, you know. There was a knife used on one occasion, a carving knife, a tray, the old steel trays. She collared my old man with a tray and he threw cups about and stuff like that, and so what I'd do when that situation happened, I used to have two or three escape routes and use one of them a lot.

II: So one of the few occasions with my mum, and being at home with my elder brothers, I was usually punished for doing something wrong. I was never really given any encouragement or a hug for doing anything right . . . We wasn't allowed to play in the garden but if he ever came home from work and we were (and, obviously, this is just me thinking that it's me getting it in the neck all the time) but I used to be singled out, as if I was some way in charge of the football game in the yard, and it would be me that would be penalized—having to go to bed early, punitive measure of retribution. It used to instill dread fear in me.

> LJ: I was abused, sexually and physically abused, constantly. And I was in hospital for eleven years with polio and they only came to see me once.

Routes from Rejection to Violence

What they said about their own violence suggested two different possible links to their disastrous childhoods. One route would trace back to their childhood the creation of needs, desires, and emotional states so strong that they would overwhelm either self-interest or the moral restraints. The other would see their childhood rejection as stunting the growth of the moral restraints themselves.

Looking first at the overwhelming of self-interest and of the moral restraints, two possible causal accounts emerged. One is that they responded to childhood rejection with anger, which found expression in violence. The other is that their childhood experience left them with unmet emotional needs, which they tried to satisfy through their peer group by winning recognition for their toughness and violence. If they had managed to develop to any degree the human responses of sympathy and respect, these were not enough to protect their victims. Such moral resources as they had were overwhelmed by the strength of their anger and of their hunger for recognition.

Responses to childhood rejection may have inhibited the development of the moral restraints themselves. One response was to grow a defensive shell, which involved avoiding any feelings of sympathy for others. And how they were treated made some feel guilty. This, together with the lack of recognition, did not help them develop a good sense of their own identity and worth.

Overwhelming the Moral Restraints: Anger and Emotional Needs

Anger

The simplest route from childhood rejection to violence goes through anger. An angry demand for attention could be expressed in childhood itself.

> IQ: And so I wasn't shown no affection, and it actually got to me because the first day I was taken to school by my mother,

and then after that she actually left me to come home and that. And I couldn't understand why all the other parents were coming and picking their kids up . . . Why don't I get picked up? . . . that's what I must have felt, because I used to, on one occasion I smashed all the milk bottles to draw attention from all them other people.

A similar need sometimes lay behind anger later in life, and often it was generalized beyond those who originally caused it.

Did you have a kind of anger you were getting out?
NB: Um, yeah.
Why were you angry?
Um, because I felt ignored, I felt lonely.

OA: I didn't used to feel guilty because I had too much hate inside me to feel guilty, against anyone.
Against everyone?
Against everyone.
Even people who haven't done anything?
Even against people who haven't done nothing to me, yeah.
Why do you think that was?
Because they had what I wanted and I didn't have it, so I was feeling angry because they had it.

Sometimes, in their minds, the victims of their adult violence seemed to stand in for those who had abused them.

LJ: My effects on other people must have been terrible. From my crime. I'm in for rape.
Yes.
I've done a lot of heavy work in groups. And the only conclusion I can come to at that time was that the guy was my brother and the woman was my mum. Because on that day I was driving up towards my parents' place because I was going to kill them. And that's where my head was. I was just going to wipe them out all together. I thought the anger might go away then.

Did you care in those days about hurting people, or not really?

Oh, yeah, I cared, yeah. It used to hurt me very much myself, when I had a nice relationship going and it split up. I'd curse myself all the more because it was down to me. It was never down to my partner. It was always down to me.

So you did care about other people and how they felt?

Of course I did, yeah.

But the anger sometimes just overcame that?

It did, it did, it took over. It took over, you know. It was her, she just wouldn't leave me alone.

Your mother?

My mother, she just wouldn't leave me alone, one way or another. And I couldn't, like I said, I couldn't talk to people about it. I carried it all the time.

This was sexual abuse?

Yeah, sexual abuse. Even when I wasn't at home, when I left home and went down to London to live, she was there sometimes. I might be in a relationship and going through perhaps a difficult patch, which would be nine times out of ten down to my fault. And it would be her, you know.

She'd be in your mind?

She'd be in my head. Saying that I was rotten, I should kill myself, and I don't deserve to live and all the rest of it and that sort of stuff.

When you—you don't have to answer any questions if you don't want to but—when you raped a person was that anger, or was it . . .

It was anger.

It was anger. Anger against your mother or anger against . . . ?

Yeah, anger against, it was my mother and my brother, in my head that night.

Emotional Needs and Deprivation

In ethics and political philosophy, there is a strand of thought that gives human needs priority over other desires. The claim is that making well-off people better off should matters less than removing the poverty of people who lack shelter, enough to eat, clean drinking water, or basic health care.

The view has obvious appeal, but questions have been raised about how to draw the line between needs and other things that people want. On one account, the needs that should have priority are for those things—like food and some health care—that are necessary simply to stay alive. Others want a more generous account of human needs, including not only what's essential to staying alive but also what's needed for a good or flourishing life. This has appeal, but one cost may be the blurring of the line between what people need and what they just want.

Perhaps the more inclusive view of needs inevitably blurs the boundary a bit. But a childhood of violence and rejection, as seen by those who experienced it, is important here. Many in the small group interviewed had this sort of past. There was the one child in the family left out because there was not enough love to go round, the only boy never collected from school and who smashed the milk bottles, the one never given a hug but often unfairly punished, the one constantly abused physically and sexually and visited once in eleven years when in the hospital, the one who had escape routes from the family violence with the steel tray and the carving knife, and the one whose mother was in his head saying that he was rotten and that he should kill himself. It is hard to avoid the thought that there are human emotional needs as well as physical ones. For some interviewees, these needs were unmet, and this contributed to the violence. They spelled out some of the needs.

The Need to Be a Somebody

Often the rejection and humiliation generated a need for recognition and respect, a need that readily found expression in violence. Sometimes the anger would combine with this.

> QA: With the anger, with how cocky I used to be, with the beer—it boiled up and boiled up and I was just like an animal. People was frightened of me and I loved that. I loved it.
>
> *Why did you love that?*
>
> I don't know. It was stupid.

Perhaps recognition is a more basic need than respect. Respect has to do with acknowledgment of your status or worth. One of the other interviewees starts off talking about status and honor, but when I ask about respect, he corrects me and emphasizes recognition, the need to be a somebody rather than a nobody.

> IQ: I mean, I, it was a big bravado thing, because I'd done a lot of armed robberies and I never got caught. So there was plenty of money about and fast cars and that, and I was living, you could say, extremely in the fast lane, very fast. And I felt people were looking up to me . . . [talking of when he was younger] And I had a lot of violent things done to me, like initiation into Teddy Boys meant you had to have your legs cut and things happened with knives and stuff like that . . . But to me that was bravado, that was like badges of honor . . .
>
> *You're saying you wanted respect. Is that right?*
>
> Not so much respect, but I wanted recognition. Yeah. I suppose I felt, thinking about it, I felt I was a nobody, but being with these people, I was a somebody.

Others needed to be at the center of things rather than on the margins, and to be well known or to have a powerful reputation.

> II: I burgled chemists from an early age (just under 16) for many years quite successfully. I had no qualms of who bought it, where I took it . . . Then, all those years ago—I felt good for being able to walk into someone's house and the whole thing would revolve around me—two shillings for this—and it gave me a sense of identity. I was quite well known in the area.

> OA: I used to go to nightclubs looking for fights, looking for people to fight to enhance my reputation. I used to go looking for people who had reputation, to take their reputation away from them and add it to mine . . . I didn't used to get a lot of sleep because I was on speed, but I built up a reputation for myself. If there was a fight, come and get me.
>
> *Was that reputation enjoyable?*
>
> Yeah, it was necessary for me at the time to have that reputation.

Why was it necessary?
Because [of] the lifestyle I was leading. I couldn't afford to get trampled over.

Sometimes the need for respect merges into the need to do something that is worthwhile from the point of view of the person himself and the importance of contributing something to others.

What would you like about the life of a doctor?
NB: Um, you can help people, get respected. You've got a title. Hello, Dr. So and So. You feel important and people see you as, that's a doctor, I need some help, let's go and see Dr. Black.
Do you feel that respect is something you are a bit short of?
Um, I, yeah. I feel as though I'm not important enough to anyone or anything, and I'm just, I think it's because of the way my parents treated me as a child. When a child grows up thinking that they're not allowed to count for enough, he, they go around attention seeking, which is what I did, I attention-seeked . . . I'd like to be a doctor, not just because of that but because, um, I've always liked the idea of being a nurse, surgeon, doctor, working in casualty departments. It's helping people. It's a good strong job to be in. It's good pay, you meet different people, you're helping people, and you feel as though you have achieved something at the end of the day when you go home. You know you've done a hard day's work, and you've achieved something. You've helped someone out.

The Need to Be Needed and Wanted

As well as needing to be noticed and to be looked up to, people need bonds with others. Sometimes this is just a matter of having a group that gives a sense of acceptance and belonging.

I was interested in what you said, if you haven't been to prison, you've never lived . . .
OA: Blacks go round in groups. Most white men don't. Most white men go with one or two mates and then don't stick

together, but Blacks do. When you're in prison, it's different. You stick together. You find people from your area, you go to the gym with them, you'll eat with them, you'll communicate with them. You're around them all the time. There's a bond there because you come from the same area . . . so you become good friends. More than that. You become—I don't know what's the word—but you become soul mates . . . I never went into the army. I always wanted to. But I suppose it's like that.

Why did you want to be in the army?

I've always been . . . I always wanted to go in the army because I felt it was something that I wanted to do. It was a profession. It was more than that. It was like joining a gang, I suppose.

But acceptance and belonging are only part of the story. There is a need for something warmer: to be needed and wanted.

OA: By the time I get out my oldest—or my eldest—will be 18, so they can make their own decisions on what they want to do. When my kids become 18, whether they want to know me or not, it's up to them. It's their decision. I won't push it on them. I would love to see them but they're adults.

Have they kept in touch with you?

No, only the oldest. But it's then up to them. It's their lives. If they want to know me, that's fine. They've got to live their life in their way and I don't want to be—if they say: "Oh wow! We've got to go and see Dad." I don't want that. I want them to say, "I want to go and see my dad."

But you would like it very much if they did?

Yes, I would. Yes, I would.

When you look back on the person you were before, what do you think you had missing?

IQ: I think the biggest thing is to be needed. Needed for myself, not for what I was. I mean I went in the pub, if I had a lot of money, people needed me. Or I thought they did, but it wasn't the case.

Stunting the Growth of Sympathy

Childhood rejection created needs that overwhelmed the moral restraints. But the interviews also suggested that it had stunted the growth of the moral restraints themselves. The growth of sympathy is linked to being open to others: being responsive to them and to how they feel. This can be obstructed if the response to rejection is a defensive shell against being hurt by others. Even people who have developed the capacity for sympathy can deliberately switch off sympathy for others out of resentment about rejection and other hurts.

The Fear of Rejection and the Defensive Wall

A number of the interviewees reported having stayed behind defensive barriers because of a fear of being rejected or derided.

> *I'm very grateful to you for telling me such a lot about yourself, about how you think about things.*
> QA: Well, I couldn't years ago, and I wouldn't years ago. I was in a shell and I wouldn't come out of that shell.
> *Why do you think you stayed in a shell?*
> Well I thought that, if I come out and blossomed, everybody would have thought I was being funny or something.

It is a preemptive strategy that refuses emotional closeness, rejecting other people first before they can hurt you again with more rejection.

> IQ: Ridicule comes into it as well. I got a lot of ridicule when I was a kid . . . How it's possible, I just don't know, but I turned from an extremely quiet placid person, frightened person, to an extremely violent person. You know.
> *Was that linked to ridicule, was it escaping from ridicule?*
> Yeah, yeah, 'cos, when I, after I got attacked, I thought that's it.
> *So really it was a kind of defense?*
> Oh, yeah.
> *Having been ridiculed, having been not loved very much?*
> That's right, you build up this defensive wall and you don't let no one or nothing into it.

Another version of the same strategy is to do things aimed at alienating people so that closeness is not offered.

> II: I spent twenty-five, twenty-six years in relationships that are very shallow. I've moved around the country, known people for a few months. One or two of the—if they've developed into more of an emotional tie, I've usually said something or done something absurd and turned them away from me as a prelude to—well, don't get too close because I don't want to be hurt by you—and I've anticipated that by being stupid.

(The impressive thoughtfulness and self-knowledge here is one instance of a strand that recurs surprisingly often in the interviews.)

Sometimes an exception would be made to the general strategy of preemptive rejection. An offer of openness, a rare crack in the defensive wall started in childhood, could lead to a positive response going against the pessimistic expectations.

> *Was it a long time before you found people you did make any emotional bonds with?*
>
> IQ: Um, oh, yeah, yeah, I mean I had a lot of relationships. At one stage I had three relationships going at once. But I think that was to prove myself, prove that you know that I was wanted or needed to a degree . . . I've known a young lady, a lady, for four years here and she's moved on now . . . but we struck relations up and I was quite surprised you know, how open I was with her. I mean, I've never discussed my offenses with anyone, especially patients and that, and as I felt the relationship was getting to grips, I sat down and said look, this is what I've done, you know, I'm not giving any excuses, this is how it is. And I was waiting for a rejection, and I didn't get it. In fact, it bonded [us] even better and to the point that actually we got engaged last Christmas. You know, that's how strong it was. And I was quite, I think, all through my life you know I've had a lot of rejection at home, and things, and I was expecting rejection,

so what I used to do, rather than people reject me, I'd get in first.

Empathy, Sympathy, Putting on Blinkers

The picture of the classical Cleckley psychopath, who has some defect that makes him unable to experience life as a normal human being does, might suggest an inborn inability to empathize with the victims of his violence. This picture does not fit the account the interviewees gave of themselves. They see themselves as having the capacity to imagine the feelings of their victims. Anger or a general resentment against other people led them in one of two directions. Either they were aware of hurting other people but simply did not care, or they avoided their own possible distress at the suffering they caused by deliberately blanking out their awareness of it.

The response of knowing but not caring was openly described.

You say you've changed your philosophy since coming in here.
IQ: Yeah, yeah.
What was it before?
I'll be honest with you, I didn't give a shit about anything or anyone. What I wanted I got, sod [damn] the consequences.

When you hated people, you probably did things against them sometimes. Did you know how they felt about it, or not?
PL: I suppose at the time I didn't really care.
You knew but didn't care. Is that right?
Yeah.

QA: I always honestly and truly believed no matter what I said was right—which it wasn't. It wasn't. I was just big-headed, didn't listen, didn't care. Sod him.
When you said "Sod you," did you not care about—if you hurt some people, you didn't care?
No, I didn't care.
Why do you think that was?
I don't know.

> *Because you do care now, don't you?*
> I think it's just being cocky. I wasn't bothered.
> *But you knew they were being hurt, but you didn't care. Was that right?*
> That's right, yeah. I didn't care about people. I used to be just born free—that's how I used to feel. Nobody could hurt me. Nobody could touch me. But I found out I was wrong.

Sometimes, through resentment, knowing about the hurt shaded into aiming for it.

> *When you were doing whatever it was you did, did you know it was wrong at the time or did you not care about that?*
> OA: Didn't care, didn't care.
> *Did you think you were hurting anyone else?*
> Didn't care. No, not at all.
> *But you knew that you were hurting them and didn't care?*
> I knew I was, I knew I was, yeah.
> *And you didn't care for what reason?*
> They had hurt me, so I was trying to hurt them.
> *Right, I understand that.*
> Except my hurt was extreme. I went to extremes.

The other response was to "put on blinkers." Some of the interviewees had developed this technique to blank out horrible childhood memories and also applied it when they hurt other people.

> LF: There's loads of my childhood I've blanked out, I mean years and years. Um, and if I don't want to face up to something, over a period of time, it just didn't happen.
> *I think we all do that to some degree.*
> I think I've relied on it too much, or got too good at it, or . . . and I suppose it's sort of, I get to a stage where I just put on blinkers, you know, I just put on blinkers . . . I just wade in.
> *When you put on blinkers, it's not thinking about the results, or . . .*
> Yeah.
> *When you're doing that, do you remember it's been a disaster previously, or not?*

> No, I don't think about it. It's always afterwards when I sit back objectively and I look back.

Respect, Reciprocation, and Identity

Another key moral restraint is respect for other people. Respect is recognition of a person's status or standing.

One kind of respect is esteem: to respect Seamus Heaney as a poet is to think highly of what he wrote. Another version is recognition of someone's status in a hierarchy, a respect linked to politeness and sometimes to deference. Soldiers express the deference version by saluting an officer. But esteem and deference are not the central moral restraints. Morality often calls for respect for people we neither esteem nor defer to.

There are displays of less forced and more equal versions of respect. We recognize someone as a person we know by greeting them in the street. With people we do not know, conventional politeness signals recognition of their standing as human beings. We recognize people's legal or moral rights by not assaulting them, not stealing from them, respecting their privacy, not humiliating them, and so on.[1]

Both conventional politeness and respect for rights can express a deeper attitude. Children, used to the way they themselves bulk large in their own lives, can be struck suddenly with a vivid awareness that all other people, just as much as themselves, have a life to lead and a point of view of their own. The concerns of another person are as desperately important to them as mine are to me. The thought is a platitude, but its dawning can be an important part of growing up. The view of other people guided by this awareness can be called "the deep attitude of respect."

At moments the same awareness can be vivid to adults. In the Putney Debates in 1647, Colonel Rainsborough argued for government only by consent: "For really I think that the poorest he that is in England hath a life to live as the greatest he; and therefore truly, sir, I think it's clear, that every man that is to live under a government ought first by his own consent to put himself under that government." And George Orwell, expressing his revulsion at having experienced an execution, spoke of "the unspeakable wrongness of cutting a life short when it is in full tide." He expressed the horror of walking along with the condemned man: "He and we were a party of men walking together, seeing, hearing, feeling, understanding the same world; and in two minutes, with a sudden snap, one of us would be gone—one mind less, one world less."

Some Kinds of Respect and Not Others

Some interviewees had respect for people high in the social hierarchy. ("Because it's the Queen's property . . . It's the way I was brought up, respect the Crown, respect the uniform, respect the royal family.") Some had the respect shown in politeness. ("I don't swear in front of females . . . I'm respectful. I mean I believe in opening doors, and if a female is walking along, be it a patient or member of staff, I let them go through the door first.") And respect for rights was prominent in their moral landscape. ("Disabled people have rights just like normal people . . . I respect their basic rights.") Occasionally the reasons given for respecting rights showed awareness of the perspective of those whose rights were violated. But respect for rights was more often rule-governed than rooted in awareness of others' perspectives.

What was mainly missing was the deep attitude of respect. For George Orwell, execution meant one world less and this made for the unspeakable wrongness of cutting off a life in full tide. The absence of any of this is part of the shallowness of some of the interviewees' thoughts on capital punishment. ("I just look at England. There's no spaces, there's prisoners everywhere, there's criminals hanging around and that, and I reckon that if there was execution then, more execution than normal, I think it'd be a more quieter world to live in.")

Respect and Reciprocation: "Not Very Real to Themselves"

Rejection can make people hungry for recognition and respect. It can also prevent them from developing the recognition of the inner lives of others that grounds the deep attitude of respect. It is plausible to see all this as being reciprocally based. People learn the deep attitude of respect for others partly through being respected themselves. It may need some reciprocity for its emergence.

At an early stage of the project Dr. Gwen Adshead and I were discussing the people—many were her patients—we were about to interview. Thinking about their capacity to harm others, I wondered whether other people and their inner lives seemed fully real to them. She thought my doubt might be right, but said, "Sometimes they aren't very real to themselves." I was intrigued by this but not sure what it meant. One possible link between a diminished sense of the reality of other people and a diminished sense of one's own reality could come from childhood rejection. "Other people not seeming fully real to them" can describe a lack of recognition of others' moral status. And "not being very real to themselves" could describe another consequence of rejection: the failure to develop a robust sense of their own identity and worth—the failure that creates such hunger for recognition and respect.

One feature in "Factor One" of the Hare Psychopathy Checklist is a "grandiose sense of self-worth." Some of those I interviewed seemed to want to give the impression of being really somebody. But behind this often seemed to be the *need* to be a somebody. And the phrase "not very real to themselves" often seemed to resonate with things they said.

> *Do you have a picture of the sort of life you want to lead when you are out?*
>
> LF: I've never had a normal comfortable time when everything's solid all around me, the people are solid all around me, just that, just simple, you know what I mean?
>
> *What do you mean "people are solid"?*
>
> Er, my family let me down, all let me down . . . This is just one example. I came off [drugs] and I hadn't had none for about six months, then my mum, it's a strange relationship, 'cos at the end of the day she's "Mum," y'know what I mean, all that sort of thing, and then she says, "You done really well, I think you deserve a treat," and then . . . I just can't, I know it's not right. So it just confuses, confusing. And that's how it's been for a long time.

Here, someone solid can be relied on, trusted not to let you down. Perhaps feeling this solidity in other people is part of developing a sense of your own solidity and worth.

Moral Identity and Agency

Most people, without using the phrase, have a sense of their own moral identity. They have a picture of the sort of person they are and some rough idea of the sort of person they would like to be. For the very lucky or the very self-satisfied, the two overlap quite a lot. For most of us there are gaps.

Not every aspect of what we are like contributes to the sense of *moral* identity. Our age, height, hobbies, and preferences for some kinds of food, sports, or music are usually less relevant than our picture of how far we are honest, generous, law-abiding, brave, kind, a good parent, or a good friend. The same goes for the sort of person we would like to be. Some ideas about that (being a good swimmer or having a less chaotic desk) may have little moral import. Only hopes or wishes charged with deeper values are part of the sense of moral identity.

Moral restraints include these value-charged pictures of how we are or what we would like to be. Here ideas of the sort of person we do *not* want to be are important. "I am not the sort of person who takes bribes." "I do not want to be a disloyal friend."

Identity and agency are linked. What we are and what we do are interwoven. We are all shaped partly by things outside our control. The kind of person we are depends on genes, parenting, the culture we grow up in, and many other factors we ourselves did not choose. But many people also play a part in shaping the kind of person they are. This self-creation takes different forms.

There is the mainly unconscious kind of self-creation Aristotle noticed. We freely choose to act in a certain way, and these actions shape our habits; in turn these habits harden into our character. Then there are choices that, usually unintentionally, shape us by influencing the personal world in which we live. These include choices of whom to marry or live with, choices of what job to do and where to live, choices about having children, and many more minor ones.

And there is conscious self-creation. Many people do this with minor goals: aiming to change what they are like by losing weight, by their choice of clothes or hairstyle, by assertiveness training courses or by reading books about how to make friends and influence people. A few have more major, consciously self-creative projects that may engage them for years or a lifetime: finding self-understanding through psychoanalysis, becoming an Olympic athlete, becoming a good Christian or Muslim.

The value–charged pictures of ourselves, as we are and as we might become, obviously influence the more conscious kind of self-creation. But they also influence the other kinds, by encouraging or discouraging some actions that may shape habits and then character, or by guiding our choices of friends, partners, or jobs. If we lack such pictures, we have less power of self-creation and lose a central part of being in charge of our own lives. How far did the men I interviewed have these pictures?

Shallow and Deep Conceptions of Identity

> Adjusted to the local needs of valleys
> Where everything can be touched or reached by walking,
> Their eyes have never looked into infinite space.
>
> —W. H. Auden, *In Praise of Limestone*

Some answers to the questions about the sort of person they would like to be were shallow, concerned only with what skills, talents, or job they would like.

> *Do you think most people have an idea of the sort of person they want to be? One of the things . . . people say is "I don't want to be the sort of person who does that kind of thing."*
>
> ZC: In some cases, I sort of like talented people. I'll give you an example—Bruce Forsyth. Such a great entertainer, you know. He can play the piano. He can do all kinds of things. I wish I was like him, talented.

> *Do you have a picture of the sort of person you are? Do you have an idea of either what you are like or what you would like to be like?*
>
> JF: I know what I would like to be like.
>
> *What would you like to be like?*
>
> I'd like to be a gangster.
>
> *Would you? Why would you like to be a gangster?*
>
> I would. I would like to be like the Kray twins.
>
> *Would you? What's good about that?*
>
> I dunno. I just would. The Kray twins—back in the sixties, the Kray twins used to stop all mugging and rapes on the street and kept the streets clean . . . they got to know celebrities and things like that. And they gave the money to charity.

Do you have a picture of the sort of person you'd like to be?
CQ: I'd like to be myself, er, working in restaurants, train to be a chef, that's what I would like to be . . . Or work for the Council or road works, do digging up road pavements . . . things like that, you know.

The shallowness is partly mentioning only jobs and not more value-charged personal characteristics. There is also the impression of little thinking behind the choice of ideal jobs. The choices of being a chef or doing road works do not seem to reflect ideas about personal suitability for a type of work or the satisfaction of the job. They seem pulled at random out of a list of jobs. Or as Penney Lewis has suggested to me, they may reflect the thought that *any* kind of normal job is better than detention in a secure hospital. Either way, the lack of reference to a value-charged picture suggests a weak sense of moral identity.

By contrast, some interviewees gave answers suggesting that they had thought about personal development at different stages of life. One man was acutely aware that long-term incarceration had blocked his chance to develop.

Would you be willing to say something about the sort of person you think you were before, and the sort of person you think you are now, what's in common and what's different?
QL: Well up until my index offense that brought me into Broadmoor in 1971, I lived basically [on] one level. I've worked, worked hard, got a pay packet, met my mates at the end of the week, got drunk, went to pubs and clubs and sometimes indulged in some petty thievery, you know. Other times, occasionally got into a fight, drunken fight, and that cycle repeated itself every week, for years, until one day I killed somebody and wound up in Broadmoor . . . I'm completely bored with institutional life . . . One day's the same as the next, you know, I'm fed up with everything that the institutions have to offer. I need life's experiences outside, you know, to develop. I haven't really been given a chance, you know . . . I'm 54 years old now, you know, if I was outside now, I'd tend to associate with people who are in their

mid-twenties, which was the age I was locked up originally, you know . . . But the trouble is that people in their mid-twenties now are not the same as the people in their mid-twenties when I was in my mid-twenties. I find it hard to get on with my own age group.

Do you know why you find it hard to get on with your own age group?

Well I've missed out on all the development stages, you know, I mean people have, during the time I've been locked up, people have had these experiences, they've got married, they've had children, they've had mortgages, they've had holidays abroad, cars, money in the bank, holidays. I've never had any of these things, you know.

Another had thoughts about moral development at different stages of life, and his comments also suggested a fairly deep sense of moral identity that he recognized to be in conflict with his past actions.

BF: You can't get an idea of right and wrong as a little kid. A lot of that involves, sort of, "Don't shout at your parents," or "You will eat all that food up before you go to bed" or something, which is a basic grounding, but . . . as you go through adolescence, it's no use. You got to learn new rules.

When you say learn new rules, is it learning rules, or is it thinking about what you really care about, or what is it?

I think that, um, you see how you want to fit in. You learn to behave appropriately, to maintain that position. And, er so I think, er, the impetuousness of childhood has to give way and maybe initially then it is a question of learning rules . . . but that stops becoming conscious quite early. I think you become what you want to become. This is me, this is how I want to behave, this is what my conscience tells me because this is where I want to be.

Do you have a picture of how you want to be?

Um, yeah, I have ideas of how I'd like to be in society and how I'd like to respond to people. I mean my own self. Er, I think at times my, er. I've been ignorant, I didn't react with a

> conscience as it were and, I'd like to undo that really and behave as a more er, humane person all the way round really.

Some gave answers whose depth or shallowness was hard to classify.

> *Do you have a picture of the sort of person that you think you are? If you were to describe yourself . . . what would you say about yourself?*
>
> NB: Um, the sort of person that thinks about other people before myself . . . I worry about other people before I worry about myself . . . So that tends to leave me as a, very down because I tend to use all, all, what I've got inside me to give to other people and leave myself with nothing. Um, er, I'm very well spoken when I want to be. Um, I use eye contact when someone's speaking to me. Um, and I'm a pleasant, bright young person.
>
> *Yes.*
>
> I have a side to me where I don't like bullies. I don't like bullying people. I don't like authority. Because, to a certain extent, um, I don't like to be pressured . . . I like a lot of space round me.

This account, while drawing on the value-charged characteristics relevant to moral identity, also has hints of shallowness. There is such a strong sense of being a self-sacrificing altruist that one wonders how much critical thought is behind it. There is a hint of randomness in the comments about eye contact, being pleasant and being well-spoken. Some sense of moral identity is expressed, but in ways that raise doubts about the speaker's self-awareness.

Stunting the Growth of Moral Identity: Guilt and Self-Hatred

Are there any clues about why the sense of moral identity sometimes fails to develop or develops only in stunted form? Where does a shallow sense of self come from? Some of the interview replies have suggested that being shown respect matters for developing a robust sense of your own identity. But being denied respect is not the only thing that holds it back. Being made to feel guilty, to feel bad about yourself, can also play a part. Some of the interviewees had experienced a lot of guilt.

What sort of things were you made to feel guilty about?
II: Well—excuse me—masturbating and things.
So you were made to feel guilty about that?
Very much so.

Sometimes even as victims they were made to feel guilty.

> LJ: I hated myself for the things my mother did to me and step-brother. Um, I thought it was all my fault. That I was the one that was doing the wrong.

Being made to hate yourself is hardly a good basis for developing a sense of moral identity. This load of childhood guilt also raises a question about the "lack of guilt" in the Cleckley picture of the psychopath and in the Factor One list of personality traits in the Hare Psychopathy Checklist. Does this overload of guilt in childhood deaden the capacity to feel guilt later in life? Or is the adult absence of guilt more apparent than real?

Some felt bad enough about themselves to feel accused even for things they have not done.

Do you ever feel guilty about things?
NB: I do, all the time, yeah.
Really?
Um, if someone kicks in a locker in the dining room or someone writes something on the walls, and because no one knows . . . who done it, I sit there feeling guilty, thinking I hope they're not all looking at me.

The interviewees gave very different accounts of whether they had felt guilty when they had committed their crimes. Some did fit the Cleckley-Hare picture of being guilt-free. But they gave different reasons for this. Some felt that their crimes were victimless and therefore they did not feel bad about what they had done. They suggested they would have felt guilty if they had harmed someone.

Do you ever feel guilty about something you have done?
NB: Um, [hesitation] No, no.

You wouldn't feel guilty about it? You wouldn't feel bad about having done something?

I suppose I don't feel guilty because I've never committed a crime where I've literally affected someone, like I've broken into someone's house and stolen everything . . . Because I've stolen from an office block . . . it's not actually affecting anyone, it's just because it doesn't belong to anyone, it's not stressing anyone out.

Others said that any guilt was overwhelmed by the hatred they felt.

Some people think that the way your conscience tells you something is wrong is that you feel bad about it. But other people think that what you feel guilty about is just a matter of the way you were brought up.

OA: Yeah, I think it's true on both accounts. It depends on the way you were brought up, what you were brought up for . . . hmm . . . it's . . . yeah . . . I mean, I didn't used to feel guilty because I had too much hate inside me to feel guilty, against everyone.

Others said they felt a lot of guilt later, through having to confront the hurt they had caused, but at the time had avoided guilt by putting on blinkers.

OA: I mean if you don't know the person, d'you know what I mean, you justify it, well you don't justify it, you don't see them.

Yes.

I mean I remember when I hurt this bloke in prison and his Mum was in court and she was crying and that, I felt, it was horrible, I felt so terrible. 'Cos she was there and I could see what she was doing. But, um, it's like a blinker thing, you don't look.

When you acted you were, as you put it, blinkered, you didn't think about the consequences for people?

But kids when they first start doing that, like if they break in somewhere and nick . . . they should face the people, 'cos

> there is nothing worse than being shamed right up to someone's face. I mean no one likes that, it's horrible.

Some said they had felt guilty at the time but had not admitted it.

> QA: In the case of actually murder, I would agree with hanging. I have killed twice—two people, and I never forget it. I didn't only hurt them. I hurt their family mentally, not physically but mentally, and their loved ones. I took them away from their families and everything . . . I felt guilty but I wouldn't admit it. I was too proud. I used to go away and say: "I was out of order there" to myself but I wouldn't say it to anyone else, but now I do.

One interviewee expressed strong feelings of guilt now, but said he had not felt guilty at the time. On his account, at the time he was full of conflict. Although he denied having felt guilt, he said he had tried to stop and had felt disgusted with himself.

> LJ: Then the act of rape is violent enough, for Christ's sake, you know. But even when I was doing that I stopped suddenly, you know. What the, what I'm doing here? What's going on? You know. I tried to make feeble apologies to the woman, stupid ridiculous apologies to the woman, you know. And I drove up to one of the motorway stations and parked in front of a police car, which was sat there. And that was it. I was just totally disgusted with myself. I didn't get a damn thing out of it. I mean, sexually, it didn't do anything for me at all. Thank God. But now, I think to myself, well you know, I mean I've tried to, all I can hope for is that, the woman, well the woman's not still agonizing about it. Hopefully, she's been able to get on with her life and put it to one side. Obviously, she'll never forget it . . . I mean it's not just affected her, it's affected her family and friends and stuff like that. These things, you don't think about. I didn't think about them anyway. I do now. I mean, there was times when I wished I could see her again.

Self-Creation and Lack of Control: The Good Side and the Bad Side

Some interviewees felt they had been very much in charge of their own lives.

> IQ: I always used to feel that there's three categories of people in prison and these establishments. There's the sad, the mad, and the bad. I also feel that you fit into one of those, and I always class myself as the bad. Not the sad, not the mad, but the bad . . . I mean, I chose the route I've took, solely myself. I mean, no one says to me, "Joe, you've got to do this, you got to do that." I've chose it, so really my destiny as such was laid out by me. It wasn't laid out before and said, "Right, your destiny is to end up in Broadmoor in thirty years' time. I mean I actually walked the road that led me here. You know, no one pushed me along.

But reports of quite often not feeling in control were more frequent.

> JF: Sometimes in my predicament, I know I'm doing wrong, even when I know I should be doing right. Even though I do wrong, I can't stop it.

> *You knew that other people were hating whatever it was. You didn't want to know about it. What pain were you protecting yourself from?*
>
> II: It almost happens with me anywhere—I get a psychological impression, feelings may not be right, and it's just a helplessness. It's a feeling that would lead to some sort of intensity, that it would push me over the edge. I wouldn't be able to cope.

> LF: I don't, I mean I know that's what I am supposed to, I mean I don't necessarily do it myself, because I always tend to make loads of mistakes and mess up . . . I know really when I look back at these things, I know what I done was wrong, but leading up to it I don't always make the right, I don't even think, so, I don't think there's decision-making there . . .

> *And you feel you don't know what you want?*
>
> No. I do know what I want, and I, it just doesn't seem, er, a sort of reality. Doesn't seem as though, you know, I can get there.
>
> *It sounds as though you want to be kind, but sometimes have a little trouble in controlling . . .*
>
> Yeah, I know, this is the thing, I know what I'd like to be, and know how I should act, but it all seems to just go out of the window.
>
> *It seems to me that you've got quite a strong sense of right and wrong, but it isn't always easy to apply it in your life.*
>
> But putting it into practice, I'm not, I know what's what, but I don't, I can't, I'm not very capable of putting it into practice.

Interviewees indicated that actions they took in haste or in a moment of rage could take someone else's life and ruin their own.

> BF: It all happens in episodes, but . . . although we're in here for a reason on the whole, er its not as though . . . the reason took up most of our lives. Sort of, instances of a minute, five minutes, at most or something bring us here.

One reported taking decisions hastily and then acting on them much later but without any further thought intervening.

> *Are these very hasty decisions taken in a mood of strong emotion?*
>
> LF: Yeah, also, hasty decisions that have spanned sort of days or weeks, d'you know what I mean? It's a hasty decision, although sometimes you expect a hasty decision to be like, two seconds later you go out and do it, you think, then you go and do it. But I can make a hasty decision about something and then sort of do it two weeks later. D'you know what I mean? Without, and not, in between thinking about . . .

Some of these accounts of not being fully in control have resonance outside this group—"I know I'm doing wrong even when I know I should be doing right" is an experience most of us have—but taken together the comments suggest a much stronger sense of being defeated in an internal battle: "It all seems to just go out of the window," "doesn't seem as though I can get there," a helplessness that "would push me over the edge—I wouldn't be able to cope." A strong form of this sense of internal struggle and defeat was found in one interviewee who saw himself as having a good side and a bad side, and saw loss of control as the victory of the bad side over the good.

FV: My head—its all messed up and I got like a good side of me that's talking to you now, and then there's a bad side of me, and when that side comes out I don't feel guilty or anything.

So, although there's two sides of you, which side is the real you?

The one you're talking to now.

Is that right? So if now you could dump your bad side, you would do so?

Yeah. Because I'm like an animal. Like I say, I attack people for nothing.

And when you're on the other side, will you dump your good side?

It's like a battle. When I stabbed this girl, about ten minutes before I did it I was having this big battle in my head going on and on—don't do it, do it, do it, do it—and like that. It went on and on and in the end I did it. But after I did it, it was like a buzz, you know what I mean. "He sorted the bitch out" and stuff like that.

I see—you sorted the bitch out and it gave you a buzz. So the bad side likes that kind of buzz.

Yeah—the bad side likes violence—getting my own back and stuff like that. The good side—it just wants a normal life. But it's like a big battle. Sometimes I lose, because I had a fight a couple of weeks ago and the bad side was taking over a lot and the nurses saw it as well.

But you don't think the bad side is the real you, then? Where does it come from?

I don't know.

It is all very far from successful self-creation. Some interviewees, using psychiatric help in attempting to change themselves, found it a struggle against immense odds.

> AO: I know some of the thoughts I have are wrong and some of the things I've thought about and said and want to do are wrong. So I know that I'm thinking wrong, or doing wrong.
>
> *What makes you feel guilty about it, or what makes you know that it's wrong?*
>
> I don't think it's that I feel so guilty. It's more that—I can't get it off my mind, for starters. Initially, obviously, it won't go away and I can't sleep. It makes me restless. It just plays on my mind . . . It worries me that eventually I will do these things and I don't want to particularly want to—difficult for me actually to say "no" to them.
>
> *Are you having thoughts about attacking people or about sex?*
>
> They involve kidnapping, rape, and violence, and murder, so . . .
>
> *If you could choose not to have these thoughts . . .*
>
> I am trying to. That's a choice that I've already made, that I'm trying.
>
> *It must be very difficult to do that.*
>
> Yeah. At the moment I'm trying chemical castration, to work on the fantasies, which will do away with the sex and the murder/violence fantasies that I have, but I ain't having a great deal of success with it.

Sometimes an interviewee, despite the inner conflict and the terrible things done in the past, did have a sure sense of moral identity: a belief that their good side was the real person, even if in the past it had been occluded.

> *You say what you would like. You would like to look after your mum. You also say that you would like to have—you say, room to be me.*
>
> OA: Yeah, room to be me.

What does it mean?

OA: (laughs) What does it mean? Believe it or not, I'm a very sensitive and loving person. I would like to be able to show somebody that I can love and look after them.

Do you think you've always been a very sensitive and loving person?

It's always been there. I've just denied it. I've just hidden it, shall we say.

4

Interpreting This Landscape

> How can you responsibly and reliably make anthropological generalizations from this one place? Why should anybody else in any other part of the world be interested in your little patch—why is it anything more than a few humps and bumps?
>
> —Matthew Johnson, *Ideas of Landscape*

There are some obvious methodological problems for these interviews. First, how far can the answers given to the questions be accepted as truthful? Second, if my interpretations of what the interviewees said are right, how far is the psychology described special to people with their diagnosis? Third, if my descriptions *do* succeed in capturing something distinctive about this group of people, are there really any more general lessons to draw about psychiatric interpretation?

(There is also a fourth, very deep, question: What is the appropriate attitude to have toward this group of people? Their tragic lives evoke sympathy in an interviewer. But also they have done appalling things to other people who are not present to win sympathy. Is there an emotional balance between the harshness of ignoring the sadness of the patients' own ruined lives and a sentimental sympathy that blanks out what they did to others? These issues will be put aside here until Chapter 25, "Character, Personality Disorder, and Responsibility.")

The Question of Trustworthiness

Central to the Cleckley account of the psychopath is the picture of someone conning and manipulative. This reputation extends to those in the broader category of antisocial personality disorder. So there is an obvious methodological problem: Can things said in the interviews be trusted?

Normally a decision about whether to trust what someone says draws on two sources. There is an intuitive "reading" of the person, based on such clues as eye contact, demeanor, tone of voice, and choice of words. And there may be independent evidence, either about what is said or about the person's trustworthiness.

In these interviews an intuitive reading was not always easy. Regarding some of the interviewees, I felt that their cold, impersonal responses gave no clue about their trustworthiness. (Unless this kind of response is itself a sign of their untrustworthiness, but that does not seem obvious.) Occasionally the voice of the therapist seemed audible. Sitting opposite a very tough-looking man, it can be disconcerting to hear him talk about now being more in touch with his emotions.

For the most part I did get intuitive impressions. But first there was a barrier to break through. Arriving at Broadmoor, I get a large bunch of keys—to the locked perimeter gate and to the locked doors on the way to the wards. Arriving at the ward, I go to the nurse. He calls the patient and takes us both to the interview room. So I appear, like a jailer with a jangling bunch of keys at my belt, in the company of someone probably seen as an authority figure. Compared to many of the people I interview, the way I talk may reflect differences of social class and education. It may remind them of past encounters with schoolteachers, lawyers, or judges.

I try to break down the barrier, but it takes time. Before leaving, the nurse may have said briskly, "Robinson, you have got a research interview. Get into the interview room." When we have sat down together, I say, "My name is Jonathan Glover. I am happy to be called Jonathan. Would you like me to call you Mr. Robinson or Frederick?" Usually the reply is along the lines of "Fred will do." The interviewee has seen a brief account of the project and has consented to the interview. But I spell out that I have not come to ask about his criminal offense. I have come to ask about how he thinks about some questions about right and wrong, and that he does not have to answer anything he does not want to. But so far little has been done to reduce the height of the barrier.

Usually the atmosphere gets better during the hour or so of the interview. I ask questions in a way I hope is both friendly and respectful. To some extent the interviewees seem to warm to being asked about how they think and how they see things. With luck, it may come across that I really do find what they say very interesting.

I put my tape recorder on the table between us and switch it on. Because I am inept with such things, after a minute or two I say, "Let's just check if this thing is working." Sometimes I find that nothing has been taped and then fiddle with the recorder rather incompetently. The man opposite looks at me with increasing incredulity and then says something like, "No, no, not like that. Here let me do it," and then arranges it as it should be. This is not something I could (or would want to) set up deliberately, but its happening helps things along.

As the barrier breaks down a bit, I start to get some intuitive impression of the person. Occasionally I think I hear a false note in what is said. When this happens, it is usually linked to a sense that the person speaking believes, wrongly, that making a good impression on me may help his progress toward release. (If he does believe this, it is despite explanations that I am not attached to the Broadmoor staff.)

For the most part the interviewees' eye contact, facial expressions, and tone of voice suggest genuineness. It is quite hard to get a few of them to speak at any length. They seem very inarticulate, or else disconcerted by the novelty or apparent oddity of the questions. Or there is the possibility that their fluency of speech may have atrophied in their years of confinement. None of this seems like a deceptive pose. But these are a minority. Most of the others come to seem quite pleased to be asked these personal questions about their values and their point of view, and to like being listened to. They often override what I have said about the interview not being about their criminal offense. Sometimes they seem eager to discuss it, as if there is something they are keen to express. And often, without being asked, they pour out things about their childhood. With all this, what sometimes comes across is a driven quality in what they say. It seems emotionally charged rather than calculated.

Of course, the brilliantly deceptive Cleckley psychopath might come over like this. There is a danger of being too influenced by the Cleckley picture of the manipulative con-man. This may make it impossible for anything ever to count as evidence against it. Signs normally suggesting a liar are taken to confirm the dishonesty. But signs normally suggesting honesty are taken to confirm the brilliantly manipulative acting. At various points in this book similar questions will be raised about the framing effects of other diagnostic categories. There is a general problem in psychiatry that traditional diagnoses can exclude in advance interpretations that count against their validity. The abstract checklist can obliterate the psychological complexity apparent when people are *listened to* with fewer preconceptions.

If the Cleckley picture is to be vulnerable to possible evidence against it, there has to be the possibility of an interpretation that sometimes takes signals suggesting genuineness at face value. We all face the problem of other minds all the time. We all "read" each other, and we never know with absolute certainty that any particular reading is correct. But a lot of the time we have fairly good reason for our interpretations, despite the fact that we sometimes disagree about when this is so.

With the people I interviewed, there is sometimes independent evidence. One obvious Cleckley-type thought is about the accounts they gave of their desperate childhoods. Making up stories of this kind could be an obvious ploy to gain sympathy and to excuse themselves from responsibility for the terrible crimes they have committed. But psychiatrists working in Broadmoor—not a group many would suspect of lying to improve their patients' reputation—have said in conversation that the huge majority of their patients, 80 percent or more, have had such childhoods.

For much of what the interviewees say there is no available check using independent evidence. Intuitively, the things said seemed mostly—but not always—genuine. Such interpretations are to some degree subjective, and those reading the answers quoted sometimes may prefer their own interpretations over those suggested here.

How Far Is the Psychology That Emerges Distinctive of Antisocial Personality Disorder?

In interviewing these men I was trying to glimpse the parts of their inner lives that have to do with their values, morality, and conscience. Even if the picture I present here is roughly right, how different are these men's inner lives from those of many other people? I have suggested that their inner lives include a command morality, ideas of primitive fairness, anger, shallowness of moral thinking, a shallow conception of themselves, a tendency to put on blinkers, and the building of a defensive wall against being hurt or humiliated by other people. But each of these characteristics is found in many people who have no psychiatric diagnosis. What are the implications of this for the usefulness of the account that emerges from the interviews? And what are the implications for the usefulness of the category of antisocial personality disorder?

Take one of the apparent features of their inner lives. One of them said, "You build up this defensive wall." But is this really a distinctive response of this group of people? The poet Ted Hughes wrote something in a letter to his son Nicholas that may find an echo in many people. He mentioned a sense of inadequacy people have, the sense of not having a strong enough ego to cope with inner storms. He linked this to the vulnerable child still inside each of us:

> Everybody tries to protect this vulnerable two three four five six seven eight year old inside, and to acquire skills and aptitudes for dealing with the situations that threaten to overwhelm it. So everybody develops a whole armour of secondary self, the artificially constructed being that deals with the outer world, and the crush of circumstances. And when we meet people this is what we usually meet . . . That's how it is in almost everybody. And that little creature is sitting there, behind the armour, peering through the slits . . . Every single person is vulnerable to unexpected defeat in this innermost emotional self. At any moment, behind the most efficient seeming adult exterior, the whole world of the person's childhood is being carefully held like a glass of water bulging above the brim.[1]

Of course, the testimony of Ted Hughes does not guarantee that *everybody* develops a defensive wall—"a whole armour of secondary self"—but if many of us respond to his thought with some recognition, this suggests that the defensive wall may be protecting far more people than have the diagnosis of antisocial personality disorder. To find out how many other people, and to find whether the wall is more common or is stronger in those with the diagnosis, needs subtle empirical investigation, including a follow-up study using a control group of violent criminals without the diagnosis.

Even in such a controlled study there would still be difficult issues of interpretation. If the defensive wall is invisible, how strongly does this suggest it does not exist? Or how strongly does it suggest the skill with which the wall itself can be defensively concealed?

Diagnostic Boxes or Dimensions?

The question of whether the psychology described here is characteristic of antisocial personality disorder raises an alternative. There may be advantages in moving away from seeing a diagnosis as a separate box that someone either does or does not fit into. The main alternative is to see people with psychiatric disorders in terms of their positions on various psychological dimensions.

The strong tradition of psychiatric boxes is influenced by seeing conditions such as bipolar disorder or antisocial personality disorder as being all-or-none: something like mumps, which a person either does or does not have. Those with these diagnoses inhabit separate boxes, largely cut off from variations found in "normal" people. Many psychologists hold the alternative view that there are "dimensions of personality"—that each of us can be placed somewhere on a continuum between, for instance, emotional stability and manic depression. On that view there is some arbitrariness in the cutoff point for psychiatric disorder.

This account of the contrast sharpens it by some simplification: we have left out the qualifications that bring the two approaches closer to each other. Not all "standard" medical disorders are so all-or-none. And on a continuum some groups may cluster at the extremes. But there are real differences of emphasis. Supporters of the continuum view may accuse the others of making psychiatric patients more alien than they should be. Supporters of the all-or-none view may say the continuum approach downplays the distinctiveness of psychiatric disorders. As in other parts of medicine, each approach may fit some disorders better than others.

Questions about antisocial personality disorder remain. Is it a useful category? If so, is it "separate" or is it at the extreme of various continuums? The defensive wall is just one of the features that may be distinctive. If Ted Hughes was right, individuals with this diagnosis are far from unique in having the defensive wall. But they might still build the wall more often, or build a higher and more fortified one.

These unknowns leave the category of antisocial personality disorder up in the air. Some psychological clusters seem particularly common among the interviewees. If this is true of most people with the diagnosis, the category may have substance. But I also came away with the impression that the diagnosis, with all its Cleckley associations, gets in the way of talking to these men, of hearing what they say, and of seeing them as the people they are.

5

Shakespeare Comes to Broadmoor

> I have heard that guilty creatures at a play
> Have by the very cunning of the scene
> Been struck so to the soul . . .
> . . . the play's the thing
> Wherein I'll catch the conscience of the king.
>
> —William Shakespeare, *Hamlet*

Helping this group of people contain or outgrow their violent impulses is a complex affair. Most of them are people whose moral and emotional growth has been stunted. By their own accounts, this was to a great extent because they were not loved as children. Much of the damage cannot be undone. Nothing will bring back the people some of them killed. Nothing will remove the physical or psychological scars left on those they attacked or raped. And for themselves, nothing will wipe out the childhood rejection, followed by society's rejection after their crimes, or the fact that so much of their lives has been spent in confinement.

Reviving and Nurturing Moral and Emotional Growth

But some of the stunted psychological growth may be possible to revive. The stunted parts include empathy and sympathy, as well as the ability to move from shallowness to depth. There is a need, for instance, to develop the respect for other people that goes beyond letting women through the door first and other conventional politeness. They also need help with building up a coherent moral identity, a sense of who they are that will enable them to live outside in the world and to live at peace with themselves.

Some of these kinds of growth are linked, if it is true that "other people not being very real to them" is bound up with "not being very real to themselves." Perhaps empathy, sympathy, and respect for others would have been learned in childhood through reciprocation: through having, themselves, been shown empathy, sympathy, and respect. And being shown these same things may be important for the growth of a sense of moral identity and the related move from shallowness to something deeper.

These conjectures suggest two approaches. One is to try to draw out deeper emotional responses, which also may stimulate them to reflect on themselves and on their values. Part of this may be encouraging them to look at their defensive wall and what lies behind it. It also means reaching deep inside them. (There may be a question about whether this justifies the possible distress involved.) The second, related strategy is to help them engage in relationships that draw out reciprocal emotional responses and mutual respect. All this may need something different from professional detachment.

This would be an effort at *trying* to revive their emotional growth, because success may be quite limited. Perhaps capacities atrophy when sensitive periods for their development are missed? Young children can pick up a new language with a perfect accent that adults usually find very hard or impossible. Are there similar key early periods for parts of emotional and moral development? If there are, then perhaps it is too late to make good all that has been lost. But just as adults can still learn languages, emotional late starters might do some catching up. The only way to find out is to try.

What is involved in helping them move toward deeper emotional responses and engage in relationships? Who would give this help? How would they set about it, and in what context? Would they be "paid friends," with the manipulation and lack of genuineness that implies? This doubt is not marginal, and perhaps no strategy or technique will completely get around it. But experimenting with various different "nonstandard" psychiatric approaches may indicate how far each succeeds or fails. Here we will start with the defensive wall.

Geese Go to Prison: Masks as Metaphor

Some approaches, once nonstandard, such as art therapy and drama therapy, are now a visible part of the mainstream. Even if there is an element of the paid friend about the drama therapist, there can still be real benefits. Peter Brook, in *The Empty Space,* laments that for many people the theater and other arts are not a necessity but an optional extra. He contrasts this with the ability of drama therapy to sometimes meet the needs of psychiatric in-patients. Themes suggested by the patients, dramatized with the help of the therapist, can draw both those who act and those who watch into discussing issues they all share. Taking no view about whether this helps treat mental disorder, Brook says the shared experience slightly changes how they get on with each other. "When they leave the room, they are not quite the same as when they entered. If what has happened has been shatteringly uncomfortable, they are invigorated to the same degree as if there had been great outbursts of laughter . . . simply, some participants are temporarily, slightly, more alive."[1]

Drama therapy can sometimes give physical embodiment to metaphors that are more important in people's lives than they may understand. The people I interviewed in Broadmoor had various metaphors for their defenses against others. "It's always been there . . . I've hidden it, shall we say." "I was in a shell and would not come out." "You build up this defensive wall and you don't let no one or nothing into it." Ted Hughes used the metaphor of armor, with the child behind, peering through the slits. Of a family of related metaphors, the mask lends itself most to theater.

The Geese Theatre works with offenders and people at risk of offending. They use masks to help participants reflect on what they are hiding, and how and why they are doing so (Figures 5.1 and 5.2). When the theater group returns later to a prison where they have led drama therapy, the inmates remember the masks more than anything else.[2]

Audiences are encouraged to request of a character, "Lift your mask." This is a literal request but also a call to say what he or she is thinking and feeling behind the mask. The audience quickly understands the vulnerabilities and insecurities often revealed. Comments quoted on the Geese Theatre website suggest that the experience can go deep.

> The masks really played on my mind a lot. In a very good way . . . Especially with lifting the mask. It is something I'll take with me for the rest of my life. (Participant, H.M. Prison Morton Hall.)
>
> I even saw a couple of so-called "hard men" letting their masks down. (Prisoner, HMP Leeds)

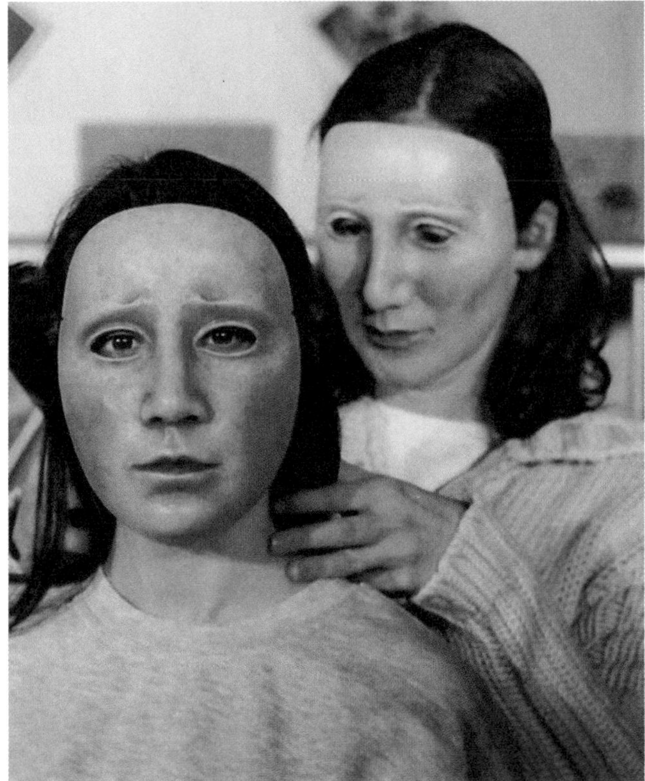

Figure 5.1: Masks at the Geese Theatre Company. Copyright © Geese Theatre Company.

I felt emotionally drained afterwards and I can't stop thinking about it. The masks were excellent—I've worn all of them in my time. (Prisoner, HMP Maidstone)

Playing Shakespeare In Broadmoor

Above all we address ourselves to the deadened organ, the imagination. It's like the doctor's art, or the courtesan's. The doctor can't love every patient, the courtesan can't love every client. It's common humanity that keeps you going. In this sense, every actor has signed an unwritten Hippocratic Oath.

—Simon Callow, *Being an Actor*

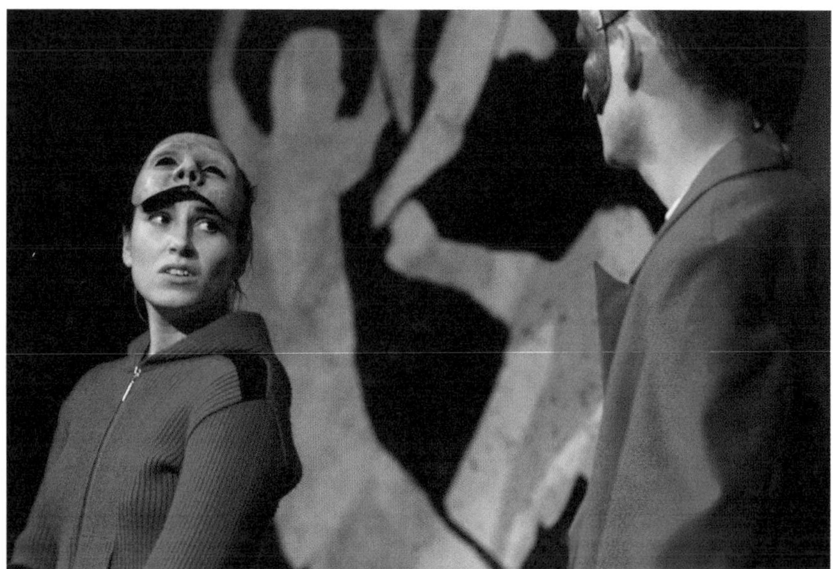

Figure 5.2: Masks at the Geese Theatre Company. Copyright © Geese Theatre Company.

The approach now to be described gave patients a chance to see powerfully acted plays that go deeply into things that have darkened their own lives. More than a decade before the interviews in Broadmoor described in this book, the hospital hosted a remarkable series of theatrical performances. Between 1989 and 1991, the Royal Shakespeare Company, the Royal National Theatre, and other groups took to Broadmoor some of Shakespeare's tragedies: *King Lear, Hamlet, Measure for Measure,* and *Romeo and Juliet.* Because so many of those confined in Broadmoor stay there a long time, it is likely that some of the people I interviewed were in the audiences. Even if not, the audiences will have included people similar to those whose values and history I have tried to sketch. These performances, and their reception, suggest some unconventional approaches to nurturing moral and emotional growth.

This chapter's title is borrowed from the title of Murray Cox's striking book *Shakespeare Comes to Broadmoor.* (In this chapter I draw hugely on that book, as well as on another of his books, *Shakespeare as Prompter.*)[3] Murray Cox was a consultant psychotherapist at Broadmoor. He had retired some years before I went there for the interviews, but people working there still sometimes lit up at the mention of his name.

Mark Rylance, then playing Hamlet, met Murray Cox at a symposium in Stratford. Over coffee he suggested, "It would be good if we could bring *Hamlet* to Broadmoor." So *Hamlet* became the first in the series of plays performed at the hospital. Nearly a quarter of the patients applied to attend. Despite the decision not to risk psychological damage to patients who might be too vulnerable, none of those who applied were excluded. The audience also included some of the nurses and other staff. After the performance the cast and the audience mingled and talked together. A few months after *Hamlet* came *Romeo and Juliet,* to be followed by *Measure for Measure* and finally *King Lear.* After the final performance some of the audience chose to stay on for a workshop in which they shared their experiences with the cast.

Reaching Deep Inside

GERTRUDE: Thou turns't my eyes into my very soul.

Both psychiatrists and actors testify to the way the plays sometimes reached deep inside the patients.

Rob Ferris, a consultant forensic psychiatrist, said that the psychiatric attempt to help the patients gain insight into their violent acts often fails. In contrast, he said, "What strikes me is the power of the theatre, the power of the performance to get them, to approach them, to communicate with them." He said that years of therapy sometimes have little obvious benefit, "yet in a single afternoon I can feel the power of that performance to reach them, and their capacity to respond."

The actors were sometimes aware of the special emotional charge given to the occasion simply by its being in Broadmoor. Brian Cox, who played King Lear, expressed this: "Lear was a rough production from the word go, and its life depended on its audience. If it was a dead audience, it was a dead performance, because we couldn't resuscitate something that wasn't there. We couldn't give life to something that wasn't there. In Broadmoor you didn't have that problem because the whole event is theatrical. To play to a bunch of psychiatric patients is a theatrical thing to do."

The actors' own feeling for what is there in the plays sometimes gave them ideas of what their performance might bring to the patients. Brian Cox reflected on *King Lear:* "It's about death, it's about accepting your end, accepting that in my beginning is my end; that you reap what you sow, unless you make amends quickly and make amends in terms of yourself. Actually it's about finding our own peace, which it must be for those tragic people at Broadmoor."

One patient had a response that came very close to this hope: "When Lear died I felt an overwhelming sense of loss, and tears riding down my cheeks. I desperately wanted to go over and hug Lear's corpse. I felt the sense of union in death between Lear and his daughters. Also the sense of peace and wholeness in the deaths . . ."

The plays did reverberate with the patients' awareness of their situation and of their own history. Brian Cox noted some responses to Lear: "When I said, 'Is there any cause in nature that makes these hard hearts?' one little girl sadly shook her head from side to side in a very painful manner." "In the mad scene: the audience laughed, with a particular quality to it which was quite thrilling. It was the line which begins, 'What! Ar't mad? A man may see how this world goes with no eyes . . . None does offend, none I say, none.' And it was extraordinary when I said that line." "When I said, 'Oh let me not be mad,' the way the phrase reverberated round the room was extraordinary."

The patients themselves spoke of the links they made with their own lives: "Hamlet, the person could also have been my mother, brother, sister and even just a friend—and how they felt at learning that I, their brother, had done what I had done—so it did have a lot of meaning . . . I hope you understand this."

Did making these links stimulate reflection on themselves? A consultant told Brian Cox that more than one patient of hers said things along the lines of, "I did so envy the ability of Cordelia and her father to have a farewell . . . it made me think about my own situation, particularly before I murdered my parents."

Some comments showed thoughts deeper and more serious than the shallow conventionality audible in some of the "Socratic" interviews: "One of the knife scenes reminded me of an incident when I threatened an ex-girlfriend, and it brought home to me the fear she felt . . . simply because I felt afraid watching the same. It also brought home to me how we compound our miseries through our own destructive feelings of bitterness and vengeance . . . If only we could learn not to act on impulsive urges of revenge we would so lessen the amount of tragedies in this society."

Actors and Audience: Giving Something Back

> To play to a large and sympathetic audience is like singing in a room with perfect acoustics. The audience constitutes the spiritual acoustics for us. They give back what they receive from us as living, human emotions.
>
> —Constantin Stanislavski: *An Actor Prepares*

A relationship started to develop between actors and audience. Things happened when they were just mingling before or after the play. Georgia Slowe (who played Juliet) saw what happened when a patient offered Jenny, who was playing the Nurse, a cup of coffee: "She turned absent mindedly and stroked him on the arm: 'No thank you, darling.' I was behind watching the man, and it was his expression that struck me, when this lovely maternal woman stroked him and called him 'darling' in an absent minded way; it was just a wonderful expression. In that moment it struck me that had he had Jenny as his mother, he might never have been in there; his whole life might have been very different."

After one performance Ron Daniels, who directed *Hamlet,* was told by a patient that this was not how Shakespeare was normally done. "'No, I know it's not,' I said, 'but it's based on a central idea of one of my family who had schizophrenia and who killed himself at the age of 23.' This patient, this man put his arms around me and hugged me and said 'it will be all right.' He was looking after my pain and I thought what was happening here wasn't just us giving, it was us receiving as well."

But mainly the relationship came from sharing the experience of the plays that resonated so strongly with the patients. Brian Cox found playing Lear easier in Broadmoor than anywhere else: "It was the most releasing performance that I have ever had, because it suddenly had a point to it. Because I suddenly felt that I was doing it to a bunch of people that actually understood what Lear's pain was about . . . They knew, because their imaginations were so acute."

The performances gave the patients the rare chance of reciprocity, to give something back to the actors, which the actors in turn appreciated. Clare Higgins, who played Gertrude, noticed, "The audience were responding in a way that I long for audiences to respond—in a feeling way and in a very open way. As we came towards the end of the play, I picked up feelings from that audience that I never usually pick up in the theatre.

They simply seemed willing to cross the stage line, and to be part of the play: there was a lot of grief in the room, and sorrow and regret, and they seemed to be pushing the play to its conclusion with us. I found it extraordinary, because I don't think many people in that room were intimate with the play, or knew how it was going to end. But they seemed just to roll with it, with us, to the end. It was a beautiful feeling. I have never had that with an audience before—that all of us together were seeing the play through."

Mark Rylance talked about his own response to an interjection during Ophelia's funeral, a response in which actor and Hamlet are merged: "There was an amazing moment when I said to Laertes, 'I loved Ophelia. Forty thousand brothers could not with all their quantity of love make up my sum.' And one of the patients stood forward and said, 'I believe you.' My heart really choked up and tears flooded into my eyes, and I thought—Oh I really needed someone to say that . . . I didn't realize how much I needed to be believed . . . I felt yes, only someone like you would understand. Perhaps that is part of why I wanted to go—or Hamlet in me wanted to go; a feeling that people would understand."

As well as this giving back, there was also some mutual respect. Mark Rylance hoped that the very fact that the actors had come might send a signal: "I imagine it was something in itself just to feel that we came and gave that performance to them. If I was somewhere like that and someone came and did that for me, I would feel that perhaps there was something good in people or that they thought I was worth it."

One patient said the shared experience led to friendship: "Actors and actresses came here as unknown people and leave firm friends. The reason . . . is that we share an intimacy and oneness that can never be experienced elsewhere. Having killed and abused ourselves, we are able to understand the madness and violence . . . in Shakespeare's tragedies because it is close to our heart. We don't have to guess what it [is] like to kill, maim, and feel absolute despair. Most of us have been there ourselves."

Paid Friends? The Worry about Inauthenticity

What about the "paid friends" issue? Is there something manipulative or inauthentic about deliberately using a performance of a Shakespeare play to reach things deep inside the patients? The emotional reciprocity and mutual respect that started to grow out of the sharing of deep experience count against this.

In advance some of the actors did worry about being manipulative or patronizing. Mark Rylance expressed this: "I was very frightened that I would be patronizing them . . . You know—they would think, well, who are these actors coming here pretending to be mad or pretending to murder or to rape and to get into that place where I have actually been and where I have actually suffered all this pain because of being there. I suddenly got very frightened about what I was doing. What right had I to come here and portray things like this to people who had perhaps experienced these things in their lives?"

But this awareness itself made for authenticity: "That feeling is like a fire that burnt away any excess of ego and all the tricks you would rely on, and I just felt I have to be absolutely honest here. The Hamlet must be absolutely acid, honest . . . It was one of those wonderful moments which I chase after all the time, when you feel you are a conductor and something is coming through you, rather than you are doing anything. And I didn't feel that I had played the part at all. I felt they played it. Something collective came through me, through the words. There was very little 'doing'; the 'doing' got burnt away and there was more being."

At one point he spoke the words "Foul deeds will rise, though all the earth o'erwhelm them, to men's eyes": "I said this line to a man who I didn't know, but who had looked at me with such clarity, with nothing but an absolutely straight gaze. It just felt immediately as if there was a very sensitive group of people there, that one had to tread very carefully and not abuse, not take advantage, just give them it as simply as one could."

Much the same thought inspired Rebecca Saire's playing of Ophelia: "Usually a part of me stands to one side, judging myself and the audience's response to what I am doing. At Broadmoor, I found that observer's part of me sucked back in. Confronted with so much truth in respect of the people we were performing in front of, subconsciously I realized I needed 100 percent of my own truth to answer them. It was as if I was playing Ophelia for the first time."

Helping People Break Down the Defensive Wall

The voices quoted here are only a few from an audience containing nearly a quarter of Broadmoor's around 240 patients. It's likely there were some who responded less. There must be a whole psychology of why some who have done terrible things are more reachable than others. In his autobiography *Beside Myself,* Antony Sher describes talking to two murderers, released after prison, as part of preparing for playing *Macbeth.* "Mark" had been a gambling addict and killed his best friend rather than admit he had gambled away the money for the electricity bill. He was sensitive in a way that suggested "no outer layer of skin"—raw, trembling, nervy, haunted by his crime—and he saw himself afterward as "Alone. Naked in the world. Always." "Jimmy" was "a Glaswegian hard man, brought up on crime." He had killed a suspected informer. "If Jimmy hadn't been caught, you sense he wouldn't have given it a second thought." He hardly remembers his crime but resents everything about prison. Mark and Jimmy both came to see *Macbeth.* Mark did not like it and wished Macbeth himself had been more heroic. Jimmy walked out after the play saying nothing. Antony Sher wrote, "I fear the worst again. Then I get a letter. In stumbling phrases [Jimmy] says repeatedly how *moved* he was."[4] It might seem strange that the play reached, not the raw sensitive man with no outer skin, but the hard man. Perhaps hardness is the defensive wall, and Shakespeare's tragedies may reach the vulnerable person peering through the slits?

The varied responsive voices after the Broadmoor performances show that patients could "give back what they receive from us as living human emotions." It is hard not to see signs of revived emotional growth in the way the plays reached inside them to evoke feelings and reflections, and in what the audience gave back to the actors.

The project was a new model of how to help people whose world was glimpsed in the "Socratic" interviews. That world is confining. They are locked into a narrow and rigid morality of retribution, convention, and authority. Prominent features in their world are emotional rejection, lack of recognition, blinkers, and the defensive wall. The Shakespeare performances may have reached "the deadened organ, the imagination," making the confinement a bit less oppressive.

The model has limitations. Not every psychiatric hospital can call on actors, certainly not of this quality. What happens when they have gone? It would be rare for four plays to turn someone's life round, even when the plays are by Shakespeare and are acted at this level. The project is particularly impressive, but it is not a magic wand.

There is a need for many nonstandard approaches to reviving moral and emotional growth. Few will have all the aspects that made the Shakespeare project succeed. But it is worth mentioning some key features. The actors showed respect for the patients by performing for them. Actors and audience discussed on equal terms, creating reciprocity. Not everything was organized. Contact in loose bits of unplanned time led to some of the best moments: the actor saying "No thank you, darling" as she stroked the patient's arm, and the patient's hug when Ron Daniels mentioned his son. (Erving Goffman, in *Asylums,* said that "our status is backed by the solid buildings of the world, while our sense of personal identity often resides in the cracks.")[5]

Perhaps two things counted most. Choosing Shakespeare's tragedies, not lighter or less relevant plays, meant going deep. And the patients had the chance to give something back. Some of this can be generalized. Other projects go deep, such as the Geese Theatre's work on masks. And reciprocity should be possible too. Ted Hughes says most of us peer through the slits of our armor. Perhaps people with and without "antisocial personality disorder" can help each other take off the armor and smash holes in the defensive walls.

PART TWO

On Human Interpretation

Still, we have the theoretical idea of the two histories, each complete in its own terms; we might call them the physical history and the personal history . . . Each story will invoke its own explanatory connections, the one in terms of neurophysiological and anatomical laws, the other in terms of what is sometimes called, with apparently pejorative intent, "folk psychology," i.e., the ordinary explanatory terms employed by diarists, novelists, biographers, historians, journalists and gossips, when they deliver their accounts of human behaviour and human experience—the terms employed by such simple folk as Shakespeare, Tolstoy, Proust and Henry James.

—P. F. Strawson, *Scepticism and Naturalism: Some Varieties*

I have not always been a psychotherapist but was trained, like other neuropathologists, to use local diagnosis and electroprognosis. And I myself still find it strange that the case histories that I write read like novellas and lack, so to speak, the serious stamp of science. I have to console myself with the thought that the nature of the object rather than my own personal preference is clearly responsible for this; local diagnosis and electrical reactions are simply not effective in the study of hysteria, whereas an in-depth portrayal of the workings of the inner life, such as one expects to be given by novelists and poets, together with the application of a few psychological formulas, does allow me to gain a kind of insight into the course of a hysteria.

—Sigmund Freud, in Sigmund Freud and Joseph Breuer, *Studies in Hysteria*

6

Hopes for the Future of Psychiatry

My interpretation of the Broadmoor interviews, like all interpretation of people, has limitations. This has some striking ones. On the basis of meetings that lasted perhaps an hour or two with each person, I have given an interpretation of their values and of how their childhoods may have shaped them.

Longer interviews might have brought out more, or corrected some of the impressions given here. If I had lived for a month with the people I talked to, I would have developed a deeper sense of what they are like. Even in interviews, other questions might have been more revealing. Other interviewers asking the same questions might have elicited different answers. Perhaps most of all, different interviewers, even given identical answers, would in some ways interpret them differently. Are some interpretations better than others? If so, why, and how can we tell?

We face problems of interpretation in everyday life with other people. These problems arise acutely for psychiatrists trying to understand people they hope to help. Someone with a psychiatric disorder is a person, with beliefs, hopes, emotions, human needs, values, and an idea of his or her own self: a personal approach to the world and a whole inner life worth trying to understand.

How should we try to understand another person's inner life? This part of the book is about the often underestimated role of our human interpretation of other people. It is triggered by obvious questions about the reliability of interpretations of the kind given of the interviews. But it also has broader purposes as part of a discussion of psychiatry. Borrowing from psychology and neuroscience, I will outline some of the mental equipment we draw on to get an intuitive feel for another person. One aim is to suggest that intuitive interpretation, inevitably part of psychiatry, is more reliable than is sometimes feared. Also, spelling out some of our processes of interpretation may help us understand how they go wrong in psychiatric disorders.

The discussion starts, in this chapter, with hopes for the scientific side of psychiatry. The power of computers to organize vast bodies of information may give a more fine-grained view, either supplementing or replacing Procrustean diagnostic categories. This view should improve our patchy understanding of the causes of disorders. Another hope comes from attempts to restructure diagnosis on a biological basis: rethinking psychiatric disorders as failures in genetic and neuroscientific systems. These give grounds for optimism.

But their success will still leave out the intuitive human interpretation that is the other side of psychiatry. The following chapters discuss what this human interpretation is, and why its development should also be one of the hopes for the future.

Wandering Diagnoses and Colonial Boundaries

Many psychiatric disorders are less bad to have now than they were in the past. Over recent decades more powerful medications with less severe (though rarely negligible) side effects have been developed. Even so, many disorders are contained, not cured. Is this simply because research still has a long way to go? Or are there flaws in the framework of psychiatric thinking?

The dominant classification of psychiatric disorders is in the *Diagnostic and Statistical Manual of Mental Disorders.* This has been developed and refined in successive editions (from *DSM*-1 to *DSM*-5). The whole project has been predictably controversial. Do some of the categories wrongly medicalize what are just parts of the human condition? Do the *DSM* categories reflect external pressures from health insurers? Are they influenced too much by the pharmaceutical industry?[1]

Along with these ethical and political issues, there are questions about whether the categories are scientifically arbitrary. A hint that this may be so comes from the problem of "wandering diagnosis": symptoms can change in ways that suggest that one disorder is morphing into another and perhaps back again. "It did look like bipolar disorder at first, but now it looks more like schizophrenia. Perhaps it is schizoaffective disorder. We will see more clearly as it runs its course." Wandering diagnosis raises questions about the distinctness and usefulness of the diagnostic categories.

Why *these* categories? Where do they come from? They are not obvious natural kinds, as the elements of the periodic table are. The categories can seem like the colonial boundaries in Africa: lines drawn from outside, sometimes uniting very different tribes in one territory, sometimes dividing a single tribe between different territories. These problems are real. Even so, *DSM* or some alternative is important for research. Without standard categories, research would be blurred. *Any* systematizing account may be better than none.

I will use the standard psychiatric categories as starting points for discussion, but with more than a tinge of skepticism. The crude map of the colonial boundaries needs to be replaced by a finer grid. This grid will be partly biological. But a view of psychiatry as being 80 percent neurobiology has its own conceptual rigidity. There is a need to reflect the complex two-way interplay between our biological and social dimensions. The conceptual map needs to be more fine-grained, and also to reflect the fluidity of how actual people change and develop.

The Need for a Finer Grid

The power of computers to analyze vast amounts of information may help us keep the gains of *DSM* for research without its arbitrariness. An enormous database can go beneath the diagnoses to more fine-grained information: not about "people with schizophrenia," but about "recently bereaved women who hear voices saying they are worthless." Time and cost may limit how detailed a history can be. But the well-resourced ideal psychiatry of the future would aim for the most detailed and precise description possible of likely relevant factors.

Although we do not know in advance what factors are causally relevant, any description has to be selective. "Her sister is taller than she is" *could* be relevant, but without some special clue it is doubtful that it is. The obvious questions include the ones of a standard case history: symptoms, the narrative pattern of the developing disorder, relevant genetic and neuroscientific information, medical treatment and the person's responses to it, and his or her personal history, including family, work, and social relationships. If available, evidence about the person's temperament and general psychological characteristics could be relevant, as could their interests, their religious or other beliefs, their values, and their hopes and fears.

Particular symptoms are more fine-grained than diagnostic categories—"having delusions" rather than "schizophrenic." Some symptoms are more fine-grained than others—"hearing voices" rather than "having delusions." Knowing what the voices say is more fine-grained still. And obviously some narratives are more fine-grained than others. "Violent and emotionally labile" is less informative than "He was emotionally warm arriving at his mother's house, saying how much his old room meant to him, and telling her about his new job, but only an hour later he was crying and he killed her cat."

A huge, fine-grained database may highlight patterns impossible to see when research is limited to the broad diagnostic categories or based on the limited experience of individual psychiatrists. There is a hopeful parallel with the way computers warn general practitioners about dangerous drug combinations when they are prescribing medication. It is good not to have to rely on what one doctor has noticed through experience.

Multiple Genetic Disruption: The Promise of a Biology-Based Framework

The wandering diagnosis problem may partly reflect something deeper in the biology of psychiatric disorder.

In the early days of mapping the human genome there was optimism that there might be simple causal links between genes and psychology. Some had hopes of discovering "the gay gene" or "the" gene for autism. That picture was far too simple.

The first complication comes from gene expression. Every cell in a person's body has the same DNA. But in different organs, such as the liver or the heart, different parts of the DNA are expressed, or turned on. Epigenetics is about this "turning on." Epigenetic changes alter which parts of the DNA are expressed. Causes of these changes include childhood abuse. Some causes come before birth. If a pregnant woman is stressed by her partner's violence, this can cause epigenetic changes in her child, and changes in the receptor for the stress hormone cortisol might still be found in the child in adolescence. Some epigenetic changes are temporary; others can last a lifetime.[2]

In the case of schizophrenia, the early optimism was linked to the hope for a "magic bullet" to counteract "the" gene responsible. The shooting image can run both ways. It was hoped that the magic bullet would eliminate the single sniper whose own firing caused schizophrenia by disrupting normal neurochemistry and psychology. This was again too simple. So far each genetic variant that has been found relevant to schizophrenia explains only a very small part of the disease's genetic component. More than a hundred variants have now been found. The single marksman has been replaced by more than a hundred different snipers, each making different contributions to the disruption.

And some of these genetic variants also increase the risk of different psychiatric conditions, such as bipolar disorder. One response to this is to ask how "different" these conditions are: "The biology of psychotic illnesses may fail to align neatly with the classic Kraepelinian distinction between schizophrenia and manic-depressive illness."[3] In the United States the National Institute of Mental Health has set up a "Research Domain Criteria Project" aimed at moving psychiatric research away from traditional diagnostic boxes. The new focus is on possibly interacting "domains": genetically influenced neurobiological systems whose malfunctioning may lie behind psychiatric disorder.[4]

Some of our current boxes may turn out to match the underlying reality no better than the medieval "humors." But this approach will not necessarily eliminate all the diagnostic boxes. Some of them may turn out to reflect real clustering of affected people on a number of the biologically based dimensions. In such a case the traditional diagnosis would be vindicated, although the details coming from the dimensional approach would give a finer-grained understanding of the causal mechanisms.

Brute Force and Intuition: The Comparison with Chess

The huge fine-grained database of the psychiatric future may well enable both social context and personal history to be integrated with the key neurobiological dimensions. Does this mean that computer psychiatric diagnosis and treatment will surpass the human version, as computers now defeat chess grand masters?

Thought about this can draw on the competitive history of supercomputers and human chess-playing skills. In 1996 the supercomputer Deep Blue lost to the grand master Garry Kasparov. But in 1997, when IBM had doubled the processing capacity, Kasparov lost to Big Blue. He says that the ten years from 1994 to 2004 were a chance to study the relative strengths and weaknesses of computers and grand masters.[5] They were the years of serious contest. Before, computers were too weak. Later they were too powerful.

Computer chess strength comes from seeing the outcome of every possible first move, followed by the outcome of every possible second move in each scenario, and so on as possibilities proliferate with more moves. Seeing all the possibilities down each branch goes far beyond what a person can do. With only twenty possibilities for each move, a depth of five moves on each side (twenty to the power of ten) gives over ten trillion outcomes. Computers spot disastrous outcomes a grand master may not. The massive predictive power can be enhanced by a huge database of moves and consequences in past games.

Computers at this level win by brute force of processing capacity. No intellectual subtlety or imagination comes into it. As Kasparov puts it, they are good where we are weak, and vice versa.

The ten years of serious contest were used to investigate human chess skills pitted against the computers. Kasparov set up, and played in, games of "Advanced Chess." Two human contestants each had access to a computer and a database of millions of games. This made some things easier. The players shed the burden of having to remember previous outcomes of a move. The computer warned of tactical blunders, leaving the players free to think creatively about strategy. The exclusion of issues about memory and tactical blunders made strategy even more decisive.

In a 2005 "freestyle" chess tournament, teams could be any combination of people and computers. People with computers—sometimes just laptops—defeated even the strongest computers alone. The best teams mixed human strategy and computer tactical acuity. The winning team was not a grand master with a massive computer, but two amateurs with three computers, each "coached" to go deeply into the possibilities of different key positions. As Kasparov put it, good process was more important than the quality of the chess player and of the computer combined.

This outcome is cheering to those of us whose tribal loyalty makes us want our team, humans, to win against computers. Human intelligence devised the coaching strategy that defeated the brute force of more powerful computers.

But we should be cautious. Many have tried to show that there are things we can do that in principle machines cannot. Computers have already surpassed some of the supposed limitations. Perhaps such limitations do exist: the biologically evolved human brain may have properties that cannot be replicated by any combination of hardware and software. But this is not obvious. It will be still less obvious as we insert biological material into computers, blurring the boundary between them and us.

Chess-playing computing has developed beyond brute force to include elements of human strategic intuition. Brute force examines every one of the branching tree's billions of moves, despite almost all of them being nonstarters. To add elements of human strategy to computer tactical power, the branching tree must be pruned. The vast number of absurd moves should be discarded, leaving room for deeper scrutiny of promising ones.

When should moves be discarded or kept? Obviously the impact on both players has to be assessed. How should we evaluate an outcome of a move as good or bad? Some approaches use general criteria: the number of moves left open, the chances of making a capture, and how well defended the position is. One alternative sets up a module for each of a set of objectives, such as taking a particular piece. The module scans the database to see which moves have previously brought the objective closer. Then more strategic choices about pruning may come in. Should different modules be activated in different stages of the game? What chances does a move give of a capture at an acceptable cost, or of checkmate?[6]

There are two ways to improve computer chess-playing. One stays with brute force but increases the calculating capacity. The other copies human intuitive strategies, pruning the branching tree in the light of increasingly sophisticated rankings of outcomes.

The Role of Human Interpretation

That brute-force computers can surpass humans is hardly more interesting than that cars can surpass the fastest runners. We know that human strategy using weak computers can defeat stronger computers. We also know that computers can be enhanced by many—perhaps all—human strategic skills. One day they may reproduce even our human skills of interpretation. As with much artificial intelligence, one of the most intriguing questions is what the process of replicating human strategies in computers can tell us about the nature of our own intuitive thought. Our intuitiveness is, at least for now, a distinctively human form of intelligence.

In psychiatry, as in chess, brute-force computing may be powerful. Perhaps one day researchers trawling the huge fine-grained psychiatric database will find ways to prevent or cure severe mental disorders. If so, the brutish method will not worry us. For now we have nothing like the near-complete neurobiological and psychological knowledge required. As in chess, the best strategy usually needs the fluidity of human interpretation as well. Gail Silver, diagnosed with borderline personality disorder, expresses a thought still likely to be echoed for many years: "The Registrar goes up on the old pedestal!! HE is going to sort out all this mess and muddle AND make me all better! Well, actually he is not. He hasn't got that magic pill or that magic wand I *so* want him to have. What he has got is the ability to help me begin to understand what is going on for me and the patience while I struggle to talk."[7]

7

"A Skill So Deeply Hidden in the Human Soul"

> Isn't the eye part of the mind?
>
> —David Hockney

> The schematism by which our understanding deals with the phenomenal world . . . is a skill so deeply hidden in the human soul that we shall hardly guess the secret trick that Nature here deploys.
>
> —Immanuel Kant

We are not the only interpreting animal. The fox interprets the sounds and smell of hounds as a threat, the hawk interprets the mouse's movement on the ground as food, and so on. But no other species on our planet has developed any serious competitor to the discriminating powers of human language or to our scientific powers of interpreting the natural world. And we are unique in the subtlety of our interpretation of ourselves and each other.

The Myth of the Innocent Eye

> For me, a landscape does not exist in its own right, since its appearance changes at every moment; but the surrounding atmosphere brings it to life, the air and the light, which vary continually . . .
>
> Other painters paint a bridge, a house, a boat . . . I want to paint the air in which the bridge, the house, and the boat are to be found—the beauty of the air around them . . .
>
> To me the motif itself is an insignificant factor; what I want to reproduce is what lies between the motif and me.
>
> —Claude Monet

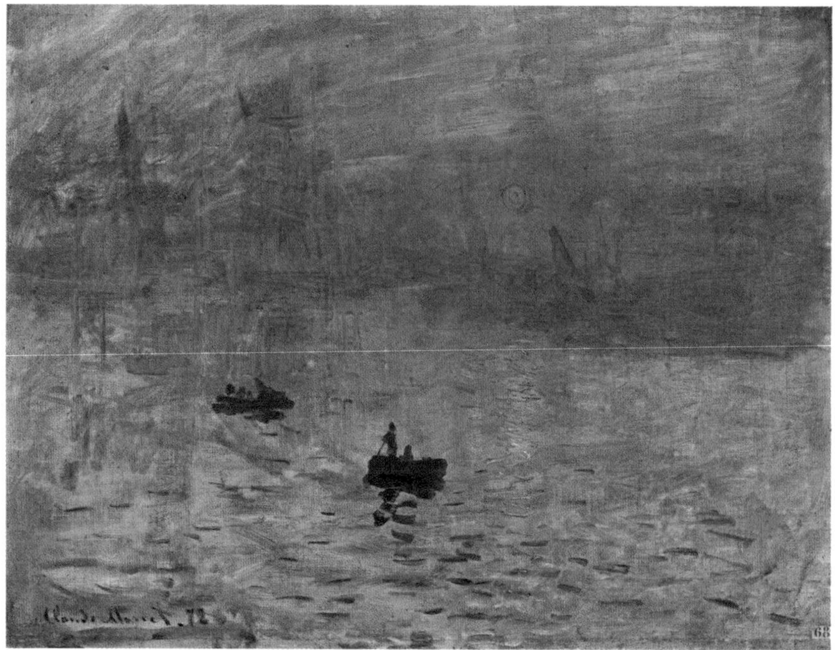

Figure 7.1: Claude Monet, *Impression au soleil levant,* 1872. Paris, Musée Marmottan. Copyright © 2012. Photo Scala, Florence.

The Impressionist painters hoped to strip off our framework, to show "what lies between the motif and me": our fleeting glimpses of the world before we interpret them. The innocent eye saw a world of light and colors washing into each other, without the sharp edges of imposed categories: bridges, houses, and boats (Figure 7.1).

But a blind person given sight would not see the world as a painting by Monet. Seeing the world as intense patches of color where air, light, and water blur together can be wonderful. But it is still an interpretation. Ernst Gombrich said, "The innocent eye is a myth."[1] Some painters agree. David Hockney knows the limits of photographs in reflecting experience: "I've always assumed that the photograph is nearly right, but that little bit by which it misses makes it miss by a mile . . . Picasso and Matisse made the world look incredibly exciting: photography makes it look very, very dull . . . the camera sees geometrically. We don't. We see partly geometrically but also psychologically . . . Isn't the eye part of the mind?"[2] The innocent eye is a myth because we see psychologically. Our experience is permeated with active interpretation.

Immanuel Kant saw the huge question this raises. *How* does the mind impose categories and concepts upon the flow of experience? Despite his own philosophical work of genius on the question, he was pessimistic about unraveling a skill so deeply hidden in the human soul. The question is still daunting. But luckily philosophers guessing at Nature's secret trick are no longer on their own. The mechanisms of interpretation are yielding a bit to cognitive psychology and neuroscience.

When Experience and Interpretation Come Apart: Agnosia

How much we interpret our experience is shown by visual agnosia. In this cluster of neurological disorders, people still see colors and shapes but have problems interpreting them. Varieties of agnosia bring out the complexity of the processes of interpretation.

We see an object from a particular angle. Knowing how it will look from other viewpoints is part of recognizing it as a cup or a hammer. This depends on integrating the seen shape and color with remembered experience of the structure of objects. Sometimes what is impaired is this ability to "construct" an object such as a hammer from its shape and color. Tests show that people with this problem have trouble recognizing things photographed from unusual angles and recognizing letters or pictures from incomplete images.[3] Cases of total agnosia are rare: a person may be able to tell mammals, birds, and insects apart, but not be able to discriminate within these categories. Or there may be problems with recognizing animals but not with recognizing flowers.

People with agnosia may come closest to the "innocent eye." One such person, "John," was left with visual agnosia after a stroke.[4] He has difficulty describing his experience, but his visual world does not seem the same as that of an impressionist picture: "The nearest description I can get to is to say that everything is slightly out of focus, though not to my eyes you understand, but to my brain . . . although I can recognise many food items seen individually, they somehow seem hard to separate en masse. To recognise one sausage on its own is far from picking one out from a dish of cold foods in a salad: a case of 'can't see the trees for the wood'?"[5] This was given some support by one test he was given. He was shown a large letter made up of a string of repetitions of another letter in smaller size. For instance, a sequence of the small letter *s*, laid out in the shape of a large *H.* He was quick at seeing the *H,* but—not seeing the trees for the wood—he was slow seeing the smaller letters that made it up.

In the other major (though very rare) type of visual agnosia, the hammer is seen as the three-dimensional object that it is, but the ability to interpret its "meaning" (a tool for driving in nails) is lost. One person with this type of agnosia who was shown a stethoscope could describe its shape (a "long cord with a round thing at the end") but thought it might be a watch. Asked to show what one might do with it, he treated it as a watch.[6]

Not all neurologists have agreed that what is disrupted in these conditions is recognition. Norman Geschwind once claimed that most classical forms of agnosia are disturbances of naming, caused by parts of the brain that receive the visual input becoming disconnected from the speech area. People with this disconnection may be reluctant to admit they cannot answer a question. The responses they confabulate may give the misleading impression of a perceptual problem.[7] But this model of a naming problem does not fit all cases. John, mentioned above, was bad at recognizing pictures of famous faces. But he said that the Queen, the Duke of Edinburgh, and Princess Anne were politicians. His problem is about recognition, not just naming.[8]

Geschwind thought it was a mistake to accept a special class of "defects of recognition" somewhere between defects of perception and defects of naming. He argued that "recognition" is not a single function, but is seen whenever someone makes an appropriate response. This may be words, gestures, drawing, and so on. He claimed that "this view abolishes the notion of a unitary step of 'recognition,'" and that we need to think in terms of the whole pattern of responses and of their failures.[9]

It is hard to dispute that a proper account of someone's problem needs this fine-grained analysis of particular responses. But might there also be a behaviorist dogma here? Recognition is normally *manifested* in words, actions, and so on. But even when it cannot be manifested, it may still exist. (There are many ways to show you have heard something. But there is still such a thing as hearing.) We do recognize things, although doing so is more fine-grained and variegated than we once thought. Kant's "skill so deeply hidden in the human soul" is coming into view as neuropsychologists unravel the implications of impairments caused by different kinds of brain damage, and use electrodes and neuroimaging to map the mechanisms of interpretation as they function in the undamaged brain.

Interpreting Movements as Actions

Members of some other species can tell whether another animal's movements are goal directed or random. Dog owners notice that a dog may react strongly to movements specifically aimed at getting hold of the dog's leash. Primates make such interpretations. If a capuchin monkey sees two people, each with an opaque box, one moving a hand randomly inside the box and the other moving a hand inside the box as if making an unsuccessful attempt to reach inside and get something out, it will go to the second box but not the first one.[10]

What are the processes involved in recognizing actions? Motor cells, neurons firing when bodily movements are made, often have specific links, some to hand movements; others are finer-grained, linked only to grasping, tearing, holding something, or taking food to the mouth. Studies of macaque monkeys with electrodes in their brains showed some of these motor cells firing when *someone else* made a particular movement. A passive monkey seeing another monkey grasp something would have a burst of firing in a "grasping" cell. It is claimed that, in humans, these "mirror neurons" are involved in recognizing intentional action.

The claim is controversial. Human brain lesions that disrupt the motor processes used in sign language do not disrupt *recognition* of sign messages.[11] And there is a problem about describing actions. There are different levels at which the "same" action can be described: squeezing a trigger, firing a gun, assassinating an archduke, starting the First World War, and so on. What exactly is it, to "recognize an action"?

Some mirror neurons generalize from one sense to another. Those firing when we kick a ball also fire when we see or hear a ball being kicked. Some make very subtle discriminations. Those firing when someone else is seen to grasp something also respond when a graspable object is seen "in person"—but not when its image is seen on a screen. They fire only when the object is near, and more strongly if it approaches fast. In a monkey, some of these neurons fire only when it sees the two-finger grasp used for small objects. Others fire at the sight only of the whole-hand grasp used for large ones. They do not fire when the action is mimed without the object. If the "object" is out of sight, firing is affected by memory of whether or not it is actually there.[12]

Although the link between mirror neuron firing and "action recognition" is still controversial, the selectivity does suggest that there is a link between their firing and recognition. Despite the many actions a physical movement may embody, these cells seem to discriminate between some intentions. Grasping something to eat and grasping it to put it in a box may look the same. But some cells fire only when food is grasped to eat and others fire only when it is grasped to put it into a box. Possibly the mirror neurons' response is not the key neurological basis of interpretation but instead draws on interpretations or memories in some other brain region.[13] Either way, this sensitivity to intentions goes beyond interpreting events as movements. A boundary is crossed, and movements are seen in terms of minds and actions.

Interpretation of Other Minds: Reliable Enough, or an Impenetrable Shadow?

Philosophers discuss the classical problem of other minds. How do we know other people are conscious? Could they not be unconscious robots, programmed to behave as if they have experiences as I do? As a teacher of philosophy, I find this question fascinating. Outside philosophy, sane people no more worry about it than they worry about whether the physical world is a figment of their imagination. Philosophers do not disagree with the sane view on these questions—they take up the intellectual challenge to explain why it is right.

Although sane people are not anxious about whether other people are conscious, they do sometimes care about a more everyday "other minds" problem: How much do we really know what other people are thinking or feeling? People disagree about how easy or hard it is to understand other people. There is a continuum of views, which can roughly be said to stretch from Gilbert Ryle to Marcel Proust.

Gilbert Ryle wrote: "The ascertainment of a person's mental capacities and propensities is an inductive process, an induction to law-like propositions from observed actions and reactions. Having ascertained these long-term qualities, we explain a particular action or reaction by applying the results of such an induction to the new specimen . . . These inductions are not, of course, carried out under laboratory conditions, or with any statistical apparatus, any more than is the shepherd's weather-lore, or the general practitioner's understanding of a particular patient's constitution. But they are ordinarily reliable enough."[14]

Marcel Proust was more skeptical. His own view was reflected by his autobiographical novel's narrator. The question arose in his childhood: "When Françoise, in the evening, was nice to me, and asked my permission to sit in my room, it seemed to me that her face became transparent and that I could see the kindness and honesty that lay beneath. But Jupien . . . revealed afterwards that she had told him that I was not worth the price of a rope to hang me, and that I had tried to do her every conceivable harm." He realized he could never know for certain whether Francoise loved or loathed him. This shock to his view of her made him have more general doubts about the pictures we form of other people:

> And thus it was she who first gave me the idea that a person does not (as I had imagined) stand motionless and clear before our eyes with his merits, his defects, his plans, his intentions with regard to ourselves (like a garden at which we gaze through a railing with all its borders spread out before us) but is a shadow which we can never penetrate, of which there can be no such thing as direct knowledge, with respect to which we form countless beliefs, based upon words and sometimes actions, neither of which can give us anything but inadequate and as it proves contradictory information—a shadow behind which we can alternately imagine, with equal justification, that there burns the flame of hatred and of love.[15]

How far are our interpretations of other people's mental states reliable? What is the right place on the continuum between Ryle's inductions that are "ordinarily reliable enough" and Proust's "shadow which we can never succeed in penetrating"? What resources can we draw on in making these interpretations?

"A Pretty Thick Shadow"? Intuitive and Reflective Interpretation

> All gaps in actual knowledge are still filled with projections. We are still almost certain we know what other people think or what their true character is. We are convinced that certain people have all the bad qualities we do not know in ourselves or that they live all those vices which could, of course, never be our own. We must still be exceedingly careful not to project our own shadows too shamelessly; we are still swamped with projected illusions. If you can imagine someone who is brave enough to withdraw these projections, all and sundry, then you get an individual conscious of a pretty thick shadow.
>
> —Carl Jung, *Psychology and Religion*

We have seen how our experience is permeated with interpretation. We see a spoon or a hammer only through complex and subtle unconscious interpretation. The complexity and subtlety increase when we turn from things to people.

Our intuitive interpretation of people is not something we think through, but an impression that forces itself on us. These involuntary intuitions can be important in criminal trials. In a trial discussed by Janet Malcolm in *The Journalist and the Murderer*, the jury heard a recorded interview by the person accused of murder. One juror is reported to have said, "Until I heard that, there was no doubt in my mind about his innocence. All the evidence had just seemed confusing. But hearing him turned the whole thing round. I began to look at everything in a whole new way. There was something about the sound of his voice. A kind of hesitation. He just didn't sound like a man telling the truth."[16]

Of course we can go beyond these intuitions to more reflective interpretation. A skeptically minded juror might wonder about the reliability of the intuition about the accused person's voice. One way of testing it might be to question some of the "confusing" evidence. Does the defense story seem coherent? Are there facts it does not fit? How well established are these facts? How well does the prosecution case do on these tests? And so on. As well as "external" tests about forensic evidence and alibis, there is the question of the relative psychological plausibility of each of the two cases. What motives and beliefs does each ascribe to the accused? Which version of his psychology makes more sense?

In this contrast, there may be a blurred boundary between intuitive and reflective interpretation. There may be unease about the intuitive hearing of the false note in the man's voice. This might be the residue of basing earlier misjudgments on how people sounded. And the carefully reflective interpretation of the evidence may rest partly on beliefs about psychological plausibility that are more intuitive than rational. The intuitive-reflective contrast may be more of a continuum than an unbridgeable gulf. But here, with this in mind, we can consider the differences between interpretations toward each end of the continuum. Starting at the intuitive end will lead into reflective interpretation.

8

Intuitive Interpretation

> As most of the movements of expression must have been gradually acquired, afterwards becoming instinctive, there seems to be some degree of a priori probability that their recognition would likewise have become instinctive.
>
> —Charles Darwin,
> *The Expression of the Emotions in Man and Animals*

> He notices the blue or red of a child's frock; the way a horse shifts its tail; the sound of a cough; the action of a man trying to put his hands into pockets that have been sewn up. And what his infallible eye reports of a cough or a trick of the hands his infallible brain refers to something hidden in the character, so that we know his people, not only by the way they love and their views on politics and the immortality of the soul, but also by the way they sneeze and choke.
>
> —Virginia Woolf, on Tolstoy: "The Russian Point of View"
> in *The Common Reader*

Intuitive first impressions of people we meet are often helpful clues. We are not Tolstoy, and Virginia Woolf consciously exaggerated in calling even his brain infallible. But we have layers of interpretation behind our intuitive understanding of people. Our brains, like Tolstoy's, can refer a trick of the hands to something hidden in the character.

Talking to children about how to write poems about people, Ted Hughes spoke of these first impressions, "which we cannot pin down by more than a tentative, vague phrase. That little phrase is like the visible moving fin of a great fish in a dark pool."[1] Where do these first impressions come from? How can they sometimes give us a revealing glimpse of the fish in the pool?

Reading Faces

First impressions often start with what we think we see in someone's face. Babies look at faces more than other things. Even among drawings, they look more at ones that are like faces.[2] We all know the role of the face in recognizing people. Prosopagnosia, in which certain brain lesions disrupt recognition of faces, helps us map the neurological basis of this recognition. Faces also help us "read" people. The processing networks used in recognition are different from those involved in seeing in their faces what people are like, or what they are thinking and feeling.[3]

If human interpretation is important for psychiatry, reading faces must also be. Someone I know with Asperger's syndrome is unusually good at understanding autistic people. I once asked her what it was that she was able to intuit about them that the rest of us fail to see. She said that people with autism or Asperger's syndrome often cannot read people's faces: "Imagine how your world would change if people had no faces."

In faces we get glimpses of minds: both of present thoughts and feelings and, more generally, of character and personality. But notoriously, people can put on an act. A deceptive face is often important. Duncan, lamenting his betrayal by the Thane of Cawdor, says, "There's no art / To find the mind's construction in the face. / He was a gentleman on whom I built / An absolute trust." A note of skepticism about our interpretations is right. How far do we really see character in faces and how far do we project it onto them? Marcel Proust's narrator, obviously reflecting the author, notices the complexity even of recognizing another's face. He adopts a skeptical view of interpretation as being mainly projection:

> Even the simple act that we describe as "seeing someone we know" is to some extent an intellectual process. We pack the physical outline of the person we see with all the notions we have already formed about him, and in the total picture of him which we compose in our minds those notions have certainly the principal place. In the end they come to fill out so completely the curve of his cheeks, to follow so exactly the line of his nose, they blend so harmoniously in the sound of his voice as if it were no more than a transparent envelope, that each time we see the face or hear the voice, it is these notions which we recognise and to which we listen.[4]

Obviously some interpretations of faces are highly loaded with the projections of our own preconceived ideas. Hostile facial caricature is part of the history of racism. And sometimes we may be misled, as Duncan was, by a generous interpretation. There are questions for psychology. How often and how far do readings of faces get someone right? How far are they Proustian projection?

You say to the group, "Someone here must have been reading my private letters." One person blushes. It is not proof, but perhaps it is worth following up? Blushing is a crude indicator, signaling only current feelings of guilt, shame, embarrassment, or sexual response. There are more subtle indicators of long-term attitudes and character. Perhaps it is too strong to say that there is *no* art to find the mind's construction in the face. How far are some people more acute than others in their readings? If there are people whose interpretations are more accurate and perceptive, are their skills teachable?

As a source of information, reading faces is like memory, which we also rely on heavily. We all know that memory is highly fallible. We repress, we forget, we misremember, we distort. But we could not survive the obliteration of the past entailed by total skepticism about memory. We have to trust memory, and although it lets us down at the margins, mainly it rewards our trust. Psychology may show how far reading faces can or cannot compete with memory for rough general reliability. In advance of that, there are reasons for modest optimism, some coming from the way painters have created ways of representing what they have seen in people's faces.

Rembrandt's Face

Rembrandt was 22 in 1628. Around then he painted the self-portrait you see in Figure 8.1. It depicts a young man, at that moment carefree and laughing. The portrait, which must have taken days or weeks to paint, manages to capture a movement of face and head that probably lasted a second or two. If you know it is a self-portrait, you know he was a gifted painter. But otherwise it tells you little more about him than this wonderful carefree moment.

Now look at his self-portrait from 1640, when he was 34, and try to "read" what is expressed in the face (Figure 8.2). The well-dressed man

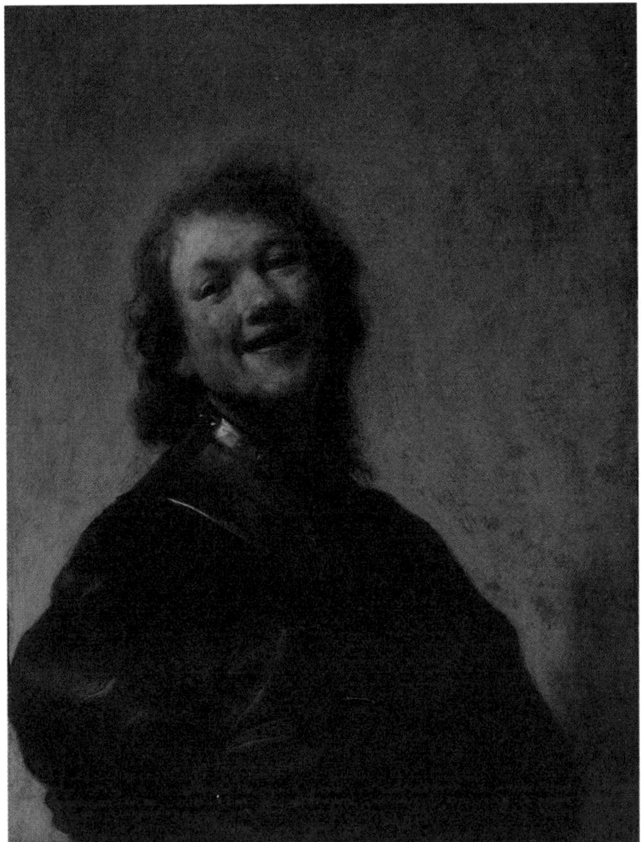

Figure 8.1: ***Rembrandt Laughing*****. J. Paul Getty Museum. Digital image courtesy of the Getty's Open Content Program.**

looking at us has an alert, penetrating gaze, a look of intelligence, with a touch of overconfidence, perhaps even arrogance. This man in his mid-thirties might be a good deal less approachable than the laughing young man of twelve years earlier. He does not look like someone who would meekly accept criticism without demur: he has the air of someone well aware of being exceptionally good at what he does. Of course, if you paint as well as this, if you are Rembrandt, it can be said to be justified confidence rather than overconfidence.

Now read the face in his self-portrait when he was 63, which he painted in 1669, the year he died (Figure 8.3). It is plausibly the aged face of the younger man in the laughing, youthful portrait. This face records the physical changes of aging: the grey or white hair, the lines, the less

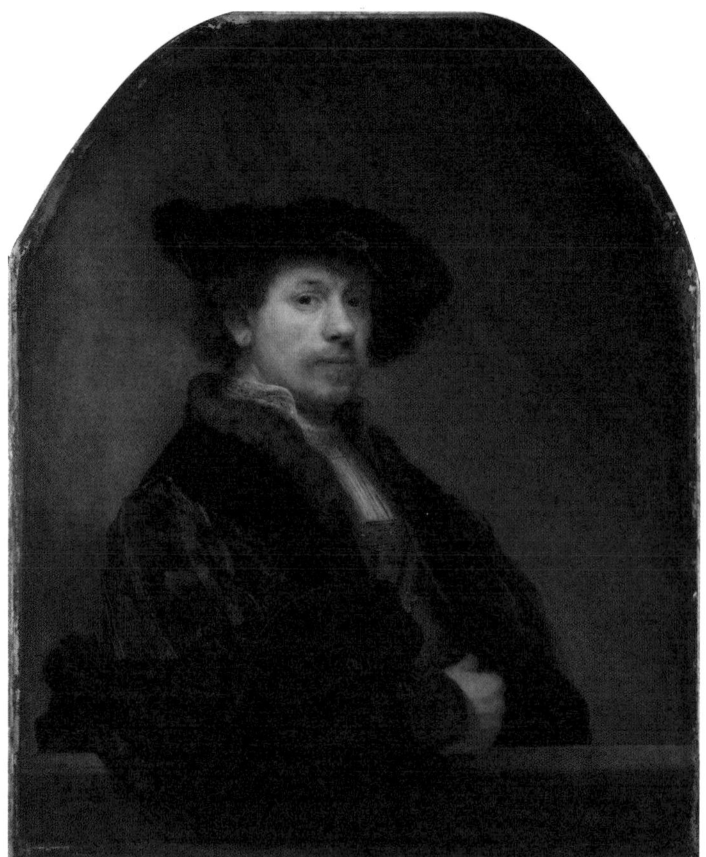

Figure 8.2: Rembrandt, *Self Portrait at the Age of 34,* 1640. London, National Gallery. Oil on canvas. Copyright © 2012, The National Gallery, London/Scala, Florence.

firm contours. But it also seems to record psychological changes. The touch of overconfidence or arrogance in the 1640 portrait is no longer visible. And there is perhaps a hint of the sadness of an old man who has seen deeper into life.

My hope is that what many people see in these faces to some extent overlaps with these readings. If we do not overlap, the overconfidence may be mine. But if most of us broadly converge in interpretation, perhaps what we "see" in the faces is there to be seen, and is not just something we project on to them.

Even with a fair degree of overlap, there are questions about our shared interpretations. Some of Rembrandt's self-portraits have been called self-conscious poses to depict a particular emotion. The paintings above do not seem like that. The last one especially seems a very honest "warts and all" portrait. It comes across as one that, by avoiding poses or

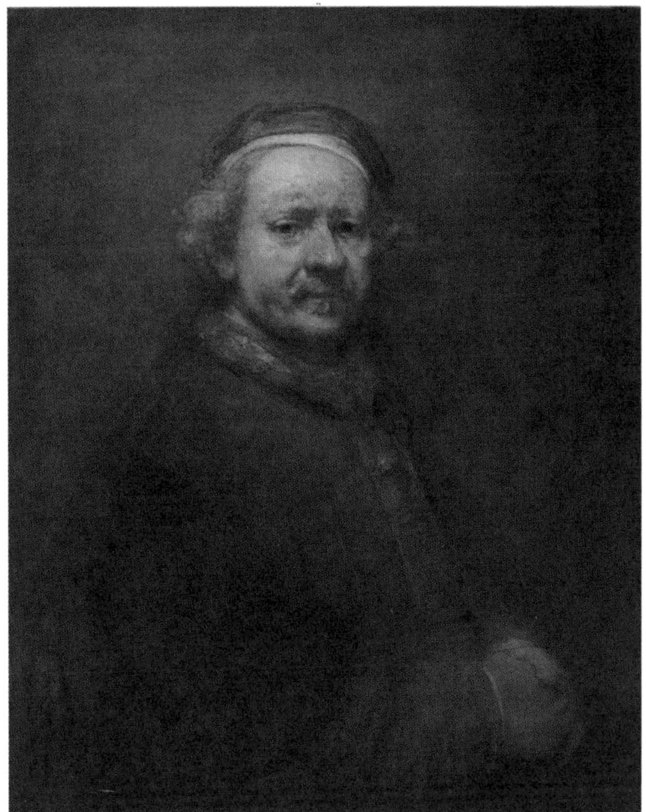

Figure 8.3: Rembrandt, *Self Portrait at the Age of 63,* 1669. London, National Gallery. Oil on canvas. Copyright © 2012, The National Gallery, London/Scala, Florence.

prettification, captures something deep. Even if we agree about this, we could still be wrong. It could be that Rembrandt used his imagination to paint a variation on how his face actually looked, expressing states not really his. There is no special reason to accept this (perhaps implausible) "insincerity" hypothesis. But those of us who are not painters may underrate the degree of art in an apparently straightforward depiction.

Francis Bacon was interested in how other painters, quite early on, might make on the canvas some random mark that could become important in the final painting. He thought this had happened in another of Rembrandt's self-portraits. In an interview with Bacon, David Sylvester said, "The thing that's difficult to understand is how it is that marks of the brush and the movement of paint on canvas can speak so directly to us." Bacon replied:

> Well, if you think of the great Rembrandt self-portrait in Aix-en-Provence [see Figure 8.4] . . . you will see that there are

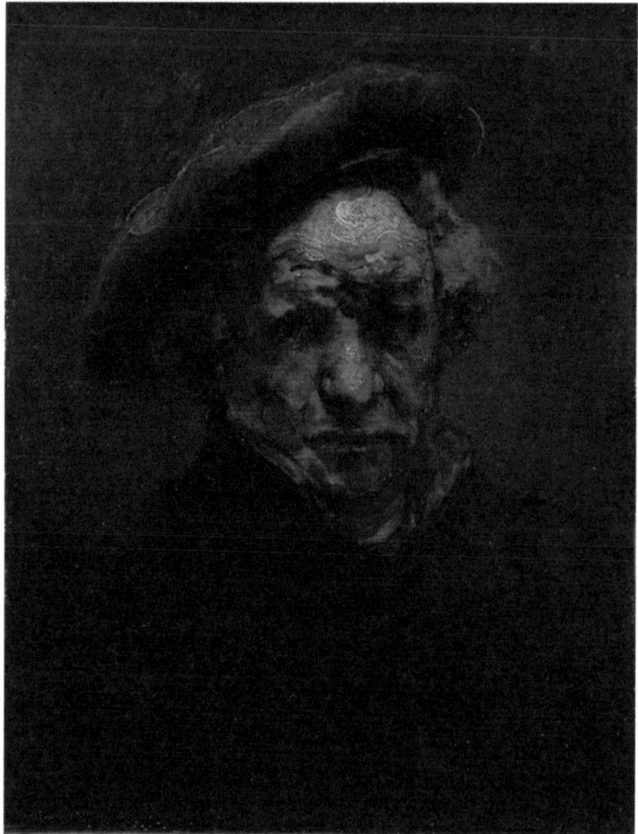

Figure 8.4: Rembrandt, *Self Portrait,* 1659. Copyright © Granet Museum. CPA. Photo by Bernard Terlay.

> hardly any sockets to the eyes, that it is almost completely anti-illustrational. I think that the mystery of fact is conveyed by an image being made out of non-rational marks . . . But what can happen sometimes, as it happened in this Rembrandt self-portrait, is that there is a coagulation of non-representational marks which have led to making up this very great image. Well, of course, only part of this is accidental. Behind all that is Rembrandt's profound sensibility, which was able to hold onto one irrational mark rather than onto another.[5]

The point of interest here is the nonaccidental part. Rembrandt's "profound sensibility," telling him to hold on to one accidental mark and not another, was linked to the shared human grammar of facial interpretation. This grammar may partly reflect the instinctive interpretation Darwin thought was probable. We also know it from shared experience, seeing how faces change when people are absorbed, or in anger, love, pride, or grief.

A representational painting is intended to convey a recognizable interpretation of what is depicted. Someone who sees a face seeming to express some of the person's inner life, and who paints that face, intends others to recognize the expressiveness. A portrait painter detects the subject's character or emotional state partly by visual clues and conveys the psychological features by reproducing these same clues. The painter conveys the expressiveness of the face because people who see the painting share the grammar of interpretation. There are extra layers of resonance when we move from a random portrait to a self-portrait by Rembrandt. We are looking at an extremely perceptive man, portrayed by a brilliant painter who knows him from the inside.

Obviously the painter's brilliance creates the powerful recognition these self-portraits arouse. But the shared intuitive grammar of reading faces is also essential. We live among people with faces. And each of us has our own face. Often we recognize an expression because we have felt it on our own face, as well as seen it on others. We know the embarrassment or boredom behind it. Because of this shared experience and knowledge, we intentionally and unintentionally communicate with each other by means of faces all the time. Martians with a different grammar (or none) would be left cold even by Rembrandt's portraits.

How Reliable Is Intuitive Interpretation?

The neuropsychological systems by which we read faces are just a fraction of the vast array of systems by which we detect and interpret things and events in the world. The visual systems by which light impinging on the retina is interpreted as color, shape, and movement are complicated enough. But we also interpret what we see as objects, and as ones we can, say, use. We go further still in recognizing a face and then seeing in its expression boredom or embarrassment. And these are just some of the systems involved in visual detection and interpretation, without starting on the subtleties of interpreting what we hear, feel, taste, or smell.

Half hidden in the depths of the English countryside are various outposts of the signal and communication detection system that feeds information to the American and British intelligence services. To anyone not knowing what they are, they look a bit strange, usually like a set of giant golf balls or huge television satellite dishes. On the outside they give little clue to the fact that inside they are bristling with the technology of detection and interpretation. The word "jihad" in a phone conversation in Bradford or in Bahrain may alert some computer in the Government Communications Headquarters in Cheltenham. The smooth exterior of the human body similarly gives little clue to the way we too are bristling with a naturally evolved neurotechnology of detection and interpretation. Our interpretations are not always right. GCHQ's probably are not always right either. But in each case powerful systems for interpretation have been developed.

Our own systems emerged during our evolution. One classical philosophical problem is whether there is any reason to expect our senses to be generally reliable rather than deceptive. One possible answer is that a species whose senses were systematically misleading about the world would probably be eaten by some other species. Similar claims can be made about the evolutionary usefulness during the Stone Age (or now) of being able to see either friendship or hostility in another person's face.

Explaining features of human psychology by their usefulness at some stage of evolution is open to a familiar skeptical question. How do we distinguish a well-supported explanation from speculation—an ad hoc "just-so story"? It is not clear that there is any general answer, apart from looking at the kind of evidence available in each case. All the same, keeping the just-so story question as a reminder about caution here, the evolutionary support for the reliability of our senses seems highly plausible. And because reading faces also provides information that is likely to be useful to survival, some parallel between the two arguments seems to hold.

9

Reflective Interpretation

> Reason . . . must approach nature in order to be taught by it. It must not, however, do so in the character of a pupil who listens to everything the teacher chooses to say, but of an appointed judge who compels the witnesses to answer questions which he has himself formulated.
>
> —Immanuel Kant, *Critique of Pure Reason*

The evolutionary approach has been extended to more cognitive predictions of the actions of others. Nicholas Humphrey noticed that the large brains of gorillas suggested minds more powerful than their simple environment called for. While wondering why they had such large brains, he was also thinking about his own personal life: "If I do this, what will *she* do? But suppose I did *that,* or if she did something else?" He thought that gorilla problems too might be mainly social. Perhaps they had evolved to interpret each other. Given the importance of society for humans, perhaps we too had evolved to be psychologists by nature?[1]

Social Chess and Social Cooperation

Humphrey used the metaphor of "social chess" to describe how relating to others requires prediction of their likely decisions, which include their responses to what we do, responses in turn influenced by their predictions of how we will react. Each move in the game "may call forth several alternative responses in the other player. This forward planning will take the form of a decision tree, having its root in the current situation and branches corresponding to the moves considered in looking ahead at different possibilities. It asks for a level of intelligence which is . . . unparalleled in any other sphere of living."[2]

Just as in actual chess (though here without the brute force of chess-playing computers to fall back on), our limited calculating powers in social chess make it urgent to prune the tree's proliferating branches. This need for pruning places an obvious evolutionary premium on human interpretation. Successful strategies, of both intuitive and reflective interpretation, need to be either programmed into us or else internalized so well that they become second nature.

Chess, being competitive, is not the only game that could be a model here. Some games, including versions of prisoners' dilemma, need cooperation for best results. To predict what will achieve cooperation, we need to understand other players. Both the competition and the cooperation in human social life should have favored the evolution of interpretation.

The evolutionary usefulness of our senses does not show that they never deceive us. The evolutionary case about social chess or social cooperation does not show that we always understand people correctly. But we are bristling with these systems for interpreting people—systems honed through the course of human evolution—so it is reasonable to expect them to be roughly reliable.

At the psychological level, how do these systems work? How do we play social chess? And how do we know enough about people to cooperate effectively?

Psychologists have started to work out some of the skills the growing child must acquire from babyhood onward to be able to do this. To grasp another person's goals and desires, the child has to interpret movements as goal-directed actions. To pick up on others' perceptual states, the child has to notice the direction of their eyes and interpret it as seeing what is looked at. There is the further step of comparing the child's own perceptual state with that of another person, which in turn draws on noticing several different things. "We are both looking at the same thing." Then, "She sees that I have seen it." Then, "She sees that I see that she sees . . ." and so on. The suggestion is that we bring these interpretative skills together to create a "theory of mind" based on obvious axioms ("Seeing leads to knowing," or "People believe that things are where they last saw them," and such), a theory that guides our interpretations of people's mental states.[3]

There are debates about whether this approach makes our readings of each other too theoretical. A person with Asperger's syndrome said to me, "I am the only one who needs a theory of mind. The rest of you do it intuitively." An alternative approach suggests that instead of having a theory, we use "simulation"—we imagine the mental states we would have if we were in the other person's position.[4] Perhaps one approach better fits some cases, and the rival approach better fits others. If the interpretative rules of a "theory of mind" can be so internalized as to be unconscious, and if the "simulation" can be guided by unconscious rules, the contrast becomes less sharp. Either way, there is a striking array of skills the child needs for even quite ordinary interpretations of others' minds.

Plausibility and Holism

Some more-complex interpretations draw on even more subtle skills. Consider the skeptically minded jury mentioned earlier, who hope to go beyond the first impression that "he just didn't sound like a man telling the truth." In evaluating the prosecution and the defense cases, they are going to have to assess the credibility of conflicting witnesses. People, as well as nature, must be interrogated not like a pupil but like a judge. As well as judging which case better fits with the facts about time, place and alibis and so on, they are going to have to assess what kind of person the accused man is. What motives and beliefs does the prosecution say he had? What is the rival defense account? Which is psychologically more plausible?

All this involves a degree of holism in the jury's thinking. Doubts about the credibility of a witness may weaken belief in the accused person's defense, but the prosecution story about his motives may seem implausible. The overall verdict has to somehow weigh these very different thoughts—and many others—against each other. The search for a plausible interpretation takes us far beyond guidelines such as "People believe that things are where they last saw them."

Our thinking, whether about people or anything else, has a degree of holism. Our beliefs are interconnected in many different ways to make up a system. Evidence casting doubt on any particular belief may have reverberations on many others.

Suppose something I expect to happen does not happen. I expected that the medicine the doctor prescribed would cure my illness. But it did not. I need to change in some way the beliefs that generated this prediction. Perhaps the doctor is not as good as I thought and got the diagnosis wrong. But this is not my only possible response.

There are alternative revisions I can make, some leaving the doctor's diagnosis unchallenged. The drug company may have supplied a poor-quality batch to the pharmacist. Or the prescription may have been made up wrongly. Or perhaps I have an unusual resistance to this medicine that works for most people.

If I do decide the diagnosis was wrong, I can give up more than my faith in this doctor. I can decide that doctors in general are no good and give up scientific medicine in favor of some alternative therapy. At the extreme I can give up belief, not just in medicine, but in scientific method in general as a way of finding out about the world. Some of these revisions are more plausible than others. But still, the falsification of a prediction leaves me a lot of free play about which revisions to make to my system of beliefs and about how extensive they should be.

One of the great twentieth-century exponents of holism, W. V. O. Quine, said the totality of our beliefs could be seen as "a man-made fabric which impinges on experience only at the edges," or as "a field of force" in which "a conflict with experience at the periphery occasions readjustments in the interior of the field."[5] When evidence seems to go against a belief, we have a choice. We may change or modify that belief. Or we may stick with that belief and instead change other beliefs in our interconnected system.

Jerry Fodor has stressed how difficult this inescapable holism makes it to understand how our thought processes work: "The more global . . . a cognitive process is, the less anybody understands it."[6] Fodor's pessimism may be right. Alternatively, even when radically different kinds of evidence are relevant, we might still be able to make progress in understanding how we assess the plausibility of rival interpretations of other people.

In the interpretation of people, as in the interpretation of anything else, the key issue is what makes one account more plausible than another. On any view, these judgments of plausibility are remarkably subtle and complex. The fact that we successfully play so much social chess shows that the skills of reflective interpretation possessed by the human brain are very powerful. Perhaps they are powerful enough to interpret even our own holistic processes of interpretation?

Self-Interpretation and Self-Creation

Many thinkers (recently, notably Charles Taylor) have stressed that humans are self-interpreting animals. Besides interpreting other people, we interpret our own actions, words, thoughts, and feelings: a running commentary on our inner and outer lives. When we are aware of it, self-consciousness may result: "I am showing I cannot be intimidated" or "I am making a fool of myself." At the lowest level, a lot of the commentary is unconscious, although retrievable if needed. Because of our conversation I hardly notice I am driving. If asked, I can say I was signaling a left turn. If asked more, the left turn is needed to avoid the road works ahead. If asked even more, the hurry is about not missing the start of the play. And so on.

A lot of our self-interpretation is not so boring. "I left because I could not bear another minute of his excruciatingly self-regarding conversation." "I refused because the voice of conscience said it would be a sin." "Taking this job isn't really a compromise. It *is* creative in a kind of way." Such interpretations, being laden with values and attitudes, may provoke others to disagree. They are also more open to our own revision.

Reflection may lead us to change attitudes or the beliefs they depend on. Someone who gives up religious belief may substitute thoughts about irrational guilt for thoughts about sin. Or the emotional tone of the interpretation may be changed by experiencing love, war, or literature, by having children, by being in extreme poverty or being bereaved. Things once important may come to seem shallow. These platitudes are important. Our interpretations change because we change.

And we change because our interpretations do. What we are is shaped by how we interpret ourselves. In addition to the moment-by-moment commentary, self-interpretation is also at the level, not of tactics, but of strategy. The boundary is not sharp, and the difference is one of degree. Hurrying to be in time for the play is tactics; thinking about the kind of husband, wife, partner, or parent you hope to be, or your hopes and plans about your work life, are strategy.

John Rawls wrote of people having life plans. Few (none?) of us are as organized as that. But there are the big, vague, and sometimes conflicting pictures at the back of our minds. "I hope we will still love each other in old age if one of us becomes demented." "I hope I am a good enough parent most of the time." "I try to push aside all this 'management' that has infected universities, hoping to keep its deadening effects from harming my teaching and writing." These vague thoughts express values we have now and hoped-for interpretations of ourselves in the future.

So I am not immune to the way I see myself. The self-interpreting part of us is not inert, but acts on other parts. The person we become is partly shaped by self-interpretation, the yeast that makes the bread rise.

Seeds and Stumbles: Experience from the Inside and Empathy

We need both reflective and intuitive interpretation. Sometimes they feed into each other. Experiencing things from the inside makes reflective interpretation more intuitive.

Because other people like or dislike such different things, we may not have enough feel for what is going on inside them. But even a moment long ago of having shared what they like may give a glimpse. As a girl Virginia Woolf used to be taken fishing. She was excited by feeling the tug on the line and then hauling the fish into the boat. One day her father, without any rebuke, said he did not like to see a fish caught: Virginia was welcome to go the next time, but he would not go along. "Though my passion for the thrill and the tug had been perhaps the most acute that I then knew, his words slowly extinguished it . . . But from the memory of my own passion I am still able to construct an idea of the sporting passion. It is one of those invaluable seeds, from which, since it is impossible to have every experience fully, one can grow something that represents other people's experiences. Often one has to make do with seeds; the germs of what might have been, had one's life been different. I pigeonhole 'fishing' thus with other momentary glimpses; like those rapid glances, for example, that I cast into basements when I walk in London streets."[7]

Sometimes we have more to go on than these momentary glimpses. Some experiences are more widely shared than the tug of a fish on the line. Part of the depth of Tolstoy's novels comes from his writing about so many different kinds of people from the inside. In *Anna Karenina,* Koznyshev (Sergei Ivanovich) and Varenka have grown close to each other and everyone thinks they will get married. They go to the woods to collect mushrooms. They both think this will be the day when Koznyshev proposes to Varenka. He goes off to another part of the birch wood for a few moments' final reflection. He makes his final decision to propose and comes back. They walk a few steps alone together:

> After a silence it would have been easier for them to say what they wanted to say than after talking about mushrooms; but against her own will, as if inadvertently, Varenka said:
>
> "So you did not find any? But then there are always fewer inside the wood."
>
> Sergei Ivanovich sighed and made no answer. He was vexed that she had begun talking about mushrooms. He wanted to bring her back to her first words about her childhood; but, as if against his will, after being silent for a while, he commented on her last words. "I've heard only that the white boletus grows mostly on the edge, though I'm unable to identify it."

More time passed with both of them knowing this was the vital moment. Koznyshev

> repeated to himself the words in which he wished to express his proposal; but instead of those words, by some unexpected consideration that occurred to him, he suddenly asked:
>
> "And what is the difference between a white boletus and a birch boletus?"
>
> Varenka's lips trembled as she answered:
>
> "There's hardly any difference in the caps, but in the feet."
>
> And as soon as these words were spoken, both he and she understood that the matter was ended, and that what was to have been said would not be said.[8]

They did not marry. Of course there can be different interpretations of this passage. One is the "Freudian" approach: Was the verbal stumbling caused by an unconscious reluctance to marry? Did Koznyshev's need for final reflection show less than wholehearted love? But still, if they had broken out of the conversational trap they fell into, they might have discovered how much they wanted each other.

We understand the grammar of a Rembrandt portrait because of our shared memories of how people look when proud or when deepened and saddened by age. We know about the stumbling of Koznyshev and Varenka, the failure to break through inhibition and polite conversation to a deeper level of contact. We understand because we have been there and know it from the inside.

PART THREE

Human Interpretation in Psychiatry

I am—yet what I am, none cares or knows;
  My friends forsake me like a memory lost:
I am the self-consumer of my woes—
  They rise and vanish in oblivions host,
Like shadows in love frenzied stifled throes
  And yet I am, and live—like vapours tost

Into the nothingness of scorn and noise,
  Into the living sea of waking dreams,
Where there is neither sense of life or joys,
  But the vast shipwreck of my lifes esteems;
Even the dearest that I love the best
  Are strange—nay, rather, stranger than the rest.

I long for scenes where man hath never trod
  A place where woman never smiled or wept
There to abide with my Creator God,
  And sleep as I in childhood sweetly slept.
Untroubling and untroubled where I lie
  The grass below, above, the vaulted sky.

—John Clare, "I Am"

10

"A Gulf Which Defies Description"

> Even the dearest that I love the best
> Are strange . . .
>
> —John Clare

We understand Koznyshev and Varenka because we have been there, stumbling in a personal encounter, blurting out what wasn't what we meant to say, and not saying what we really want to. But most of us haven't been where those with severe psychiatric problems are. We do not have the same feel for their experience, and a first-person account can be a shock.

The poet Ivor Gurney fought in the First World War and was injured in a gas attack. His diagnosis, in the language of the time, was "nervous breakdown from deferred shell shock." Later he was committed to an asylum, with auditory hallucinations and delusions of being tormented with electricity. A poem he titled "To God" both harks back to the cruelty of the war and expresses the intense horror of his condition:

> All has deserted me
> And I am merely crying and trembling in heart
> For Death, and cannot get it. And gone out is part
> Of sanity. And there is dreadful Hell within me . . .
>
> And I am praying for death, death, death,
> And dreadful is the indrawing or out-breathing of breath
> Because of the intolerable insults put on my whole soul
> Of the soul loathed, loathed, loathed of the soul.
> Gone out every bright thing from my mind.
> All lost that ever God himself designed.
> Not half can be written of cruelty of man, on man,
> Not often such evil guessed as between Man and Man.[1]

It is not surprising if people with inner lives like that do not always fit in.

Psychiatric Illness, "Strangeness," and Personal Chemistry

People with psychiatric disorders can strike others as strange. Things they do may seem unintelligible. They may look odd or have an unusual posture or gait. They may laugh at unexpected times, or stare, or say things in ways that make it hard to have a conversation with them. At times it is hard to get through to them: they can seem unreachable. And the gulf may seem as wide from the other side too, so that even the dearest that I love the best are strange.

The inaccessibility has baffled families, friends, and psychiatrists. Eugen Bleuler, the inventor of the term "schizophrenia," said that people with the disorder were stranger to him than the birds in his garden. Karl Jaspers said that people with schizophrenia were queer, cold, inaccessible, rigid, and petrified in ways that are peculiarly baffling: "We may think we understand dispositions furthest from our own, but when faced with such people, we feel a gulf which defies description."[2]

People who have been hit by schizophrenia are not birds but persons, and therefore their problems may be compounded by our inability to reach them. Normally we reach people through smiles, frowns, irony, jokes, tone of voice, touching, meeting of the eye, and so on. In a thousand ways we share experience, and signal our shared or our disagreeing responses. Some of this is a shared human grammar. Some of it is shared within a culture or within a smaller group, such as football fans, or lesbians, or members of a religion. Some of it is the private language of a couple, a family, or a group of friends. The way people bond is often thought of as a matter of their "personal chemistry" with each other. Schizophrenia can disrupt this personal chemistry, adding isolation to illness.

Understanding "from the inside" someone with this loneliness matters independently of any contribution to developing a cure. It is also a serious intellectual challenge—to psychiatry, to psychology, and to philosophy. So far our theories about knowledge of other minds have not helped us much here.

Trying to Interpret "Strange" Inner Lives

> I could tell them about school and home, and how I felt about the eating disorder, why I needed to self-harm. It was my way

> of communicating: my way of getting people to listen because I didn't know how to find words, or how to get someone to listen to me.
>
> —Anonymous: An autobiographical case study presented to a conference on child and adolescent psychiatry

A psychiatrist has three central tasks. There is seeing that someone needs psychiatric help: "not waving but drowning." There is interpreting what is going wrong. And there is seeing what may help.

Seeing that someone needs help may draw on the psychiatrist's own emotional reaction to the person. A general practitioner once said to me that "a doctor's own response is his most sensitive instrument."

There is the hope that interpreting what is going wrong may help to put it right. But there is also the hope—perhaps related—of finding an interpretation that can help break down the isolation, the "gulf beyond description." This means trying to see how people who need help see themselves, to get an idea of their experiences. First-person accounts are a key to understanding the ideas and metaphors they use to describe and make sense of their own lives.

Giving appropriate help depends a lot on finding the right interpretation. (Only "a lot," rather than "entirely." Someone with a false theory might still help, simply through sympathetic attempts to understand. But the aim should be to make contact *and* to understand.) There are different possible explanations of a person's emotional unreachability.

People who need help may not want to communicate. Depression or previous hurts may make them despair or hide behind the defensive wall.

Or the problem could be a failure of communication. Perhaps they are not interpreting other people's signals correctly. Not noticing the reactions to bizarre clothes or to sudden inappropriate laughter, or being oblivious to someone else's signals about having to leave, can all create an impression of strangeness. Or the failure can be in the other direction. Perhaps their own appearance, tone of voice, choice of words, or facial expression is sending the wrong signals to other people. Either interpretation suggests a poor sense of the small details of everyday life.

There may be remedies. Sending the right signals, and how to read signals sent back, are teachable skills. Some women with postpartum depression have difficulty bonding with their babies. It sometimes helps to show them videotape of how they and their babies interact. This can help them read and respond to the baby's body language.[3] Psychiatric "strangeness" might be helped by something like this.

Strange behavior can reflect an inner life that is hard for others to intuit. Karl Jaspers thought this: "When we trace back behaviour, activities and general conduct of life in an individual and try to *understand* all this psychologically and *with empathy* we always come up against *certain limits* but with schizophrenic psychic life we reach limits at a point where normally we can still understand . . . Why a patient starts to sing in the middle of the night, why he attempts suicide, begins to annoy his relatives, why a key on the table excites him so much, all this will seem the most natural thing in the world to the patient but he cannot make us understand it."[4]

Such a different inner life raises deep difficulties. Biological psychiatry, citing such causes as abnormalities of brain chemistry, sometimes helps to cure or contain disorders. But it gives no intuitive understanding of how people feel from the inside. We need to start from our normal framework of interpretation and see if it can be extended to fit the people we are trying to understand.

This framework could be called "Aristotelian common sense." Aristotle gave a systematic analysis of our everyday understanding of people: how beliefs and desires shape decisions and actions, how actions turn into habits, and how habits turn into character. He gave recognizable outlines of the framework—sometimes dismissed as prescientific "folk psychology"—which we still use in thinking about people and what they do.

Critics say this framework has not developed since ancient times. Our folk psychology is mainly informal and intuitive, so its growth can easily go unnoticed. Its extension by Freud is an instance. Of course, much Freudian theory is widely doubted: the Oedipus complex, the death instinct, "pale criminality," and so on. So it is easy to overlook how such Freudian concepts as unconscious motives, repression, projection, and defense mechanisms have been absorbed into our folk psychology. In his poem on Freud's death, Auden got the balance just right: "If often he was wrong and at times absurd / To us he is no more a person / Now but a whole climate of opinion." The case of Freud highlights a question. What is progress here? Unconscious motives have entered everyday psychological thinking. The perhaps less plausible death instinct has not. But there is a lot to investigate about what the constraints of plausibility are here, and what *their* claim to be accepted comes to.

Our evolved skills of interpreting other people give a good reason for taking folk psychology as a starting point. But Aristotelian physics is a warning. Aristotle created a brilliant synthesis of the science and the folk physics of his time. In the seventeenth century it came to be accepted that bodies not interfered with may either be at rest or else be in a state of uniform motion in a straight line. Aristotle's contrary view was that bodies must be at rest until some force moves them. His view, more than modern physics, reflects intuitive common sense. His commonsense psychology has not dated in the same way, but it also is challenged. Neuroscience may change our conceptual map of freedom of action and of personal identity. And common sense has difficulties with some of the complexities of many aspects of psychiatric disorder, such as delusions.

Psychiatry should be both conservative and revisionary. We need all our skills of human interpretation, *and* skepticism about some of the categories of thought they rely on. And there is a lot to learn from what people say about their own "strange" behavior.

11

Autism and Interpretation

> While I was trapped between the windows, it was almost impossible to communicate through the glass. Being autistic is like being trapped like this. The windows symbolized my feelings of disconnection from other people and helped me cope with the isolation.
>
> —Temple Grandin, *Thinking in Pictures and Other Reports from My Life with Autism*

> This isolation was not from being left to my own devices. It stemmed from the isolation of my inner world and only the unthreatening nature of privacy and space would inspire the courage to explore the world and get out of my world under glass step by step.
>
> —Donna Williams, *Nobody Nowhere: The Remarkable Autobiography of an Autistic Girl*

Autistic people do not find it easy to understand the world in ways other people do. And others often find them "strange" and hard to understand. Interpreting what they do is the first challenge their condition poses to psychiatric efforts to help them.

The Autistic Landscape

The diagnosis of autism is based on patterns of behavior rather than on genetic or other biological evidence. Large variations in the severity of the problems show that an all-or-none diagnosis of "autism" would cover a very wide band indeed. This made it natural to move to the dimension approach implied by "the autistic spectrum." It is widely accepted that this in turn is too simple and that there is at least an "autistic triad."[1] The three dimensions of the triad are (1) impaired social capacities; (2) impaired capacities for communication; and (3) limited imagination. The weak social capacities and impaired communication include difficulties with conversation, with sharing interests, emotions, and responses, and with eye contact and body language. Autistic people might make no use of gestures or facial expressions. They find it hard to relate to people and make friends. They may lack interest in people.

Limited imagination is also shown in rigidity or repetition: always taking the same routes or eating the same food, repeating speech or movements, or fixation on a narrow set of interests. People with autism can also find it hard to interpret other people's mental states. As children they are not good at imaginative play. But "limited imagination" does not mean they have no inner imaginative life.[2] In particular, other people may too readily see an autistic person's difficulties with interpretation as indicating a lack of empathy. The view from inside may be different: "I ask you, those of you who are with us all day, not to stress yourselves out because of us. When you do this, it feels as if you're denying any value at all that our lives may have . . . The hardest ordeal for us is the idea that we are causing grief for other people . . . the thought that our lives are the source of other people's unhappiness, that's plain unbearable."[3]

Research suggests there is little overlap in the genes associated with the three dimensions, which are combined in different proportions in different persons with autism.[4] As the picture grows more complicated, some have suggested that we should think, not of autism, but of *autisms,* and replace the autistic spectrum by the *autistic landscape.*

The "Language" of Autism

> The words we want to say and the words we *can* say don't always match that well . . . When there's a gap between what I'm thinking and what I'm saying, it's because the words coming out of my mouth are the only ones I can access at that time.
>
> —Naoki Higashida, *The Reason I Jump*

> Though I spoke with the words of "the world," my gestures were and remain the more important language of "my world."
>
> —Donna Williams, *Nobody Nowhere*

The incapacity and distress severe autism imposes on those who have it can be very great. They may seem to take no notice of other people. They may be largely or entirely unable to use spoken language. They may have frequent screaming fits, or for long periods make anxious-sounding noise. Patterns of self-injury include slapping themselves, pulling their hair, or continuously banging their heads.

This kind of behavior seems hard to interpret at the "human" level of beliefs, desires, and intentions. At first sight it may seem more plausible to interpret it, as was once standard, in terms of some neurological breakdown causing unmotivated bodily activity. The screaming fits, the noises, the slapping and head-banging can seem to be below the level of intelligible actions.

But there are reasons not to give up on interpretation too soon. Jim Sinclair gives some in an open letter to parents of autistic children:

> You try to relate as parent to child, using your own understanding of normal children, your own experiences and intuitions about relationships. And the child doesn't respond in any way you can recognize as being part of that system. That does not mean that the child is incapable of relating. It only means you're assuming a shared system, a shared understanding of signals and meanings, that the child in fact does not share . . . It takes more work to communicate with someone whose native language isn't yours . . . You're going to have to learn to back up to levels more basic than you've probably thought about before, to translate, and to check to make sure your translations are understood. You're going to have to . . . let your child teach you a little of her language, guide you a little way into his world . . . Approach respectfully, without preconceptions, and with openness to learning new things, and you'll find a world you could never have imagined.[5]

Problems of Interpreting the World and Other People

> The essential social problem in autistic spectrum conditions is not one of avoidance of, or lack of interest in, interacting with others . . . but inability to grasp the tacit rules that govern

> social interaction intuitively, or to "read" the facial expression, tone of voice and body language of others. Often, our own body language is odd and we do not express emotions in the same way as others. (I remember as a child that I had to teach myself how to do a "social smile" while looking in a mirror.)
>
> —Clare Sainsbury, *The Martian in the Playground*

The "strangeness" of many individuals who inhabit the autistic landscape is exacerbated by this limited grasp of the shared grammar of reading each other. Some people with less severe versions of autism, and others who have emerged from the more severe versions, have described this from the inside. They describe the autistic inner life to be interpreted and give clues about how to do it. Like any group, autistic people vary a lot in their inner lives, so there may be different "dialects" in the autistic language to be interpreted. Temple Grandin says that because autistic people often think more visually than verbally, the meaning they give to words may depend heavily on individual associations: "For example, 'French toast' may mean happy if the child was happy while eating it." And for one child "partly heard song" meant "I don't know."[6]

Donna Williams had such severe childhood autism that some thought she was psychotic.[7] She is now a successful author, artist, and singer, but she remembers her limited powers of interpretation in childhood. She decided not to sing in front of other people, but "I didn't realize for many years that they could still hear me even if I couldn't see them."[8] She could read, but could not grasp what novels were about: "It was as though the meaning got lost in the jumble of trivial words."[9] Once in class she sat next to a girl with hair in a plait: "I ran my hand down her plait. She looked around at me and I was frightened by the way that her face was joined to her hair. I had wanted to touch her hair, not her."[10] And more generally: "I could comprehend the actions of another person, particularly if they were extreme, but I had trouble coping with 'whole people'—their motivations and expectations, particularly to do with giving and receiving."[11]

As a reaction to the struggle to interpret her experience of the world, she developed defenses. Perhaps autistic rigidity and repetition are too readily seen as reflecting only a lack of imagination. Donna Williams's repetitious concern with order and system was a defense: "The constant change of most things never seemed to give me any chance to prepare myself for them. Because of this I found pleasure and comfort in doing the same things over and over again."[12] Part of the difficulty of interpreting change seemed to come from its speed. Her defenses against this must have seemed odd from outside: "One of the ways of making things seem to slow down was to blink or to turn the lights on and off really fast."[13]

Autistic Thinking and Problems of Expression

> One of the biggest misunderstandings you have about us is your belief that our feelings aren't as subtle and complex as yours. Because how we behave can appear so childish in your eyes, you tend to assume that we're childish on the inside, too. But of course, we experience the same emotions that you do. And because people with Autism aren't skilful talkers, we may in fact be even more sensitive than you are. Stuck here inside these unresponsive bodies of ours, with feelings we can't properly express, it's always a struggle just to survive.
>
> —Naoki Higashida, *The Reason I Jump*

Temple Grandin is an autistic woman whose thinking is overwhelmingly visual. She says words are her second language. Her work includes designing equipment for dipping cattle without making them panic. Other equipment she devises might use computer modeling, but she can work it out by "running three-dimensional visual simulations" in her imagination, testing designs by imagining cattle walking through them. "It is like seeing it on a videotape in my mind. I can view it from any angle, placing myself above or below the equipment and rotating it at the same time. I don't need a fancy graphics programme that can produce three-dimensional design simulations. I can do it better and faster in my head."[14]

But communication can be hard for people who have words as only their second language. Learning to express themselves to others can be painfully slow. "To talk, I first had to think the words, almost write them in my head, usually twice if I was to say a longish sentence . . . The difficulty in linking thoughts and voice made it hard to keep up if more than two people were involved in a conversation. By the time I had thought out what I was going to say, and directed my voice to say it, the opportunity to say anything had usually passed."[15]

Exposure Anxiety

From outside, the reluctance of some autistic people to be touched can seem mysterious. Naoki Higashida says how it seems to him from inside: "For a person with autism, being touched by someone else means that the toucher is exercising control over a body, which even its owner can't properly control. It's as if we lose who we are . . . There's also the dread that by being touched our thoughts will become visible. And if that happened, the other person would *really* start worrying about us. You see? We put up a barricade around ourselves to keep people out."[16]

Donna Williams could also use her defenses against other people and what she saw as intrusiveness. At a dancing class, instructions were called out, and someone might try to guide her. "Helpful invasive arms, instructing, interfering. Me looking at my feet. The walls were going up. The music was a blur. There was too much turmoil going on around me, invading my space and invading my mind. With clenched fists, I stamped my foot and spat several times upon the floor."[17]

The feeling of being invaded was linked to fear of exposing her own personality. Touching on anything personal in her writing for English classes, she would write obliquely, almost in code. Her drawings were often symbolic, "as anything too personal could never be seen unless I could create some sort of distance."[18] When she needed to ask a question, she again would do so obliquely, not looking directly at the person and then seeming to ignore the reply. "It took an incredible degree of courage to seek out an audience and talk about something I was interested in. To me, this made me painfully vulnerable. I was expressing something about my own personality and identity. The fear it inspired would simply not have allowed me to express anything personal in any other way."[19]

Imaginary friends were easier. "They were far more magical, reliable and predictable and real than other children, *and* they came with guarantees. It was a world of my own creation where I didn't need to control myself or the objects, animals and nature, which were simply *being* in my presence. I had two other friends who did not belong to this physical world: the wisps, and a pair of green eyes which hid under my bed, named Willie." Imaginary friends could become a defensive mask: "As with anything I became close to, I would try to lose myself within it. I took to sleeping under the bed and I became Willie. By this time I was three years old. Willie became the self I directed at the outside world, complete with hateful glaring eyes, a pinched-up mouth, rigid corpse-like stance and clenched fists."[20]

Masking her inner self against exposure could make Donna Williams feel that she too was getting out of touch with it: "I see that girl in the mirror, looking back at me. / I see her thinking I am crazy, for believing I am free. / Yet I can see it in her eyes that as I am staring, / She's trying to understand that I am not lying, / I am just trying to find my way back home to me."[21]

Interpreting the Language of Martians

Autistic people's accounts from the inside have made these aspects of their world available. Their difficulties in interpretation and expression, and their anxieties and defenses, are the context for interpreting their "language." Sometimes they explain what they are trying to cope with or express with their "strangeness."

Donna Williams mentions difficulty with depth perception. Dropping things repetitively makes the dimension of depth seem more real, as does rocking from one foot to another. But there is also an emotional side. Repetitive dropping expresses the freedom to let good emotions flow in and out of herself without pain or fear. Rocking from one foot to another can feel like preparing to leap over the darkness between herself and the world. The rhythm and jolting of jumping seems to help the jumble in her brain to sort itself out. Clapping can signal either pleasure or the end of something. Laughing releases tension or anxiety. Head-banging can help with tension: thudding rhythms in her head calm her down. Looking directly at things can make it hard for her to see their significance, but "staring past them" is relaxing and makes them easier to take in.[22]

What seems strangely antisocial becomes more intelligible in the context of exposure anxiety and its related worries about identity. Sometimes she would sit for a long time in her room absorbed in the wallpaper patterns. "When I needed to go to the toilet I'd get up and take a few steps across the floor before going on the purple carpet I hated so much. As time went by I became more and more aware of myself through doing this. I'd watch a puddle form and giggle as it seeped into the precious carpet. Symbolically this was 'my world' with a 'me' in it. The more I covered that carpet, the more of a 'me' in the world there was. The smell didn't worry me. The smell belonged to me and closed out other things. By the time my mother discovered what I'd done, my purpose for doing this had already been achieved. I'd called myself back out of my body into my room—a room I'd made sure belonged to me."[23]

Accounts from inside, by making autism more intelligible, narrow the distance between autistic and nonautistic life.

Ian Hacking has argued that it may be wrong to think of these individuals as describing autism "from the inside." He invites us to read these texts "not as describing well-defined experience, but as creating ways to express experiences," and suggests that they may be "less telling what it is like to be autistic than constituting it."[24] The contrast between telling what it is like and constituting it may be misleading. Could the accounts not be doing both? Perhaps all of us, in finding words to describe to others our often blurry and amorphous inner lives, impose on them interpretations that change our own experiences of those lives. Telling and constituting interact with each other, whether we have autism or not.

Hacking's objection to talking about things "inside the mind" is that it carries the suggestion that looking inside the mind is like trying to see into a closed box. So from outside we can know what someone thinks, feels, or intends only by inference from their behavior. He follows Ludwig Wittgenstein in being skeptical about the need for inference. Just as we often see, rather than infer, what a painting depicts, so we often *see* that someone is angry or intends to answer the telephone.

Wittgenstein was influenced by Wolfgang Kohler, who believed we see a whole gestalt, not separate items to be put together like a jigsaw. Kohler said that a friend looking at my face will *see* me tense up when I notice a snake. He is quite right that the friend will not have to work out an inference: "There is a snake. Now it is entering his visual field. The expression on his face has suddenly changed. Perhaps I can infer that he has undergone a change of psychological state." We do not have the innocent eye that would make such a labor of it. Instead we have all the mechanisms underlying the grammar of facial interpretation. We are not conscious of them, but their functioning lets us to see it intuitively.

None of this means that the metaphor, if it is a metaphor, of "inside" is misleading. Often we can read in a face anger, inner guilt, or love. But not always. Proust was right to be uncertain about how Françoise felt about him. And most people can't just *see* how an autistic person behaving strangely is feeling inside. Autistic grammar of expression and of interpretation is different from ours, and not intuitive to us.

If we see a girl making a puddle and giggling as the wet seeps into the carpet, the interpretation does not just leap out at us. Does this mean that the autobiographical account is not "telling what it is like to be autistic" but instead "constituting" it? When Donna Williams later wrote, "The more I covered that carpet, the more of a 'me' in the world there was," she is using metaphorical language that the rest of us might use. It seems unnecessarily skeptical to doubt that she is expressing a feeling we understand.

Temple Grandin once said, "Much of the time I feel like an anthropologist on Mars."[25] Some people on the autistic spectrum express the thought the other way around. Clare Sainsbury's book about her schooldays, *Martian in the Playground,* reflects the fact that (what she later discovered to be) Asperger's syndrome made her feel put on this planet by mistake. If we were visited by real Martians, we would expect their language to be difficult for us and would make great efforts to interpret them. The rest of us formerly did not realize that people with autism were in this way Martians, whose strange behavior was a language we could try to interpret.

It goes without saying that those autistic people who *feel* like Martians are *not* aliens. *(Homo sum, humani nihil a me alienum puto.)* Now that some of the "Martians" have managed to break through and tell us a bit about their thought and language, there is a real hope that we can start to map its outlines, its dialects, and its idiosyncratic personal differences. There may still be a long way to go, but the fundamental change has taken place. What seemed too strange to have any meaning is now potentially open to interpretation and to all that may flow from that. It is a model to bear in mind when approaching other "unintelligible" psychiatric conditions.

12

Interpreting Delusions

> She . . .
> . . . speaks things in doubt
> That carry but half sense. Her speech is nothing.
> Yet the unshaped use of it doth move
> The hearers to collection; they aim at it,
> And botch the words up to fit their own thoughts.
>
> —Gentleman (on Ophelia's madness),
> William Shakespeare, *Hamlet*

To understand delusions we need to work out the neurological or neurochemical changes linked to them. But we also need to interpret what is going on at the human or psychological level. Delusions themselves involve interpretations, although deviant ones, of what the deluded person experiences.

Delusions may be distortions of either intuitive or reflective interpretation. Perhaps there is not always a sharp boundary between the two. As with night and day, there may be dusk in which the intuitive and the reflective shade into each other. The answer to this is relatively unimportant. Nearly all of the relevant cases are clearly on one side or the other of the boundary. In at least one direction there is interaction. Intuitive distortions sometimes cause distortions of the reflective interpretation needed to back them up.

"Delusion" is hard to define. It is common to think of delusions as false beliefs, irrationally based and stubbornly held. This is not utterly wrong, but it is too simple.

Instead of attempting a watertight definition, I will outline a cluster of central features of delusions, or at least of the delusions for which psychiatric help may be relevant.

The Delusional Cluster

There are problems about how strongly some delusional "beliefs" are really held. There is "double bookkeeping." The person may say, "The staff here are poisoning my food," and then happily go off to lunch. Apparent statements of belief may be undermined by a mocking demeanor or a manic cackle.

One psychiatrist's patient claimed to have had a baby at Buckingham Palace. This claim, if persisted in by a woman with no royal connections, seems to be a false belief amounting to a delusion. However, there are possible interpretations of her saying "I had a baby at Buckingham Palace" that do not involve her believing in the statement. She could be toying with the idea that it is true, or acting out a fantasy about being a princess. It could be something said to mislead or annoy the psychiatrist. It could be some kind of joke. Things said by people seeing psychiatrists can have the ambiguities of comments by Shakespearean clowns or fools.

Even where belief does come in, there is a range of possibilities. Perhaps the person believes the delusion quite literally—or holds part of it, wavering about it at different times. There is also nonliteral "belief," again found also in people without a psychiatric diagnosis. Joan Didion described her "year of magical thinking" after her husband John died: "Of course I knew John was dead . . . Yet I was myself in no way prepared to accept this news as final; there was a level on which I believed that what had happened remained reversible." Clearing out his clothes, she found a reluctance to give away his shoes: "I stood there for a moment, then realized why: he would need shoes if he was to return. The recognition of this thought by no means eradicated the thought. I have still not tried to determine (say, by giving away the shoes) if the thought has lost its power."[1]

A woman with a diagnosis of schizophrenia had a delusion linked to vomiting. Her later account was explicit about her "belief" not being literal: "I got the idea that in taking food I was in a sense eating the body of my youngest child. I did not believe this to be the literal case, but the aversion to food was because of this association."[2] Many delusions are better described as being "on the belief spectrum" rather than simply as beliefs.

Delusional beliefs are often false, even bizarrely so. But we all have false beliefs, and delusions sometimes may happen to be true. Some paranoid people really are persecuted. What matters is whether experience or other evidence is interpreted in ways likely to produce beliefs that track reality.

We all have only limited rationality.[3] So coming to beliefs by imperfect means of tracking reality does not mark off deluded people from the rest of us. Irrationality is a matter of degree. Delusional beliefs, though, are based on *extremely* poor means of tracking reality.

Typically they involve *over*interpretation, often to an extreme. David C. Boyles describes this as part of his experience of schizophrenia: "Then the songs on the radio started to be singing directly to me. There was a messaging theme from all the songs. I was supposed to choose. I was stuck in between two worlds . . . Things in the environment were taking on new meanings. I noticed black birds flying in circles in the sky. It was a symbolism to me, of evil waiting to catch its prey."[4] When the phone rang at night, he rejected his brother's telling him it was a friend, thinking "it was evil calling, coming to get me." When he was driving at night, the brightness of the oncoming headlights was a "contact from God."[5]

What about fanatical followers of dubious religious or political systems of belief? Psychiatric delusions are only a minority of stubbornly held irrational beliefs. Delusions need to be distinguished from such beliefs coming from indoctrination or other social influences. In the psychiatric context, delusions are stubbornly held irrational beliefs that come from some personal distortion of thought. Richard Dawkins writes of *The God Delusion,* which he sees as a delusion in the sense of being an irrational false belief. He does not see it as a *psychiatric* delusion, but as one heavily influenced by indoctrination and social pressures. As his book shows, he sees it as a delusion for which the cure is argument, not psychiatric treatment.

Delusions are stubbornly held. Few psychiatrists expect to reason someone out of a delusion. If the victim of a delusion does question it, checking sometimes seems only to generate new experiences apparently confirming it: "Then I began to have the feeling that other people were watching me. And, as periodically happened throughout the early stages, I said to myself that the whole thing was absurd, but when I looked again the people really were watching me."[6]

Different kinds of delusion may need different explanations. Hearing "voices" may have different causes from delusions of alien control, where the person thinks some of his or her actions come from the will of someone else. "Thought insertion," where the person believes "This thought is in my mind, but is put there by someone else," may need a different explanation from Cotard's delusion: "I am dead."

Some delusions are only about a specific topic. Some of these are bizarre. People with Capgras delusion think a family member or friend has been replaced by an identical impostor. Some, equally specific, are much less peculiar. People with rejection sensitivity are sometimes deluded about other people's attitudes toward them: "The doctors and nurses in this hospital have all taken against me." At the other extreme are wide-ranging delusional systems, where the individual sees the entire world through a ramified system of incorrect beliefs. Some delusions last a long time; others are unstable and fleeting.

Some delusions (including thought insertion, delusions of alien control, Cotard's delusion, and others) involve distorted awareness of oneself or one's thoughts or actions. Others, such as delusions of persecution, are not about oneself in the same immediate way. Different delusions may involve different distortions of perception or thought. A single delusion may have more than one cause. And what explains the origin of a delusion may not explain its content.

Distortions of Intuitive Interpretation

Some great scientists and philosophers, including Wilhelm Ostwald and Ernst Mach, were at first skeptical about the existence of atoms. Einstein traced this back to their "stick to the facts" attitude: "This is an interesting example of the fact that even scholars of audacious spirit and fine instinct can be obstructed in the interpretation of facts by philosophical prejudices. The prejudice—which has by no means died out in the meantime—consists in the faith that facts by themselves can and should yield scientific knowledge without free conceptual construction. Such a misconception is possible only because one does not easily become aware of the free choice of such concepts, which, through verification and long usage, appear to be immediately connected with the empirical material."[7]

In this obliviousness to interpretation these thinkers are, on a grander scale, like the rest of us. Most of us do not know—or else forget—Proust's thoughts about the intellectual processes involved in such an apparently simple thing as seeing a face. We do not think about the possible role of mirror neurons in seeing what other people are doing. Few people notice how much they impose interpretations on what they see or hear. So interpretations can seem obvious, not open to serious challenge.

A Muslim taxi driver asked me what my religion was. When I said I did not believe in God, he was astonished. How I could *possibly* not believe? A large issue for a taxi ride, but I said something about reluctance to believe things without good evidence. He expressed further astonishment. How could I not *see* the evidence in everything around us? He unconsciously made the much debated assumption that order or beauty in the world must come from a designer. The striking thing was the unawareness of any assumptions or interpretation on his part. He just *saw* the work of God in all around him. Interpretation was invisible to the taxi driver as it was to Ostwald and Mach.

Often we do know about our reflective interpretations. Playing social chess, we consciously estimate other people's reactions to what we do. But intuitive interpretation, lying behind the way we just "see" things, is rarely conscious. Some people are completely unaware of these processes of interpretation. Others notice them only in reflective moments. Because interpretations usually seem to be just how things are, it is easy to be taken in by a false intuitive interpretation. And for deluded people, as for taxi drivers and great scientists, it is hard to be persuaded of a mistake.

Delusions of alien abduction are a case in point. Some people have awaked from sleep to find they cannot move. They interpret this as having been paralyzed by aliens who are abducting them. There is a plausible alternative account of their paralysis. In some stages of sleep, motor output from the brain is blocked, so that our body does not do things like lash out at people who threaten us in dreams. This sleep paralysis normally goes away when we wake up. But under some conditions there is a delay, resulting in a frightening experience of waking up unable to move.

It is very hard to change people's minds about having been a victim of alien abduction. In her study of this, Susan Clancy gives various explanations, of which the first is that "the abduction memories and the concomitant emotions *feel* real to them."[8] Why do the abduction memories feel real? The invisibility of interpretation probably plays a role. We see these people as having an experience of paralysis and wrongly interpreting it as part of alien abduction. But to them the experience presented itself as an *experience of being abducted by aliens,* with the element of interpretation hidden from view. So any skeptic seems to be denying that they had the experience that they remember so vividly. If this is right, it may be a factor in other delusions as well.

One account of delusions sees them as rational responses to strange experiences. They are thought to come from the person's trying to make sense of abnormal experiences caused by some neurological or neurochemical failure.[9] This model has been applied to hearing "voices," delusions of alien control, and thought insertion.

On this account, the "voices" people hear come from a breakdown in the brain mechanisms that let us distinguish real sounds from imagined ones. Christopher Frith suggests that some symptoms of schizophrenia reflect a disorder of self-awareness. They may come from a breakdown in the system that underlies our normal awareness of our own goals and intentions.[10] Delusions of alien control involve a failure to realize that my action was brought about by my own intention. People who hear "voices" ascribe the products of their own imagination to external speakers. And those with thought insertion do not recognize that they themselves are the authors of certain thoughts rising up in their own minds.

Christopher Peacocke has suggested that what the person lacks an awareness of might not be intentions and goals. The missing awareness may be of something more fundamental. To think a thought is a kind of action, similar in this way to physical activity, normally active rather than passive. But persons with these delusions experience their thoughts or actions as passive. This misplaced sense of passivity may be the key to both thought insertion and "alien control." The deluded person might know his or her intentions but just not realize that they are *actively carrying them out.*[11]

These are all failures in the brain's self-monitoring mechanisms that normally give rise to the sense of agency. When I decide to drink some water, the brain monitors this intention. My awareness of it accompanies my lifting the glass to my lips. This is what keeps our actions on track. If the monitoring fails, I may find myself lifting the glass, apparently without intending to do so. The idea of being controlled by someone else may seem a possible explanation of this.

This model may fit thought insertion. Having a thought can be seen as a kind of performance, again coming from an instruction that is monitored. Of course it does not feel as if a thought is preceded by such an instruction. When we see the leaves fall, a thought about Hopkins's poem "Margaret" might come to mind. We are not aware of any process coming between seeing the leaves and the thought. But as John Campbell has suggested, there must be some process, no doubt unconscious, by which seeing the leaves causes the thought. Perhaps our thoughts are kept on track by a monitoring process, as our actions are. Breakdown of the monitoring system could make a thought seem not to be under one's own normal control. As with "alien control" of actions, the sense of passivity could create an impression that the thought comes from "outside."[12]

Why are delusions so persistent, clung to so hard? Some of them have a peculiar vividness and intensity. The writer with the pen name "John Custance" was diagnosed with manic-depressive psychosis. He took from a psychiatry textbook the phrase "heightened sense of reality." This fitted times when "the outer world makes a much more vivid and intense impression on me than usual." One aspect of this he noticed was heightened visual experience. Others were rapid leaps from one idea to another, and a sense of ineffable revelation in which it seemed that "all truth, all the secrets of the Universe were being revealed, as though I had some clue, some Open-Sesame to creation."[13]

Part of the stubbornness of delusions could be that this vividness and sense of revelation give such a powerfully authentic impression that skepticism stands little chance against them.

Tagging

Our knowledge of some things about our bodies and our mental lives comes from some kind of inner "tag." I know which hand is my right one, without being able to say *how* I know. I know a name is on the tip of my tongue without understanding how. Things are tagged in many different ways. Some tags may be linked to delusions. They include tagging things as familiar or strange, tagging things as being or not being part of "me," and tagging thoughts or actions according to what I intend them to be.

Some delusions involve disturbance of our usual ability to recognize people. Obviously this could be linked to a failure of our normal systems for recognizing faces. But sometimes the explanation could involve tagging.

One component of recognition can be thought of as a "familiar/strange" tagging system. Among disorders of recognition, perhaps the most dramatic is the previously mentioned Capgras delusion: the belief that someone close has died and been replaced by an identical impostor. A related delusion is that someone's appearance has changed so they now look just like someone else. And there is the Fregoli delusion (named after an actor and impersonator) of a persecutor who turns up disguised as various other people. Perhaps a "familiar/strange" tagging system, working too hard, generates these indescribable but intense and conviction-laden experiences.

Andrew Young and others have put forward an account of a failure that could be involved in Capgras delusion.[14] There is evidence for the existence of at least two anatomically different systems involved in recognition. There is "overt" recognition, based on analysis of information about the person's appearance, voice, and so on. And there is "covert" recognition, involving an emotional response that tags the person as familiar. Young suggests that the covert system may be out of action in those with Capgras delusion, with the result that, although they know the person in front of them looks and sounds exactly like their husband, wife, or partner, the absence of the normal emotional response gives a strong tag of unfamiliarity, leading to thoughts about an impostor.

Another system that may be disrupted is the tagging of things as being or not being part of me. The idea of things being tagged as "me" or "not me" gets some support from the difficulty of describing experiences of peculiarly vivid awareness of "being me" that people sometimes have. In *The Idiot,* Fyodor Dostoyevsky draws on his own experience in describing the intensity of Prince Mishkin's consciousness just before the onset of an epileptic fit. It was "purely and simply an intense heightening of self-awareness . . . and, at the same time, the most direct sense of one's own existence taken to the highest degree."[15]

It is striking that Dostoyevsky does not specify any visual, tactile, emotional, or other feature of the experience. There is no equivalent of Proust's madeleine dipped in tea that might serve as a vehicle for this direct sense of one's own existence. The lack of such a vehicle would fit with the cause of the pre-epileptic experience being some kind of boosted functioning of an unconscious tagging system.

Gerard Manley Hopkins had moments of heightened self-awareness. He emphasized the distinctiveness of the experience. He also stressed its incommunicability—something that would be expected if it came from unconscious tagging rather than from interpreting some sensory or emotional feature of the experience. He said, "When I consider my self-being, my consciousness and feeling of myself, that taste of myself, of I and me above and in all things, which is more distinctive than the taste of ale or alum, more distinctive than the smell of walnutleaf or camphor, and is incommunicable by any means to another man (as when I was a child I used to ask myself: What must it be to be someone else?). Nothing else in nature comes near this unspeakable stress of pitch, distinctiveness, and selving, this self-being of my own."[16]

As with Dostoyevsky, the incommunicability of the nature of Hopkins's intense experience of the self suggests an unconscious tagging system. If there is such a "me/not me" tagging system, its failure or malfunctioning could be part of the explanation of the inarticulate certainty that "I am dead" found in those with Cotard's delusion.

Sometimes in dreams or imagination we make mistakes that can be seen in two ways. I dream I am having a conversation with Mahatma Gandhi, but the image of the face is of Jawaharlal Nehru. Was I dreaming of Gandhi but making a mistake about his face, or was I dreaming of Nehru but getting his name wrong? I may simply know the answer to this: "It *was* Gandhi—I just got the face wrong." The dream is mine and my sense of what was going on overrides the visual discrepancy.

There is a system of labels or tagging bound up with what I take myself to be doing. If the person was tagged as Gandhi, then that is what my image meant even if I did get the face wrong. (It is said that Warden Spooner, after preaching a sermon in New College Chapel, corrected himself: "Every time I said 'Aristotle,' I should of course have said 'Saint Paul.'" Even an eccentric preacher is the authority on what he meant to talk about.)

Normally we cannot explain what this tagging consists in by citing a feature of the experience. There is no equivalent of the caption appearing below someone's face on television. ("It may be Nehru's face, but underneath it *says* it is Gandhi.") Tagging seems to involve no conscious interpretation of any sign. Whatever goes on in the process of tagging is unconscious. All we are aware of is the end result: our conviction that it is Gandhi. No one is going to persuade us that we are wrong. If tagging is linked to delusions, they might be clung to so strongly because of some carryover of this unshakeable conviction.

Why do people cling to delusions so stubbornly? Perhaps the heightened sense of reality plays a role. So, perhaps, does the unshakable certainty given by tagging. Even if both factors are relevant, there are still unanswered questions about delusions' deep roots. When one delusion is given up, why does another often emerge to replace it? This substitution suggests a "wellspring" model, in which delusions rich in detail keep bubbling up to the surface of the mind. To say the wellspring must be some kind of unconscious mental activity is not to explain it. (Though there may be some link with whatever unconscious processes generate dreams, which also are often startlingly specific.) It is hardly news to say that there are processes here of which we understand almost nothing.

Distortions of Reflective Interpretation

Some accounts of delusions emphasize "poor reality testing"—the misinterpretation of evidence. Other accounts suggest that delusions may reflect differences of epistemological stance—distortions deeper and more central in the person's way of interpreting the world.

If delusions are partly defined as beliefs that are based on bad tracking of reality, to *explain* them by "poor reality testing" is close to tautological. To have content, the explanation has to cite fairly specific distortions of perception or thought. One possibility is that delusions come from highly exaggerated versions of distortions to which we are all prone.

"Normal" people weigh evidence in ways that are systematically skewed. When people are given a description of another's personality (shy, meek, tidy, and so on) and asked to guess the probability of his being a farmer or a librarian, they tend to see which of their two stereotypes the personality fits. They ignore the fact that there are many more farmers than librarians.[17]

Our judgment is distorted by irrelevant factors, giving too much weight to the first case ("anchoring") or to cases involving people we know or who are famous ("salience"). We more easily accept evidence fitting our preconceptions than evidence against them. We underinterpret evidence, not seeing the wood for the trees. Or we overinterpret it, jumping to conclusions, projecting patterns onto it, or seeing causes in mere conjunctions.[18]

Where "poor reality testing" seems the right account, exaggerated versions of "standard" distortions such as salience and anchoring may help to generate and maintain delusions. Overinterpretation may play a role in paranoia. There is evidence that people with delusions are more ready than others to jump to conclusions, even about things not relevant to their delusions.[19]

There are some questions left unanswered by this approach. For instance, why are delusions so specific? "Poor reality testing" does not explain this. One woman thought she was being persecuted by spectacle-wearing doctors and nurses, who used their glasses to refract too much light into her eyes.[20] She was not just overestimating the probability of this happening. Why persecution by means of light? Why with spectacles?

Another remaining question is why many delusions are so bizarre. There are thoughts that other people are robots, or that the whole world depends on me, or that my best friend has been replaced by an identical impostor. Being so bizarre, these beliefs suggest something more radically wrong than cognitive biases or unusual experiences. And the belief of people with Cotard's syndrome that they are dead goes beyond the bizarre to the paradoxical or impossible.

People's accounts of their delusions are sometimes so bizarre as to be almost unintelligible. Philosophers such as Ludwig Wittgenstein, W. V. O. Quine, and Donald Davidson in different ways have stressed the links between meaning and belief. If, on my interpretation of what you say, your beliefs come out as unintelligible or highly irrational, this raises the question: Have I misinterpreted you? If it all makes more sense on a different account of what you meant, should not that account be preferred?

John Campbell has pointed out that this kind of rationality constraint on how we interpret people raises a problem about interpreting delusions.[21] Can someone who says he is dead, despite walking and talking, really understand "dead" as we do? Can someone who claims her husband has been replaced by an impostor, and does nothing to test this by discussing past shared experiences, really understand the meaning of what she says?

In his discussion of this question, Campbell quotes a person with schizophrenia who said that his words bear two meanings: the meanings they ordinarily have and the meanings he is trying to use them to express. There is no obvious answer to the general question of whether deluded people have a proper grasp of the meaning of their claims. Perhaps "grasping the meaning" is a family of achievements, and each may admit of degrees.

Such beliefs as that other people are robots, or that the whole world depends on me, do not demonstrate simply a poor grasp of evidence. Perhaps they even more reflect some difference in the framework brought to bear on interpreting it.

Reflective Interpretation Is Holistic

People's beliefs form a system that functions in a holistic way. When predictions based on things we believe turn out to be mistaken, we have choices about which of our beliefs to change. Some beliefs may have very shallow roots. We thought it was not summer, but one swallow changes our mind. Or some belief may be tenaciously clung to, regardless of the case against it. As Cardinal Newman said of his religious belief, ten thousand difficulties did not make a doubt.

We need the right balance between responses that are too rootless and those that are too rigid. The extreme of rootlessness is having such a tenuous commitment to a belief system that all of it is destroyed by some slight evidence against any part of it. The extreme of rigidity is clinging to a belief system so tenaciously that no evidence is ever allowed to change any of it. But what is the right balance? Can we start to explore this by looking at cases where the balance has been absurdly misjudged?

There are some striking instances of how the rigid approach can explain away evidence. Confronted by the fossil evidence for evolution, Philip Gosse argued that, to test our faith, God had arranged fossils to look as if evolution had happened. His fixed point was the truth of the Bible story, and the rest of his thinking had to be skewed to fit this.

Another, political, instance comes from the British Communist Party in 1939. The Central Committee of the Party had to discuss the Nazi-Soviet pact. One of its implications was an order from Moscow that they were to withdraw support from the war against Hitler. They were to work for Britain's defeat. Many members had joined because the Party seemed to provide serious opposition to the Nazis. The new policy would make them go against their deepest political instincts.

Many of them had also adopted, as a fixed point in their system of beliefs, the idea that the Soviet Union could do no wrong. The transcripts of the debate show them agonizing as they tried to retain this fixed point in their system by skewing other beliefs. Some bending and squeezing would make it easier to see the Soviet Union as right. Suppose democracy and fascism were not importantly different. Or suppose the British Empire was as bad as Nazi Germany. Or Germany was so weak as not to be a threat. Or suppose Britain and France were worse aggressors than Nazi Germany. None of these claims was plausible, but each was adopted by some members of the Central Committee in the effort to defend the fixed point in their system.[22]

Gosse on evolution, and this response to the Nazi-Soviet pact, are two extreme cases of the holism of a belief system being exploited to protect a particular belief. In these cases the evidence is tortured by stretching and squeezing to make it fit the fixed point in the system. The implausibility is obvious. The same is true of many delusions, as with the identical impostor in Capgras delusion.

Delusions as Epistemological Distortions?

Few philosophers would be surprised by the thought that there is an overlap between philosophy and psychiatry. Perhaps less attractive is the thought of an overlap between philosophy and madness. Some people become interested in philosophical questions as their sanity starts to crumble.

The sailor Donald Crowhurst disguised his failure in a 'round-the-world race by sending radio reports of false positions to suggest he was winning. Worry about the fraud being detected, and a long lonely time in a hostile sea, may have led him to lose touch with reality. As this happened he started to write in a logbook a section headed "Philosophy." His thoughts included these: "The process we call Mathematics. The flower of basic intelligence. Ideas can be manipulated. If manipulated under a correctly formulated set of rules, they produce new results which clearly reveal aspects of the original concept which, though valid, would not have been so clearly revealed. The idea that Mathematics is the language of God, however, possesses more poetry than abstract validity." (So far, a recognizable if unenticing philosophical thought about mathematics. But a worrying note creeps in.) "It should be restated as Mathematics is perhaps the only certain common ground man TODAY occupies in the Kingdom of God." (And soon sanity is clearly lost.) "That these sentences would at first sight apparently be devoid of physical meaning is hardly surprising, for if we had a complete understanding of their meaning we would indeed have arrived at the stage it is now the object of the exercise to predict."[23]

In this Donald Crowhurst was not alone. One of the striking features of people on psychiatric wards is how much their conversation is about topics also discussed in philosophy journals. Is the physical world the only world? Does it exist outside my mind? Could other people be unconscious robots? Is there a God? Do we have free will? Is telepathy possible? The atmosphere of the discussion is different, but the topics overlap.

One thing some people on psychiatric wards have in common with philosophers is awareness that the commonsense interpretation of the world is not the only one. It can seem that people on psychiatric wards take seriously forms of skepticism that philosophers discuss only academically.

John Custance, whose "heightened sense of reality" and "ineffable sense of revelation" during his manic episodes have been noted, was also interested in philosophy. He was a striking case of someone whose sense of revelation led him to treat his belief in the significance of his abnormal experiences as a fixed point. To preserve this belief, he changed other beliefs, including philosophical ones, undeterred by considerations of plausibility.

He described one of his abnormal experiences. In one room of the hospital were framed pictures, whose glass reflected the window on the opposite wall and the buildings outside. Over a period of weeks he found that the reflections became distorted: "The chimneys left the vertical plane and moved round to the horizontal, eventually to forty or fifty degrees below the horizontal, while the reflection of the building itself became correspondingly curved, until the whole vertical structure formed a sort of inverted U. This puzzled me greatly. I don't think I was horrified at first. What could it mean? My vision was otherwise quite normal; I could play badminton, billiards, and so on. But whenever I sat in one of those chairs and looked at the prints, I could see this strange phenomenon. Certainly I was bewitched. But that was no new discovery; it did not frighten me more than I was frightened in any case. Then, suddenly, the answer came. Bishop Berkeley was right; the whole universe of space and time, of my own senses, was really an illusion."[24]

John Custance was unusual in knowing a bit about Berkeley's philosophy. But perhaps, without mentioning philosophers, this kind of strategy may be adopted by others trying to understand their strange experiences? An interesting discussion by Louis Sass links psychiatric delusions with philosophical discussions of skepticism.[25] Sass looks afresh at the much discussed case of the German judge, Daniel Paul

Schreber, who in 1903 published a notably articulate account of his psychiatric illness.[26]

Schreber had a ramified delusional system in which he heard voices and sometimes saw two suns. He had a unique relationship with God, who depended on him and who contacted him through "nerves." Schreber had the solipsistic view that the world and other people depended in various ways on his own mind. Some events were miracles that depended on him, while other people often had only a problematic existence. "The human forms I saw during the journey and on the platform in Dresden I took to be 'fleeting-improvised-men' produced by miracle."[27] But at times his grip on his own existence as the person who had his experiences seemed precarious; he would describe the experiences impersonally, as though they occurred but did not belong to anyone.

Louis Sass takes up the strand of solipsism in Schreber and compares it with Wittgenstein's discussion of solipsism. Wittgenstein suggested that solipsistic thoughts are more likely to arise when a person is passive. When we walk around, perhaps knocking things over and picking them up, we are more likely to be aware of objects' independent reality than when we are sitting still and staring. Schreber's delusions were embedded in a life that fit Wittgenstein's view. Apart from brief and reluctant walks, Schreber liked to sit still all day at the same place in the garden.

More importantly, Wittgenstein makes conceptual points about the paradoxes of solipsism. Arguments for solipsism are usually conceptual rather than empirical. The evidence for the existence of things other than me is not poor. The solipsist says that *no* evidence is enough to *prove* their existence beyond doubt. The same line is taken about proving that other people have experiences. By setting the standard of proof unattainably high, the solipsist makes it impossible to defend the view that things and experiences exist outside my mind. Wittgenstein's response is that if you make it impossible for others to have experiences, it becomes empty to say that they belong to you: "If as a matter of logic you exclude other people's having something, it loses its sense to say that you have it."[28] Sass links this up with the way Schreber's impersonal descriptions suggest only a weak sense of himself as the person having them.

Sass's application of Wittgenstein suggests a new use for philosophical discussions of the implications of deviant beliefs. These implications may suggest possible experienced consequences for deluded people who actually hold those beliefs. Perhaps this applies especially to people with a distorted sense of themselves and of their own agency. But it may be possible to build on Sass's approach by asking about more general links between philosophical beliefs and psychiatric disorder. The links could go either way. A deviant epistemology might distort the interpretation of normal experiences, or, as with Custance, the validity of a delusive experience can be defended by means of altering beliefs about epistemology. Either way, it seems worth looking at what happens to deluded people's sense of plausibility.

Loss of Plausibility Constraints

Perhaps someone with Capgras delusion has the neurological deficit that Young and others describe: when a familiar person appears, the usual emotional response is lacking. But more than this must be missing. If you are someone I usually warm to, but today I feel no emotional response to you, I may look for an explanation. Perhaps I have a hangover. Perhaps today you are using some perfume I do not like. Perhaps things said last time have left some chilliness between us. If none of these seems true, I will go on looking. But one explanation I will not be tempted by is that you have been replaced by an identical impostor. As a convincing story it ranks below the school excuse that "the dog ate my homework." Capgras delusion carries with it the loss not only of an emotional response but also of a sense of plausibility.

In delusions, as well as pressures to distort, there is not the usual restraining thought: "Surely all this is too unlikely?" To think about what may be going wrong, it would be helpful to have a clearer account of the undistorted constraints of plausibility.

We often identify delusions by their bizarre implausibility. The distortions of thinking in Gosse's interpretation of the fossil evidence, and in the 1939 Communist Party Central Committee's interpretation of the political situation, have a mainly social rather than a psychiatric explanation. They come from such strong indoctrination (or self-indoctrination) in a religious or political ideology that thinking is distorted to protect the ideology's central beliefs. Here the religious and political cases contrast with the psychiatric ones. But what the "social" and the "psychiatric" distortions of thought have in common is a disregard for the constraints of plausibility. It is this that makes such thinking a very poor guide to tracking reality.

Linking these different distortions of thought by their shared disregard of implausibility raises questions. What are the normal plausibility constraints? And why should they be respected? When is it reasonable to give up a deeply entrenched belief because of new evidence against it? When is it reasonable to use the entrenched belief as a reason to doubt the evidence? When is it reasonable to accept someone's testimony and when is it not? Should we prefer a simple and elegant theory that fits *nearly* all the evidence, or a complex and untidy account that fits *all* of it? How much evidence is needed to turn a hypothesis into a fact?

One hope has been that science and philosophy, partly by extrapolation from obvious cases, might be able to explain what plausibility is. Perhaps they might even generate rules to steer people toward the more plausible interpretations of the world. Such an inquiry might highlight misguided strategies of thought underlying delusions.

If epistemology and philosophy of science gave this clear guidance, we would have a map of the plausibility constraints on beliefs. We might then see whether a deluded person lacks the whole map or only some parts of it. But those parts of philosophy disappoint this hope. Books on philosophy of science are not rulebooks for scientists trying to choose between hypotheses.

There is the case, argued by Jerry Fodor, that the holistic nature of reflective interpretation makes it unlikely that we will find specific strategies for deciding about the plausibility of rival beliefs.[29] Reflective interpretation *is* holistic, but the conclusion drawn may be too pessimistic. It seems worth trying to approach the general question by looking at some ways in which we do draw a line between plausible and implausible beliefs.

Our minds are finite and we have to answer questions in a limited time. So we consider only some aspects of a problem. We choose between a limited number of strategies. And we consider only a few possible answers as serious candidates. Does this bounded rationality have an underlying coherence, supporting the exclusions we make against other possible ones? Or do we separate the plausible from the implausible by many different strategies, each justified by having been found to work roughly but quickly in a context that is irreducibly specific and local?

Some implausibility detectors appeal to very general parts of our system of belief. Doubts about a claimed miracle may appeal to the general reliability of scientific laws. And, as in this case, different general belief systems often influence what is seen as likely.

But other implausibility detectors are highly specific. At Paddington Station, I ask the price of a rail ticket to Oxford. The man behind the glass says it is 407 pounds but when bought on a Tuesday it comes with a lettuce as a free gift. The resulting mental alarm bells have not been triggered by the scientific worldview. The warning comes from specific beliefs about the likely costs of tickets, and about likely promotional offers. If the man then asks to borrow the pair of socks I am wearing, the plausibility of his testimony plummets even further toward zero. One of the reasons it is hard to say whether certain scenes in Dostoyevsky or in Franz Kafka are closer to dreams or to madness is that both dreams and madness escape the normal plausibility constraints.

A possible clue to the experience of delusions comes from dreams. They too combine rational thinking with tolerating the bizarre. Dostoyevsky describes waking memories of how ingeniously in a dream we outwitted our enemies: "You guessed that they were perfectly aware of your trick and were just pretending not to know your hiding-place; but again you outwitted and cheated them, all this you remember clearly." He goes on: "But why was it that your reason was able to reconcile itself to the obvious absurdities and impossibilities with which your dream was crammed? One of your killers turned into a woman before your very eyes, then from a woman into a shy and hideous little dwarf—and you accepted it at once as an established fact, with barely a hesitation, and at this very moment when your reason, on the other hand, was at a pitch of intensity and demonstrating extraordinary power, shrewdness, perception and logic?"[30]

Reasoning can persist, split off in dreams from the lost normal sense of plausibility. If this can happen in dreams, it is less surprising to find it also in madness. And, outside of either dreams or madness, reasoning and intellectual analysis can function independently from (at least some of) the plausibility constraints.

In epistemology the standard form of reasoning about beliefs is Socratic. A belief is challenged first by questions designed to make the person state it more explicitly and to give reasons for it. Then unwelcome logical consequences are drawn out from the belief or from its supporting reasons. Epistemology works by spelling out the costs of different systems of belief. Unwelcome consequences are an implicit invitation to abandon or modify a belief. But the fact that they are unwelcome does not itself come from logic. It comes from an intuitive sense of implausibility.

Logic alone is enough to exclude inconsistent belief systems, but not to choose between consistent ones. Someone with no intuitive sense of plausibility can still produce a map of the costs of belief systems. But the map on its own will not generate decisions about which costs are acceptable or unacceptable. Something extra is needed. That "something extra" is relevant to delusions.

Plausibility Constraints and Emotional Chemistry

Epistemology without intuitive plausibility weightings is inconclusive. This is paralleled by the "frame problem" in artificial intelligence. If an intelligent machine is designed to perform a simple task like fetching a package, and given access to any information it wants about the alternative strategies, it may never actually start the job. Without any way of excluding irrelevant information or questions, it will have an indefinitely large number of preliminary calculations to carry out. After several years it may still be working on such calculations as that going out of the door will not start a snowstorm in Russia, or will not make any camels die in Egypt.[31] Difficulties in designing a relevance detector for such a machine have suggested that, in people, emotional responses may function as relevance prompts. There may be no general *intellectual* strategy for seeing what is relevant. Instead, we might go by how things "feel."

Antonio Damasio has argued for the cognitive role of emotional responses. His patient "Elliot" had undergone surgery to remove a brain tumor.[32] As a result he was incapable of completing tasks on time. Asked to read and classify some documents, "he might spend a whole afternoon deliberating on which principle of organization should be applied: Should it be date, size of document, pertinence to the case or another?" Elliot's state was the frame problem come to life. His intellectual abilities were intact, except that he was unable to plan activities over time or to make decisions. Damasio concluded that Elliot's emotional coldness stopped him valuing some options above others and "made his decision-making landscape hopelessly flat."

This may be like the plausibility constraints on beliefs. The "something extra" needed in addition to logic may not be an intellectual strategy. It may depend on the emotional "feel" of an idea. (Not on the great emotions of love, hatred, anger, or fear, but on calmer passions: "There is something fishy about this"; "That sounds really cool"; "It has a good feel to it";

"I don't like the sound of that"; "There is something not quite kosher about this offer.")

Perhaps deluded people's lack of a sense of plausibility is linked to problems of "personal chemistry" in everyday life. Their intuitive and emotional "feel" for other people is often weak. And one of the symptoms of schizophrenia is having great difficulty in making decisions. The indecisiveness of schizophrenia is reminiscent of Elliot. It too may come from an emotional blankness that makes it hard to assign values to different options. The evaluative weight deluded people give to things is often bizarre. K. W. M. Fulford speaks of "evaluative delusions." One patient forgot to give his children their pocket money. He called this "the worst sin in the world," saying that he was "worthless as a father" and that his children would be better off if he was dead.[33] In addition to making it hard to assign values to options, disrupted emotional intuition could make it hard to assign plausibility to beliefs.

Beliefs and Their Weight

When thinking about plausibility, we often use the metaphor of weight. How weighty is a certain argument? How much weight should be given to this testimony? The metaphor can be used to contrast two kinds of failure in the sense of plausibility. Bad cognitive strategies can give a belief (or some evidence or an argument) either too much weight or too little weight.

Some beliefs are given great weight. There are everyday beliefs we cannot seriously give up. I have no more than two hands. Trees do not make jokes. Chairs do not leap away to avoid being sat on. These beliefs are so heavy that we cannot pick them up and move them. If I seem to experience joking trees, I will wonder whether I am dreaming, drugged, or having a psychiatric breakdown. It is right to give weight to these beliefs, as they have vast empirical support.

But a belief may be given too much (sometimes *much* too much) weight. A clear nonpsychiatric case was the belief of the British Communist leaders in 1939 that the Soviet Union could do no wrong. In psychiatric disorders, the belief "I am dead" may be treated as too heavy to move in the way that "Trees don't make jokes" is. One explanation of this heaviness could be some distortion of a tagging system whose normal operation gives certainty without supplying evidence open to conscious scrutiny.

When people think about philosophy, nihilism can be a temptation. There are so many alternative ways of thinking about the world (and so many arguments about them to evaluate) that it can seem impossible to choose among them. None of them seems to have any more weight than any other. Far from being too heavy to move, their lightness makes them both seem unreal and absurdly easy to pick up. A student in a philosophy examination who feels this lightness might choose any opinion more or less at random.

Something like this could happen to people whose psychiatric disorder has disrupted their emotional and intuitive feel for plausibility. When thinking is as "light" as this, someone may just "choose" any old version of the world, without feeling a real commitment to it. This would fit with the "double bookkeeping" of some people who have delusions. It would also fit with the sense of mockery, the sense of the person not really being serious about the belief, that sometimes comes across.

The Six Conjectures

The approach here centers around six conjectures. The first three are about the "heaviness" of distortions of intuitive interpretation. The other three are about distortions of reflective interpretation.

First conjecture: Because the interpretation that shapes our perceptual experiences is invisible, challenges to a delusive interpretation may be defeated by a strong intuitive conviction that alien abduction or whatever *was* experienced. This makes the belief "heavy" or hard to shift.

Second conjecture: The heaviness of some delusive intuitive interpretations might be linked to the heightened sense of reality that delusional experiences sometimes give.

Third conjecture: The link between heaviness and unconscious tagging delivers "certainty" without evidence open to scrutiny.

Fourth conjecture: When holism plays a strong role in our reflective interpretation, intense feelings of intuitive conviction, if treated as fixed points in a belief system, may lead to distortions in other parts of the system. These distortions could affect beliefs about standards of plausibility.

Fifth conjecture: Delusional beliefs depend on the loss or impairment of the normal feel for what is plausible.

Sixth conjecture: The failure of the plausibility constraints may itself be part of the disruption of emotional intuition so common in psychiatric disorder.

These conjectures aim at a part of the "human" interpretation of delusions that, while drawing on neurological information, is intuitively intelligible in psychological terms. The six conjectures are all empirical claims, needing empirical testing. I put them forward in the hope that they can advance knowledge—even if, as Karl Popper taught us, this is achieved most often by inviting refutation.

13

Waking Dreams

And yet I am, and live—like vapours tost
Into the nothingness of scorn and noise,
Into the living sea of waking dreams,
Where there is neither sense of life or joys

—John Clare, "I Am"

Part of human interpretation in psychiatry is trying to get an idea of what a person's disorder feels like from inside. Psychiatry textbooks and the flat prose of papers in journals can leave medical students unprepared for bizarre things they might encounter on a psychiatric ward. Even if all my conjectures were to turn out correct, what I've said so far about delusions would not do much to convey the feel of having a delusion. First-person accounts give a better idea. But people with psychiatric disorders sometimes find their inner world hard to express in words. Their art may get closer to conveying their experiences.

Here I will refer to a few paintings and drawings to illustrate certain common patterns, as well as the great variety of psychiatrically disturbed experience. This art does not have to be reducible to mere medical symptoms. It can be powerful as art, making vivid some experiences that are otherwise inaccessible. It can express totally sane moral or political responses to the person's situation. Some major artists who have had psychiatric disorders have been able to turn this experience into a positive contribution to their art. William Blake and Vincent van Gogh, for example, put to creative use disorders few or none of us would choose to have.

The Varieties of Disordered Experience: Glimpses of Inner Worlds

Sometimes people with psychiatric problems paint pictures that portray the living sea of waking dreams with such force and directness that no interpretation is needed. Laura Freeman, a university student with mental health problems, has a blog "How to Juggle Glass" reflecting this

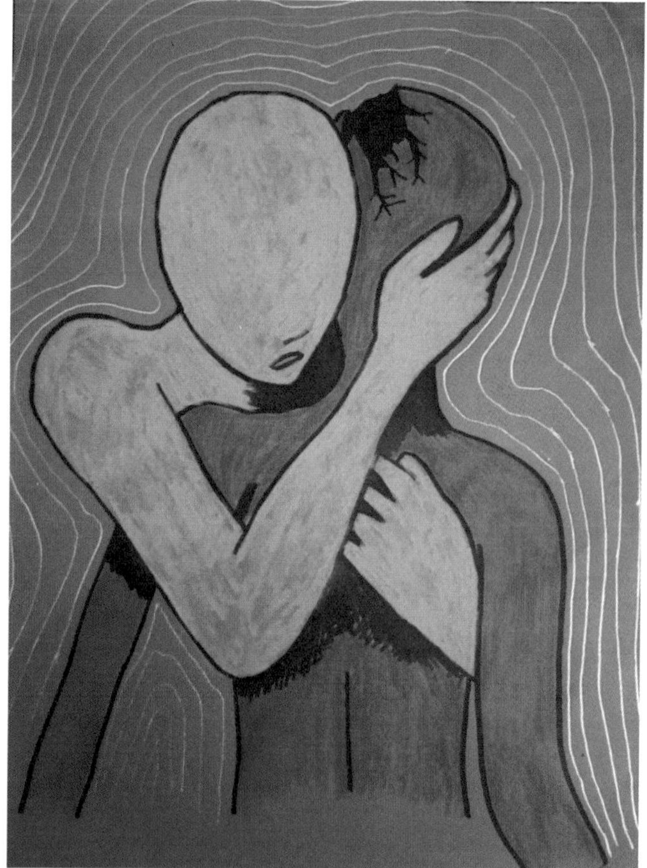

Figure 13.1: Laura Freeman, *Broken Hug.* Courtesy of Laura Freeman.

experience. Some of her paintings, such as the one shown in Figure 13.1, have an immediate emotional impact. Another of hers conveys more powerfully than words the disruption, darkness, and isolation of a state of depression (Figure 13.2). The forcefulness of these pictures dramatically reduces the "gulf that defies description." The directness is linked to being clearheaded about a psychiatric problem, with no self-deception or "lack of insight."

Not all psychiatric art communicates self-awareness of such clarity. Some paintings and drawings convey vividly but less directly the ways in which psychiatric disorder affects people's feelings and how they see things. These can have a disturbing strangeness, giving only enigmatic clues to their inner lives. Figure 13.3 shows a painting by Adolf Wölfli.

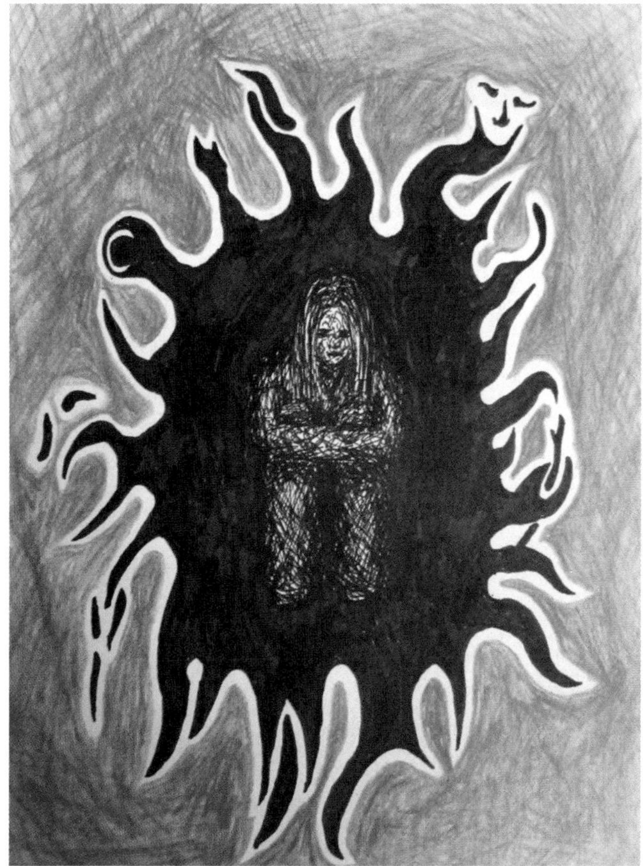

Figure 13.2: Laura Freeman, *Hiding in the Dark.* Courtesy of Laura Freeman.

The painting is powerful, but we might wonder how much self-awareness Wölfli had about the strangeness of the experience it expresses. The little bits of writing included in Wölfli's painting are one clue to its "psychiatric" origin. A lot of art reflecting psychiatric problems is filled much more with obsessive, tiny writing. This painting is mainly disturbing because of its pattern and "relentlessness." It is symmetrical, precise, and detailed. There is an insistent rigidity, with no asymmetry allowing the eye to wander to any other focus. The picture seems to force itself on us, as Wölfli's experiences may have forced themselves on him.

In Heidelberg, a small collection of paintings and drawings made by psychiatric patients, probably started by Emil Kraepelin, was greatly expanded by Dr. Hans Prinzhorn. He published his book *Artistry of the*

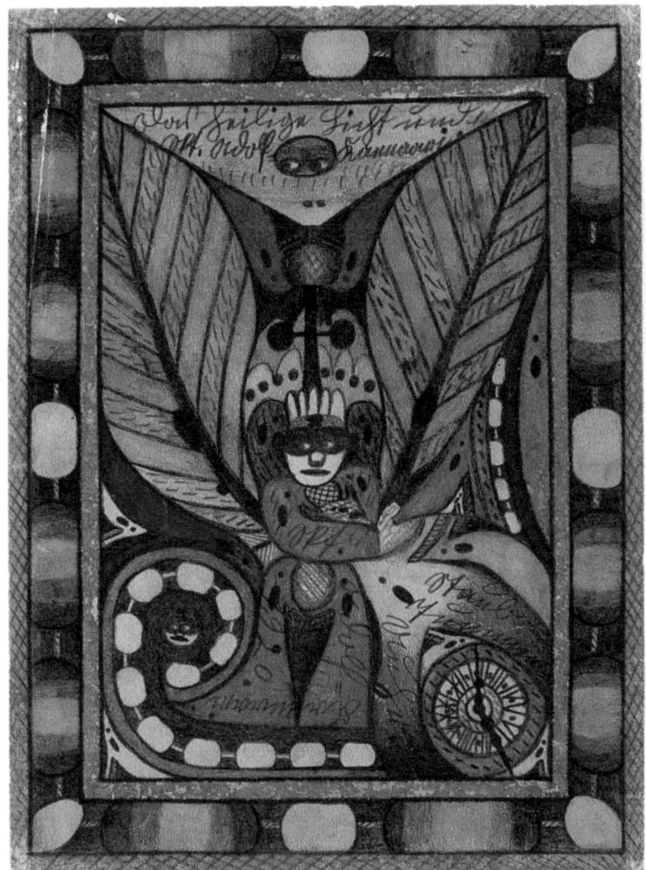

Figure 13.3: Adolf Wölfli, *Angel*, 1920. The Anthony Petullo Collection.

Mentally Ill, based on these pictures, in 1922.[1] The collection is the great source for psychiatric art in Europe from the late nineteenth century to the first quarter of the twentieth century. The year after Prinzhorn published his book, Max Ernst showed it to artists in Paris. In the 1940s Jean Dubuffet collected paintings of psychiatric inpatients under the title of L'Art Brut (Raw Art). Through these and other channels psychiatric art influenced much other painting. Because of this, some slightly later work is perhaps too self-consciously aware of what it "should" look like. The Prinzhorn artists may have been more innocent in expressing their experiences.

Sometimes the content simply depicts delusions already described in words. Jakob Mohr was paranoid. He described how transmitted electric waves turn him into a "hypnotic slave." His drawing shown in Figure 13.4

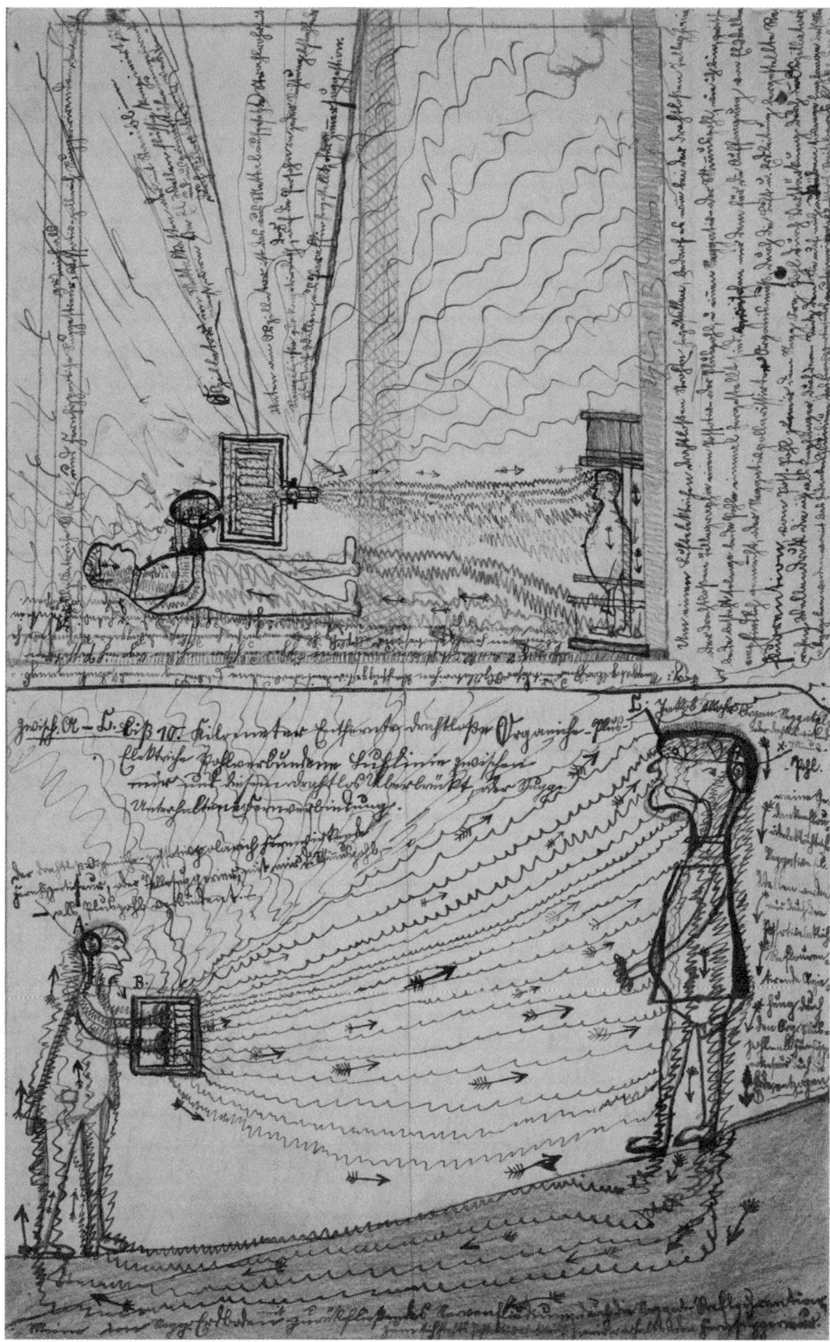

Figure 13.4: Jakob Mohr, *Proofs*. Copyright © Prinzhorn Collection, University Hospital, Heidelberg.

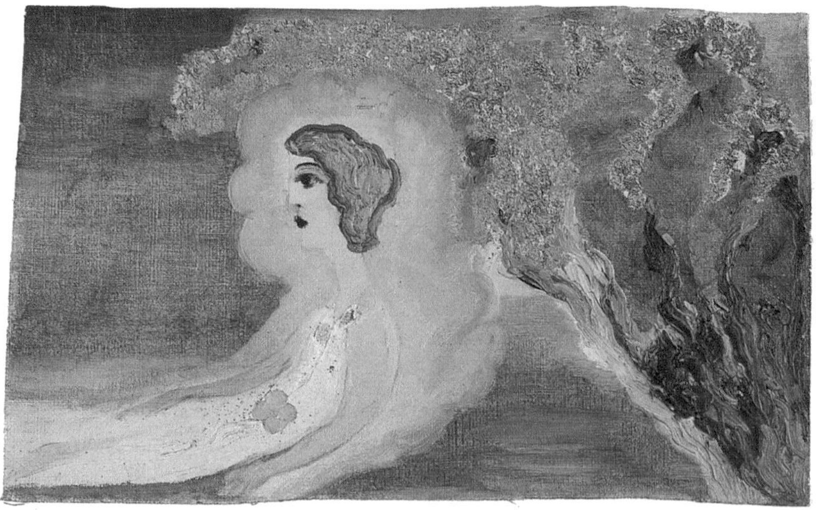

Figure 13.5: Else Blankenhorn, *Untitled*. Copyright © Prinzhorn Collection, University Hospital, Heidelberg.

is a diagram showing this influence by the arrows going toward him. (There is again the obsessiveness conveyed by the voluminous amount of minutely written text in his drawing.) The controller of the machine also extracts Mohr's thoughts and listens to them through headphones: "Waves are pulled out of me through the positive electrical attraction of the organic positive pole as the remote hypnotizer through the earth."[2] The diagrammatic detail in the drawing, titled "Proofs," may be meant to persuade others that the delusion is true.

There are recurring patterns in the work in the Prinzhorn collection, but individual artists' experience is not submerged in a collective "psychiatric" style. At the other extreme of style from Mohr, some of the work has little detail and few clear boundaries. A weirdly ethereal atmosphere is created, as in the painting by Elsa Blankenhorn of a woman surrounded by a halo of cloud perhaps blurring her view of others and their view of her (Figure 13.5).

Many other works give a vivid impression of artists' inner states. The drawing in Figure 13.6 was by Adolf Schudel, whose diagnosis was "hallucinatory insanity." Dr. Prinzhorn seems to have found it baffling: "The picture has a strange and eerie quality because of the strangeness of the details and because we find it impossible to attribute any rational meaning to it. It crumbles into numerous single motifs, each of which seems to want to say something original without finding the saving expression. For whom

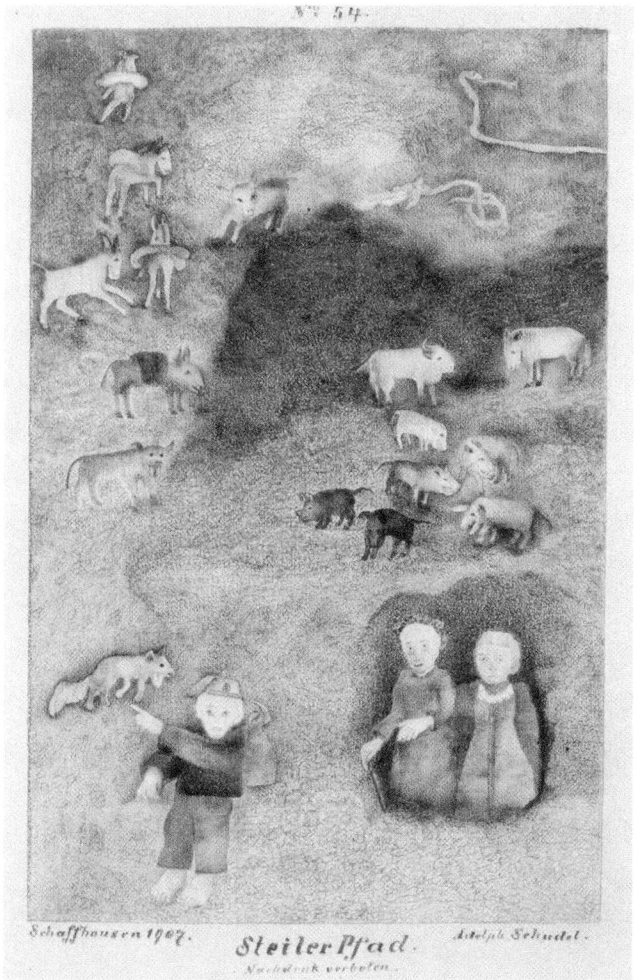

Figure 13.6: Adolf Schudel, *Steep Path.* Copyright © Prinzhorn Collection, University Hospital, Heidelberg.

is the pointing gesture of the pale dwarf intended—for the viewer or for the two women emerging from the cave? We gain nothing by posing such questions; the decisive element of this magic world lies precisely in its ambiguous impression, and its relative cohesion can be explained convincingly neither by the composition nor by any rational relationship between the figures."[3]

Perhaps the bafflement stems from looking for an interpretation at too detailed a level—at the "single motifs" and at the relationship between the figures. Seen less analytically, but as a whole, it seems a powerful

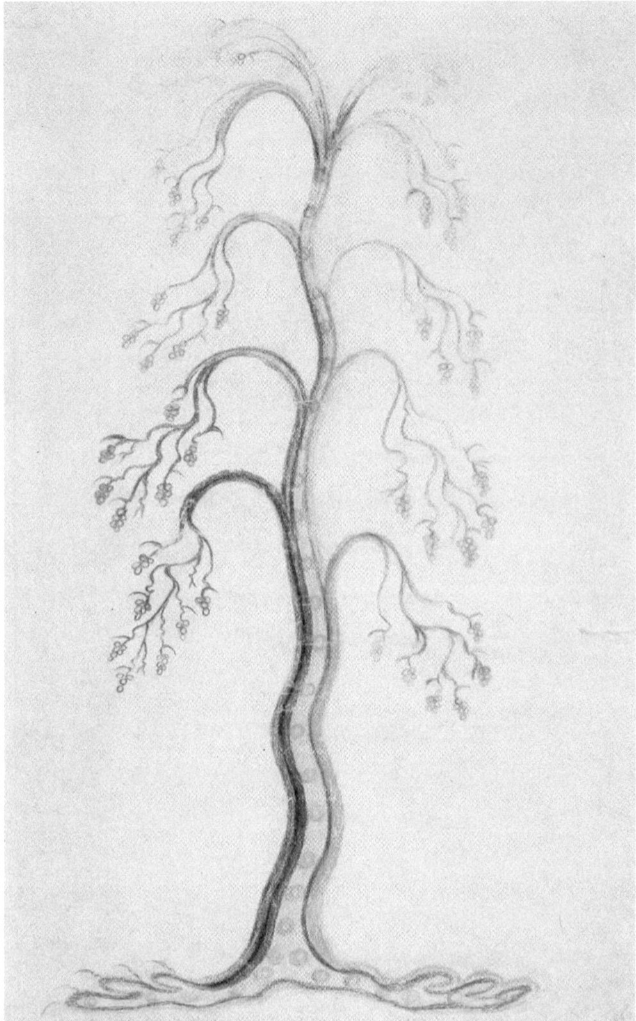

Figure 13.7: Heinrich Anton Mueller, *A Proud Earthly Tree With Little Bunches.* Copyright © Prinzhorn Collection, University Hospital, Heidelberg.

expression of Adolf Schudel's inner world. Two women emerge from some dark hole or tunnel, only to be pointed toward a steep upward path already possessed by strange and frightening animals, beyond which are snakes. Anyone seeing their own life like this has reason to despair, or at least to feel terribly daunted.

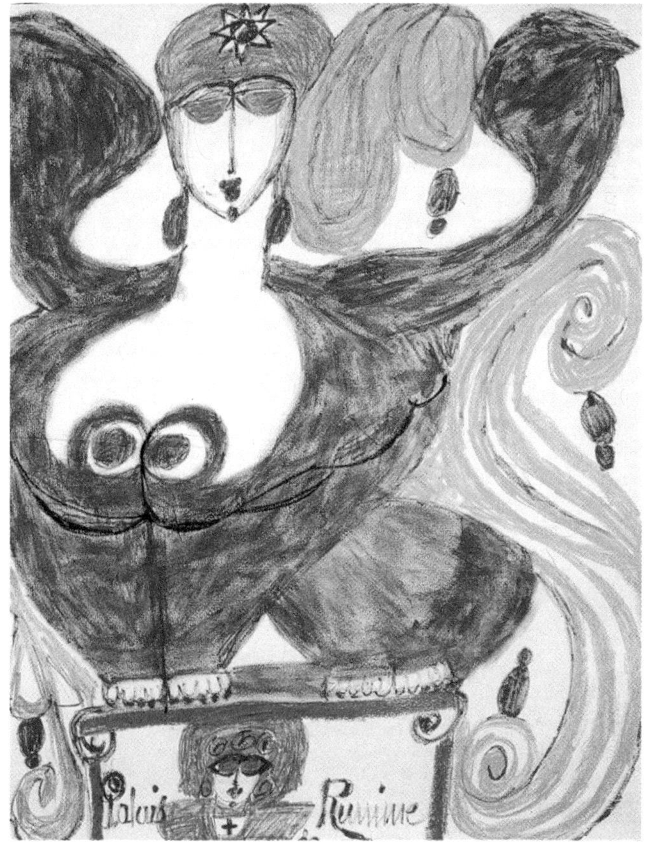

Figure 13.8: Aloise Corbaz, *Palais Rumine.* From the Musgrave Kinley Outsider Collection, The Whitworth Art Gallery, The University of Manchester.

Others express an inner world more obliquely, by showing physical objects seen differently. Curves in things normally straight, as in the tree depicted in chalk by Heinrich Anton Mueller (Figure 13.7), give an impression of a world in which firm objects become droopy and might just slither away.

Aloise Corbaz was diagnosed with schizophrenia. Her painting shown in Figure 13.8 powerfully reflects the strange and disturbing inner world of her disorder. There is the bright purple dress, which somehow flows into her breasts—not flowing into covering them, but into *being* them. It is the same with her arms and hands. The face is shaped like a stylized heart or shield. Do the strange, opaque blue eyes (or glasses?) suggest a

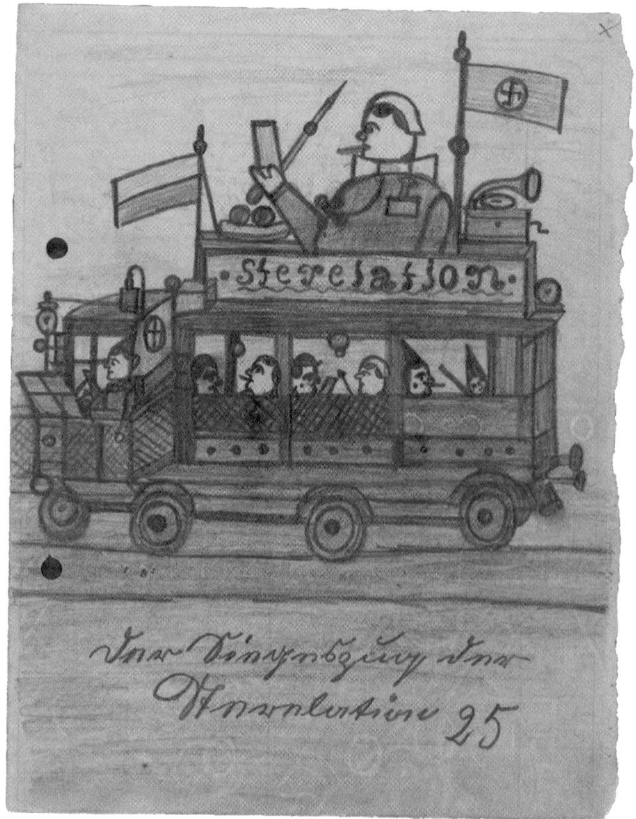

Figure 13.9: Wilhelm Werner, *Sterilization Bus*. Copyright © Prinzhorn Collection, University Hospital, Heidelberg.

barrier stopping the woman from seeing the world or a barrier preventing us from seeing inside her? Or both? On the left at the bottom of the purple dress is what looks like a pair of feet, of which only the toes can be seen. Looked at another way, these can be seen as the claws of a vulture-like bird, a view that turns the purple arms above into flapping wings. On the right at the bottom is another pair of feet with toes or claws apparently attached to the same purple "body," which suggests that the woman's head might be the front of a four-legged animal. Apart from the board at the bottom saying "Palais Rumine," the picture is all flowing curves with no straight lines or square angles, which echoes Heinrich Mueller's tree painting in creating the impression of a kind of permanent slithery motion.

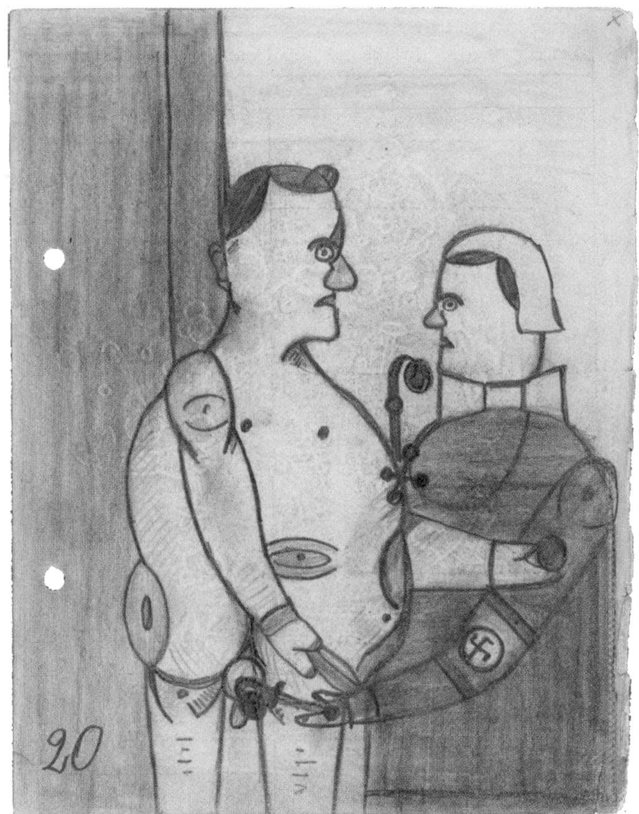

Figure 13.10: Wilhelm Werner, *Forced Sterilization.* Copyright © Prinzhorn Collection, University Hospital, Heidelberg.

"Psychiatric" Art Expressing Utterly Sane Thoughts and Feelings

Some "psychiatric" art is powerful in another way. Wilhelm Werner was a victim of the Nazis twice over. First the Nazis sterilized him against his will, and then in 1940, as part of the "euthanasia" program, they murdered him. His pictures on the theme of sterilization bring out the grim reality that contrasted with the cheery Nazi slogans fed to the public. Figure 13.9 shows a sterilization bus, with partying people inside, a Nazi flag flying, a gramophone playing music, and a nurse atop the bus holding a needle and a plate on which are two testicles.

Werner's portrayal of himself in Figure 13.10 has some of the characteristic marks of art reflecting inner disturbance. The joints of his

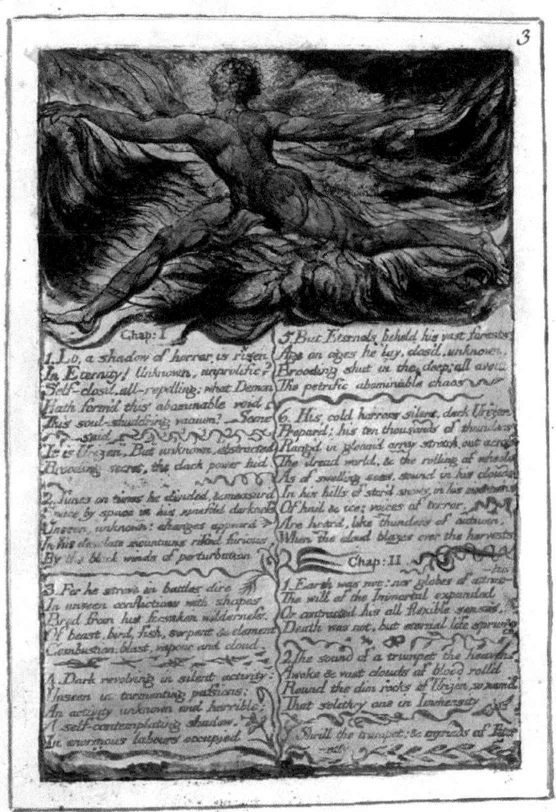

Figure 13.11: William Blake, First book of Urizen, plate 3. Lessing J. Rosenwald Collection, Library of Congress. Copyright © 2014 William Blake Archive. Used with permission.

body seem to be held in place by the heads of metal bolts. And his hands have metal pincers instead of fingers. But these "psychiatric" aspects of the picture do not in the least diminish the emotional and political power of his depiction of the steely Nazi nurse as she forces the sterilization on him.

Using "Visions" to Shape a Vision: William Blake

Few would now doubt that William Blake was one of the most creative and interesting English painters and poets of the late eighteenth and early nineteenth centuries. But it is also hard to doubt that nowadays he would

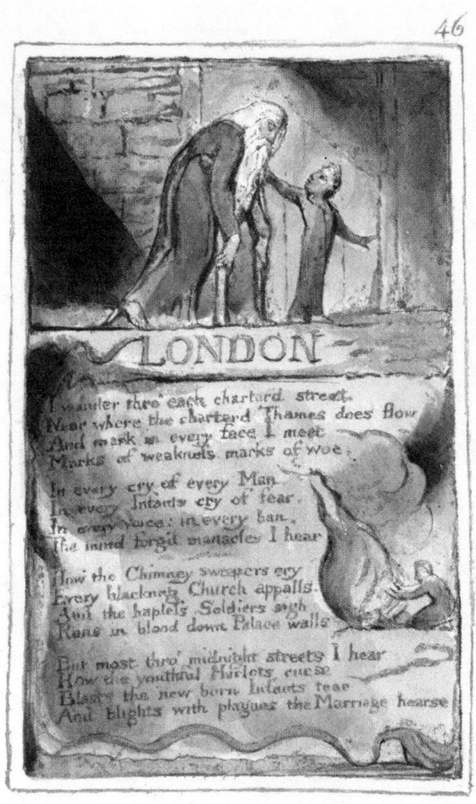

Figure 13.12: William Blake, "London," from *Songs of Innocence and Experience*. Copyright © The Fitzwilliam Museum, Cambridge, UK.

qualify for a psychiatric diagnosis. This might be encouraged by the "mad" side of his work. One way in which this comes out is in the look of some of his work and the suggestion it can convey of a private world. His *Prophetic Books* include many pages of minute writing, like that in Jakob Mohr's "Proofs" (see Figure 13.4), though Blake's calligraphy is much more beautiful. A casual glance at some of the many pages of voluminous writing about the bizarre world of Urizen, Los, and others can deter further investigation (Figure 13.11).

But Blake transcends all this. In *Songs of Experience* he expresses with anger an utterly sane vision of commercial London's indifference to victims like the soldier or the child prostitute (Figure 13.12). "Mind-forged manacles" are something close to a human universal, but they had to wait until Blake to be caught in this perfect phrase.

If Blake were alive now, another ground for psychiatric diagnosis would be his apparently psychotic experiences. He describes a complex and self-enclosed religious private world of quasi-biblical mythological people. Is this a ramified delusional system such that—as with Schreber—he literally thinks he is describing reality? Other interpretations might be that this is a consciously created fictional world like that of Tolkien, or that on the "belief spectrum" it lies somewhere between full belief and conscious invention. But the "visions" seem to have been at the "fully believed" end of the spectrum. He had no doubts about his many visions in the garden of his cottage in Felpham:

> For when Los joined with me he took me in his firy whirlwind
> My Vegetated portion was hurried from Lambeths shades
> He set me down in Felphams Vale & prepard a beautiful
> Cottage for me that in three years I might write all these
> Visions
> To display Nature's cruel holiness: the deceits of Natural
> Religion.
> Walking in my cottage garden, sudden I beheld
> The virgin Ololon and addressed her as a Daughter of
> Beulah . . .

In the catalog to his 1809 exhibition in Soho, Blake says that some of his paintings of the ancient world are copies of originals now lost. "The Artist having been taken in vision into the ancient republics, monarchies and patriarchates of Asia, has seen those wonderful originals . . . which were sculptured and painted on walls of Temples, Towers, Cities, Palaces . . . Those wonderful originals seen in my visions, were some of them one hundred feet in height."[4]

The journalist Henry Crabb Robinson reports him again speaking of his paintings as simply recording what he saw in his visions: "And when he said my visions, it was in the ordinary unemphatic tone in which we speak of trivial matters that everyone understands and cares nothing about. In the same tone he said repeatedly the 'Spirit told me.' I took occasion to say 'You use the same word as Socrates used. What resemblance do you suppose there is between your Spirit and the Spirit of Socrates?' 'The same as between our countenances.' He paused and added, 'I was

Socrates.' And then as if correcting himself, 'A sort of brother, I must have had conversations with him. So I had with Jesus Christ. I have an obscure recollection of having been with both of them.'"[5]

These delusive "visions" about conversations with Christ and Socrates are not easy to separate from the human and moral vision that gives his work much of the power that still resonates. Some of Blake's contemporaries saw this duality in him. After reading *Songs of Innocence and Experience,* Wordsworth said, "There is no doubt that this poor man was mad, but there is something in the madness of this man which interests me more than the sanity of Lord Byron or Walter Scott!"[6] Henry Crabb Robinson wrote of "the wild and strange, strange rhapsodies uttered by this insane man of genius" and asked, "Shall I call him Artist or Genius—or Mystic or Madman? Probably he is all."

Would Blake have had his human vision without his "visions"? We find it easy to warm to the vision while rejecting the "visions." But about Blake himself the question is impossible to answer with any certainty.

The issue is more general, going beyond Blake's visions to false beliefs in general. Those who are religious believers may seem, to those of us who are not, to be deluded. (Not in the psychiatric sense, but in the minimal sense of holding beliefs that are either false or at least not based on reliable means of tracking reality.) For those of us who are unbelievers, the question about Blake is paralleled by a question about the frequent goodness of character and action found among believers. These include the Quaker pacifists who have borne such impressive witness against war, Archbishop Tutu's commitment to reconciliation with former oppressors, and Pastor Trocmé's risking his life in leading his whole village in Nazi-occupied France to hide and shelter hundreds of Jews. It is possible that these good people, even without their religion, would have acted in the same way out of concern or respect for others. But surely it is not obvious that stripping away the religious basis would have left their character and actions unchanged. (Those who think unbelief mistaken—a negative delusion—have the parallel question about moral goodness linked to secular outlooks.)

Blake's visions seem so central to his whole outlook. They gave him what he saw as a secure basis for an independent religion of his own: a personal standpoint from which to criticize the scientific and philosophical movements of his day and the institutionalized churches.

Perhaps because of a heightened sense of reality they brought, the visions presented themselves to him as indubitable. In this way they provided a fixed point around which his system of beliefs was shaped. This shaping gave him idiosyncratic views about plausibility, which made more straightforwardly empirical views seem distorting and limited. In *The Marriage of Heaven and Hell,* he wrote: "If the doors of perception were cleansed every thing would appear to man as it is, infinite— / For man has closed himself up, till he sees all things thro' narrow chinks of his cavern." Newton, Locke, Voltaire, and Rousseau were among those he thought had closed themselves up, seeing only through the narrow chinks. Their conceptions of the senses were too limited to include visions like his as a source of knowledge.

This highly personal epistemology parallels his confidently personal view of how the dead and formulaic religious morality of the churches drew attention away from the suffering that really mattered. The little boy, in whose voice Blake wrote the poem "The Chimney Sweeper," who is "crying weep, weep, in notes of woe!," says his father and mother are both gone up to the church to pray: "And because I am happy, & dance & sing, / They think they have done me no injury: / And are gone to praise God & his Priest & King / Who make up a heaven of our misery."

Some modern psychiatrists think the problem with hearing "voices" is not the experiences themselves but how people cope with them. There are strategies to help reduce the disruption caused by "voices": the encouragement of self-help groups, anxiety management techniques, advice to focus on the experiences and to monitor them, to keep diaries and to engage in dialogue with the voices.[7] These strategies are claimed to help people to cope successfully with "voices" by integrating them into their lives. (In the case of horrible voices, surely this would be only a second-best strategy, for use only when they cannot be eliminated?)

Blake's integration of his "visions" into his life can be seen as an unconscious parallel to this. As his visions were benevolent rather than hostile, and he thought they were not delusions, he needed no conscious coping strategy. But the role they played in supporting his highly independent view of the world beneficially integrated them into who he was. They gave him the feeling of solid ground. And this sense of solid ground is apparent in the confidence he always displayed in the vision whose expression was the heart of his life.

"Put These Very Passions to Good Effect": Vincent van Gogh

The fame of Vincent van Gogh's "madness"—unlike that of his paintings—exaggerates the reality.

Dr. Peyron, the doctor at the asylum, diagnosed epilepsy, though that hardly seems to cover the range of "psychiatric" symptoms described by those who knew him and by van Gogh himself. Karl Jaspers thought the diagnosis should have been schizophrenia.[8] But Kay Redfield Jamison, citing the family history of severe mood instability, more plausibly suggests manic depression. She points out that in nineteenth-century France the distinction between that and epilepsy was not clear.[9]

There are obvious problems in "diagnosing" people long dead. But there is no doubt that van Gogh had a major psychiatric problem. He had recurring depressions. In his first breakdown in 1888 he threatened Gauguin with a knife, which he then used to cut off his own ear. After this and after other breakdowns he spent periods in the asylum. At these times he heard voices and, as others told him, "it seems that I gather dirt and eat it."[10] Those around him wrote to his brother expressing acute concern. In December 1888 one wrote, "I think he is lost. Not only is his mind affected, but also he is very weak and despondent." Two months later another wrote, "He has imagined that he is being poisoned and is seeing nothing but poisoners and poisoned people everywhere." He became mute and hid under the bedcovers, sometimes crying.

With all this, is it really plausible to say that the legend of his madness exaggerates the reality? These acute outbreaks of violence and paranoia were self-contained psychotic episodes. In the rest of his life he was clearheaded about them. His reaction was the opposite of Blake's endorsement of his own visions. In what Karl Jaspers called "his sovereign attitude towards his illness," van Gogh saw it as something to reject, to escape from by creative work: "It is perfectly true that last year the attack returned various times—but then also it was precisely by working that my normal condition returned little by little. It will probably be the same this time."[11]

A month later he wrote about part of his vision of his own work, and again about its role in resisting his illness: "Aurier's article would encourage me, if I dared let myself go, to risk making a kind of tonal music with colour . . . But the truth is so dear to me, *trying to create something true* also, anyway I think, I think I still prefer to be a shoemaker than to be a musician, with colours. In any event, trying to remain true is perhaps a remedy to combat the illness that still continues to worry me."[12] And three months after this he wrote, "At the moment the improvement is continuing, the whole horrible crisis has disappeared like a thunderstorm, and I'm working here with calm, unremitting ardour to give a last stroke of the brush."[13]

The letters also sometimes have a down-to-earth sanity that includes a good ear for the apt mocking phrase, whether used to puncture things overrated or applied to himself. He praises a character in Daudet for saying that, "achieving FAME is like when smoking, sticking your cigar in your mouth by the lighted end." And in another letter of the same year, in which he reports that "*large* SUNFLOWERS" are his subject matter, he says, "I'm painting with the gusto of a Marseillais eating bouillabaisse."[14]

What is mainly found in the letters is the opposite of madness. Van Gogh comes over as having had a clearheaded sanity about his periods of illness and a passionate commitment to his painting: "Strictly speaking I'm not mad, for my thoughts are absolutely normal and clear between times, and even more than before, but during the crises it's terrible however, and then I lose consciousness of everything. But it drives me to work and to seriousness, as a coal miner who is always in danger makes haste in what he does."[15]

He had a vision of what he hoped to do: "Sometimes I know clearly what I want. In life and in painting too, I can easily do without the dear Lord, but I can't, suffering as I do, do without something greater than myself, which is my life, the power to create . . . And in a painting I'd like to say something consoling like a piece of music. I'd like to paint men or women with that *je ne sais quoi* of the eternal, of which the halo used to be the symbol, and which we try to achieve through the radiance itself, through the vibrancy of our colourations."[16]

What his disorder almost certainly did contribute to his painting came from his "heightened sense of reality." John Custance's use of this phrase for his own manic episodes came in an account with strong echoes of both van Gogh's paintings and his letters. Custance describes lights being deeper and more intense, sometimes like the Aurora Borealis. And people's faces had a special quality: "I will not say that they have exactly a halo round them, though I have often had that impression in the more

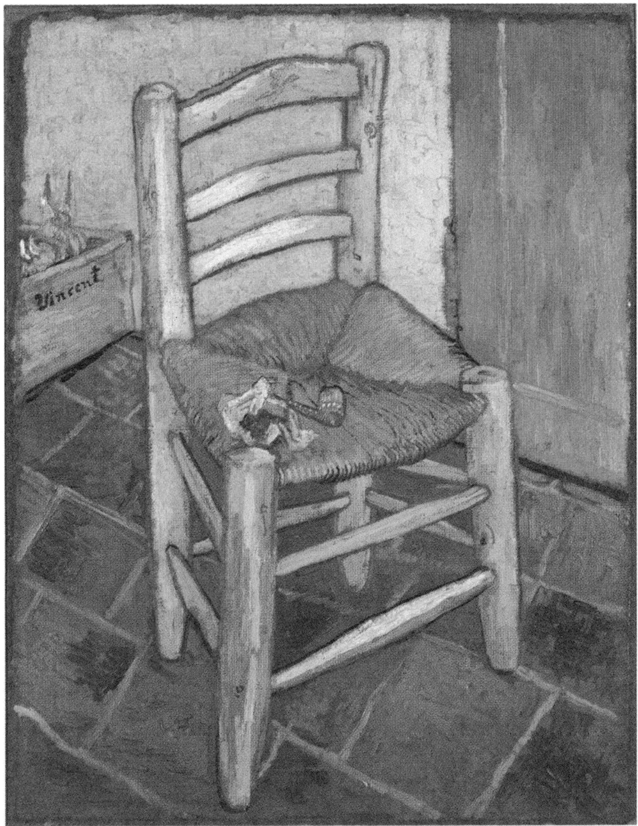

Figure 13.13: Vincent van Gogh, *Van Gogh's Chair*, 1888. London, National Gallery. Oil on canvas. Copyright © 2012 The National Gallery, London/Scala, Florence.

acute phases of mania. At present it is rather that faces seem to glow with a sort of inner light which shows up the characteristic lines extremely vividly."[17]

Aldous Huxley's description of his own heightened visual experience after taking mescaline is also reminiscent of van Gogh: "I was looking at my furniture, not as the utilitarian who has to sit on chairs . . . but as the pure aesthete whose concern is only with forms and their relationships within the field of vision . . . But as I looked . . . I was . . . back in a world where everything shone with the Inner Light, and was infinite in its significance. The legs, for example, of that chair—how miraculous their tubularity, how significant their polished smoothness! I spent

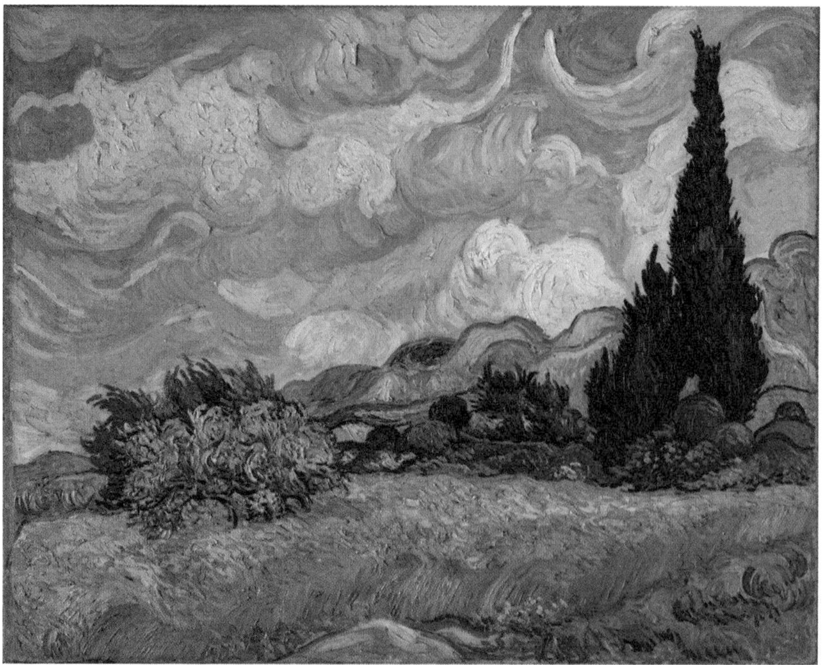

Figure 13.14: Vincent van Gogh, *Wheat Field with Cypresses,* 1889. New York Metropolitan Museum of Art. Oil on canvas. Copyright © 2012. Image copyright The Metropolitan Museum of Art/Art Resource/Scala, Florence.

several minutes—or was it several centuries?—not merely gazing at their bamboo legs, but actually *being* them." Later Huxley opened a book on van Gogh: "The picture at which the book opened was *The Chair*—that astounding portrait of a *Ding an Sich,* which the mad painter saw, with a kind of adoring terror, and tried to render on his canvas." Although Huxley thought the painting inadequate to the vision, he thought van Gogh's chair (Figure 13.13) was "incomparably more real than the chair of ordinary perception" and "obviously the same in essence as the chair I had seen."[18]

The intense sense of reality so visible in the paintings is also there in van Gogh's letters: "Ah, while I was ill, damp, melting snow was falling, I got up to look at the landscape—never, never has nature appeared so touching and sensitive to me."[19] The intensity fired his energy to work: "Today I worked from 7 o'clock in the morning until 6 o'clock in the evening without moving except to eat a bite a stone's throw away. And that's why the work is going fast . . . At the moment I have a clear head, or a lover's blindness towards my work. Because being surrounded by colour like this is quite new to me, and excites me extraordinarily. Fatigue doesn't come into it; I could do another painting tonight, even, and I could bring it home."[20]

Van Gogh's inner disturbance is *one* reason his paintings do not have the serenity of, say, Vermeer's. But it gave the blazing passion and the intensity that is part of what makes them great (Figure 13.14). As Karl Jaspers said, "The ground of the landscape appears to be alive, waves seem to rise and ebb everywhere, the trees are like flames, everything twists and seems tormented, the sky flickers."[21]

Unlike Blake, van Gogh understood his own instability and his susceptibility to madness. His response to it was utterly sane:

> I am a man of passions, capable of and given to doing more or less outrageous things for which I sometimes feel a little sorry. Every so often I say or do something too hastily, when it would have been better to have shown a little more patience . . . This being the case, what can be done about it? Should I consider myself a dangerous person, unfit for anything? I think not. Rather, every means should be tried to put these very passions to good effect . . .
>
> So instead of giving in to despair I chose active melancholy, in so far as I was capable of activity, in other words I chose the kind of melancholy that hopes, that strives and that seeks, in preference to the melancholy that despairs numbly and in distress.[22]

Both sides of van Gogh—the troubled passion and how it is put to good effect—are in the brilliant self-portraits. The tautness and intensity are visible in Figure 13.15. In his right eye (on the left) there is a glint of disturbance. But it is not an insane painting. It is a sane portrait of a sometimes tormented man by a painter of genius.

Near the end of van Gogh's life, the illness is more visible in the letters. They show despair closing in. One of his last paintings, the *Wheat Field with Crows* (Figure 13.16), may be the most powerful expression ever given to one despairing view of the world. The dark crows seem sinister. The field and sky are seen as being in violent motion and, at the

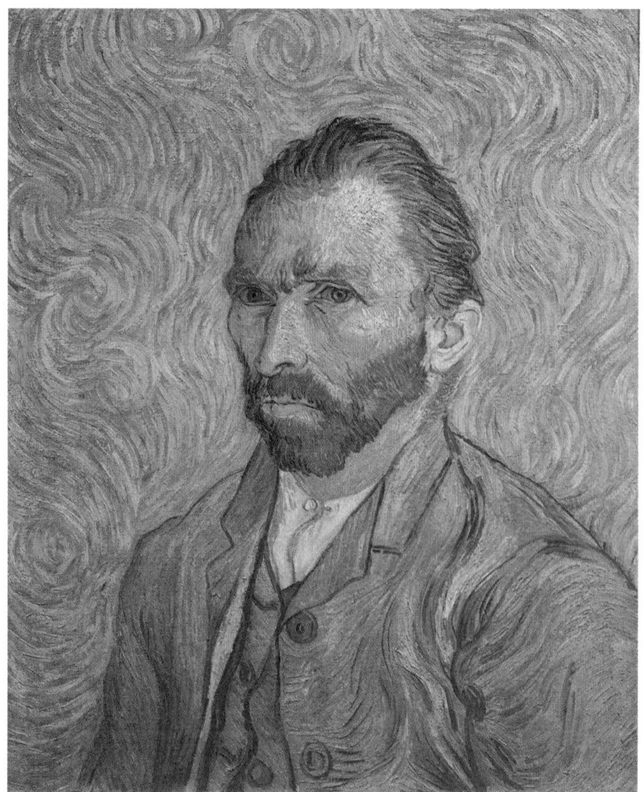

Figure 13.15: Vincent van Gogh, *Self-Portrait,* 1889. Paris, Musee d'Orsay. Oil on canvas. Copyright © 2012. Photo Scala, Florence.

same time, as claustrophobically oppressive. The greatness of the painting comes partly from its making one kind of desperate state of mind intelligible from the inside.

In a letter he wrote at the time, he said, "What can be done—you see I usually try to be quite good-humoured, but my life, too, is attacked at the very root, my step also is faltering . . . There, once back here I set to work again—the brush however almost falling from my hands and—knowing clearly what I wanted I've painted another three large canvasses since then. They're immense stretches of wheatfields under turbulent skies, and I made a point of trying to express sadness, extreme loneliness."

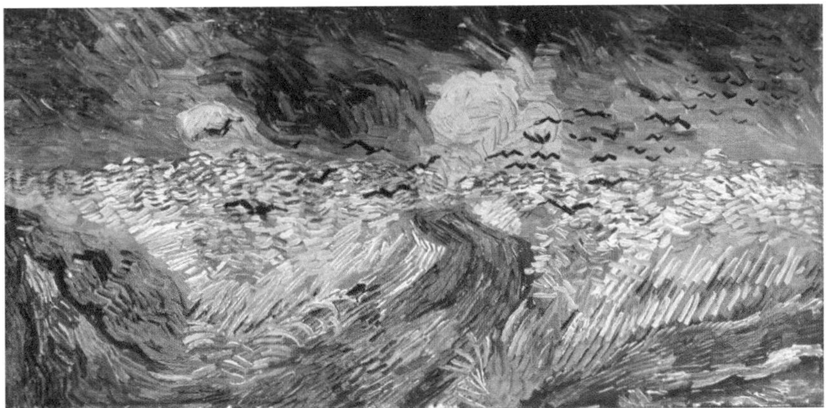

Figure 13.16: Vincent van Gogh, *Wheatfield with Crows,* 1890. Amsterdam, Van Gogh Museum. Copyright © 2012. Photo Art Resource/Scala, Florence.

Disordered Experience, Expression, and Self-Creation

These different works of art reflect the wide range of psychiatrically disordered experience, as well as the personalities and skills of the artists. Some of the pictures (those in Laura Freeman's blog, Wilhelm Werner's sterilization protests, and van Gogh's paintings) express an undeluded view of the artist's situation. At the other extreme is Jakob Mohr's diagram of how his persecutors were reading his mind and controlling him. Others come somewhere in between. Adolf Schudel's *Steep Path* or Aloise Corbaz's *Palais Rumine* reveal disturbing inner worlds. The artist may or may not be in the grip of such a world at the time of painting, but clearly has experience of it.

The pictures are reminders of platitudes that matter. Not all psychiatric disorders involve delusions or insanity. The person who does suffer from delusions usually does not experience them all the time and may produce undeluded political protests or powerful—sometimes even great—art. And the power, sometimes greatness, of the art may owe something to the person's psychiatric disorder.

The contribution of the disorder can be made in very different ways. If the account given earlier of Blake is somewhere near right, lack of "insight" about one's delusions may even be helpful. Blake's uncritically accepted "visions" and his ability to integrate them into his life may have had great importance. Their role in his quite unconscious creation of his own charged view of the world helped shape him and so his art.

If the account given of van Gogh is somewhere near right, his disorder contributed in a very different way. Between his mental breakdowns, he was entirely sane and was undeceived about his delusions. He used his painting to defend himself against insanity. He also used it to partly create himself: not numb despair but active melancholy. He had a deep need to be creative, together with ideals about the value he hoped his work would have in revealing things to others. But the role of his disorder was not just the negative thing his art was pitted against. (Though that gave to his work the urgency of the coal miner hurrying to escape danger.) Above all, it gave him the heightened sense of reality, the charged vision so many of his paintings express.

It may seem that these comments treat van Gogh's paintings as mere symptoms of disorder, and reduce a great painter to merely a person with a particular psychopathology. That is a mistake. To say that a painter is expressing his or her own experience of psychological disturbance is not to discredit either the artist or the work. Aloise Corbaz's painting gives the rest of us a glimpse of the inner experience of schizophrenia through being such a powerful expression of it. She was a considerable artist in being able to achieve this.

Having delusions, or knowing severe depression or mania, are aspects of human experience. As with fighting in war, only a minority have these experiences. But, again as with war, the experiences are often particularly intense. Someone is not belittled by being called a war artist, and it is no slight to say that someone's art expresses the experience of psychiatric disorder. Vicariously, the rest of us grow deeper in our experience and understanding through the works of painters and writers who manage to convey something of either war or psychiatric disorder.

People who are bereaved, unemployed, persecuted, humiliated, or treated unjustly, or whose physical or mental health is damaged, respond to disaster in contrasting ways. Some are diminished: becoming passive, defeated, vengeful, or bitter. Others respond with resilience, courage, generosity, or creativity. When the disaster is mental disorder, the world can be enriched. Van Gogh or Dostoyevsky might not have created their great works if some ideal cure had been available. The tension is clear. We would not wish to be without their work. But major psychiatric disorder is so horrible, we would also not wish it on anyone. Methods of prevention and cure (medication, therapy, different ways of treating children, and such) should be developed. *Of course* we do not want to retain conditions blighting lives, even if they are a stimulus to great art. But while these conditions do exist, we are right to feel pleasure—and sometimes awe—at the ways, both creative and self-creative, in which people can put these very passions to good effect.

PART FOUR

The Boundaries of Psychiatry

If the mind doctors over these last two hundred years have shown us anything, it is that our model of the human mind needs to be capacious . . . What is clear is that as we have moved through the twentieth century and into the twenty-first, an ever wider set of behaviours and emotions have become "symptomatic" and fallen under the aegis of the mind doctors. A vast range of eccentricities or discomforts that seem too hard to bear shape suitable cases for treatment.

—Lisa Appignanesi, *Mad, Bad and Sad: A History of Women and the Mind Doctors from 1800 to the Present*

Despite the recent misguided tendency by many to caricature a medical approach as being narrow, biological and reductionist, we are struck by how keen other members of staff are for themselves or their relatives to be seen by an experienced psychiatrist when mental illness affects them . . . For those with severe mental illness, to avoid medicalisation is at best confusing and at worst damaging or even life-threatening . . . These considerations about the nature and breadth of psychiatry bear upon the fundamental issue as to where its appropriate boundaries lie, and whether practitioners should try to span such a broad spectrum of skills, knowledge and interests.

—Nick Craddock, Robin Jacoby, Peter McGuffin, and 34 other Members or Fellows of the Royal College of Psychiatry, "Wake-Up Call for British Psychiatry," *British Journal of Psychiatry* 193 (2008): 6–9

14

The Need for Boundaries: The Dark Side of Psychiatry

How should psychiatrists think about the people to whom their professional skills are directed? How should they act toward them? What are the professional limits to what they should do? Some answers to these questions have been morally disastrous and humanly catastrophic. These answers have led to different, though overlapping, dark strands in the history of psychiatry.

Participation and Collaboration

Nazi Atrocities

Some psychiatrists advocated or took part in the murder of 70,000 patients in psychiatric hospitals as part of the Nazi "euthanasia" program. An early advocate was Alfred Hoche, a professor of psychiatry at Freiburg and one of the two authors of the 1920 defense of involuntary euthanasia, "Permission for the Destruction of Life Unworthy of Life." Max de Crinis, a psychiatrist at the Charité Hospital and professor of psychiatry at the University of Berlin, was deeply involved in planning the mass murder of the patients. Carl Schneider, who worked on schizophrenia (though not the Schneider who listed the "first rank symptoms" of schizophrenia) was a professor of psychiatry and neurology at Heidelberg. As well as being one of the leaders of the "euthanasia" program, for research at his Heidelberg clinic he took brains from the people killed.[1] The gas chambers used in the Nazi death camps were first tried out in the killing of patients in psychiatric hospitals.

The Soviet Union

> Solomon Volkov: I understand you couldn't trust these doctors.
> Joseph Brodsky: I think that the level of psychiatry in Russia—as throughout the world—is extremely low. The means they

> use are extremely approximate. In fact, people have no idea of the true processes at work in the brain and nervous system. For example, I know that an airplane flies, but how specifically it does that I can only dimly imagine. The situation in psychiatry is similar. Therefore they subject you to utterly monstrous experiments. It's no different to opening a clock with a hatchet, right? That is, they really could damage you irrevocably. Whereas prison—well, what is it, really? A shortage of space compensated for by an excess of time.
>
> —Solomon Volkov, *Conversations with Joseph Brodsky*

Some psychiatrists in the Soviet Union played a role in the abuse of political dissidents. Anatoliy Koryagin wrote of "the inconceivably high 'sick rate' among dissidents." He said that very few escaped psychiatric examination and that in the 1960s and 1970s one dissident in three was sent to a psychiatric clinic. Diagnosis was sometimes made without seeing the patient. Sometimes it was collective. In 1987 four Hare Krishna members were diagnosed at the same time with schizophrenia.[2]

A major center of this approach was the Serbsky Institute in Moscow, which had a political section. Pyotr Grigorenko, after criticizing what he saw as Soviet deviations from Leninism, was given a diagnosis of paranoid delusions by Academician Professor A. V. Snezhnevsky, and by Professor Daniil Lunts. Snezhnevsky, director of the Serbsky Institute and the public face of official Soviet psychiatry, tried to rebut international criticism. In 1971 he gave an interview to Izvestia about the "lofty humanism" characteristic of Soviet psychiatry and his "feeling of deep disgust" at the "outrageous fabrication" that healthy people were hospitalized in the USSR.[3]

Vladimir Bukovsky gave interviews to the Western media about his arrest for "anti-Soviet agitation" and his transfer to the Serbsky Institute to be declared insane. He was treated compulsorily in Leningrad for a year. On release he took part in demonstrations and was then hospitalized in the Serbsky Institute. He was charged with slandering the state and sentenced to three years corrective labor. After his sentence he sent detailed documentation of Soviet psychiatric abuses to the West. In 1972 he was tried for "anti-Soviet agitation and propaganda." He wanted to call as defense witnesses some of the victims of abuse. That was ruled out by the judge, who ruled that they were "insane people and their testimony would be invalid." Bukovsky was sentenced to twelve years.[4]

Joseph Brodsky, after being investigated by the KGB, was sent to mental hospitals. He compared them unfavorably with prison: "In the asylum it's much worse because they inject you with all kinds of crap and force various pills down your throat." The injections were painful only when they injected sulfur, which kept people still by making any movement excruciatingly painful. This was sometimes to restrain violence, "but apart from that, the women attendants and male nurses just got their kicks that way." There were other abuses: "You're lying there reading . . . and suddenly in walk two male nurses who pull you off your cot, wind you up in a sheet, and start dunking you in a bathtub. Then they pull you out of the bathtub, but they don't unwind the sheet. And these sheets start drying on you. It's called the 'wrap.' A nasty piece of work. Very nasty."[5] Later, without seeing Brodsky, A. V. Snezhnevsky gave him a diagnosis of schizophrenia.

Such diagnoses were made easier by the concept of "latent" schizophrenia, of which Snezhnevsky was a prominent advocate. In 1973 the *Guardian* published a letter from him and other Soviet psychiatrists defending their approach: "There is a small number of mental cases whose disease . . . can lead them to antisocial actions which fall in the category of those that are prohibited by law, such as disturbance of public order, dissemination of slander, manifestation of aggressive intentions, etc. . . . they can do this after preliminary preparations with a cunningly calculated plan of action . . . To the people around them such mental cases do not create the impression of being obviously insane. Most of them are persons suffering from schizophrenia or paranoid personality. The seeming normality of such sick persons when they commit socially dangerous action is used by anti-Soviet propaganda for slanderous contentions that these persons are not suffering from a mental disorder."[6] Those persecuting political critics for "slander" must have been glad to have psychiatrists who were helpful about diagnosing a disorder so "latent."

China

In China psychiatric abuse of dissidents goes back to the time of Mao and the Cultural Revolution. The Soviet diagnosis of "latent" schizophrenia was taken up by some psychiatrists in China and there also was used to back up the "treatment" of political dissenters.[7]

The Maoist politicization of psychiatry surpassed the Soviet practice. A psychiatric survey in 1972 went beyond political dissidents to say most mental illness came from a bourgeois outlook.[8] One of the authors, Jia Rubao, explained. "People with mental illness were usually obsessed with personal gain: The process goes exactly like this: under the socialist system, it is impossible for these people to satisfy their selfish desires and so the 'boil' cannot be lanced; at first, the normal thoughts and the pathological thoughts coexist side by side, but as the pathological thoughts gradually gain the ascendant in their minds, they begin to sing, dance and run around aimlessly, tearing off their clothes and going around naked, and sometimes injuring or killing people—that is, they become mentally ill. We see, therefore, that bourgeois worldview and methodology are the fundamental causal factors in the emergence of mental illness; indeed this is the essential nature of mental illness."[9]

Psychiatric abuse has continued in the post-Mao period. Beginning in 1987 a network of secure units for mentally ill offenders was set up. They were called "Ankang" (peace and health) hospitals and were run by the police. An encyclopedia of police work lists categories of people to be detained there, including "political maniacs" who shout reactionary slogans, write reactionary banners and reactionary letters, make antigovernment speeches in public, and express opinions on important domestic and international affairs.[10]

Treatments included psychosurgery. It has been reported that in the Ankang hospital in Tianjin in the 1980s, dozens of lobotomies and similar brain operations were performed each year.[11]

Hospital punishments for disobedience were severe. "If such and such a person was to be punished, her bed would be taken to the area between the dining hall and the workshop, and she would be tied by her four limbs to the bed . . . In the evening when we returned to the dormitory, we would watch the bed carried away, and see the empty space where it had stood. A cold shiver would go through your heart. You didn't know when it would be your turn."[12] Punishments included forcible injections that left facial muscles stiff and eyes fixed and staring, and electric current administered by acupuncture needles.

Psychiatry is used as a weapon against groups such as Falun Gong. One case was a 62-year-old man reported to be "besotted" with Falun

Gong. "He soon became solitary and untalkative, and he began giving people valuable presents for no reason. He always ate less than other people and would buy the cheapest of foods. He said that [this was because] he wanted to be a genuinely 'truthful, compassionate and forbearing' person. After the government declared Falun Gong to be an evil cult, he not only ignored all efforts to dissuade him from continuing to practice Falun Gong, but also joined with other practitioners in traveling to Beijing to 'uphold the Dharma' on behalf of Falun Gong."[13] Diagnosis: mental disorder caused by practicing an evil cult; should bear partial legal responsibility for his crimes.

British Colonial Africa

Arrangements in colonies usually include advantages for colonizers over the colonized. Psychiatric treatment in colonial Africa was no exception. In 1980, following the transition from white-ruled Southern Rhodesia to Zimbabwe, the new minister of health visited the segregated Ingutsheni Mental Hospital. Wards for Europeans had rooms with beds, with pictures on painted walls. The windows had curtains. Wards for Africans were dark and dank. Men and women alike, grossly overcrowded, "slept, barracks-style, on felt mats instead of beds, directly on top of cold cement floors." The windows were dark slits giving no view. The Africans were assigned to manual farmwork; European patients did gardening and played tennis.[14]

In the late 1930s and early 1940s there were tensions within the hospital medical staff. Doctors and nurses new from Britain complained in the press about poor facilities, dirt, rubbish, and vermin. In 1942 a Commission of Inquiry was set up.

Treatment in the hospital reflected the segregation. Between 1932 and 1938 convulsant shock therapy was given to 205 people—that is, to all the in-patients with a diagnosis of schizophrenia. Deep coma was induced by intravenous injection of Cardiazol until a major seizure occurred. For this treatment Europeans were given a general anaesthetic. African patients were not. Instead they were held down by several strong men. Dr. Kenneth Rodger, the hospital's medical superintendent, reported remarkable "recovery rates": the highest, in 1938, were 83 percent among Africans and 76 percent among Europeans. Dr. Rodger reported the treatment as "100 percent safe for Europeans," but "with the native it is different." He had to report the death in 1938 of seventy-nine African patients, many linked to this treatment. He said he regretted the deaths but felt they were "more than offset" by the recovery rates.[15]

This treatment was replaced by electric convulsant therapy (ECT), but there were problems with this too. The deputy superintendent, Dr. David MacKenzie, told the Commission of Enquiry that while he was away, Dr. Rodger—inappropriately, in MacKenzie's view—had given ECT to three African patients. When MacKenzie returned, these patients were either dead or dying. The Commission were unimpressed by his "unsolicited statements." They argued that the death rates had not increased steadily since the introduction of shock therapies, so Rodger's negligence was not proved. However, the Commission did find some things shocking: the same room was used (though at different times) for European and for African film screenings, and the yard for European women could be seen by male African staff.[16]

Dr. Mackenzie's complaints suggest decency and integrity. But they stand out against the background of dark and dank African wards, the rubbish, and the vermin. His complaints go against a culture where a doctor is relaxed about seventy-nine African deaths in one hospital in one year and claims they are "more than offset" by improved recovery rates. The culture included the Commission of Enquiry's choices of which issues to take seriously. Like other professionals, individual psychiatrists can reflect too well the values of those in power.

Local values and prejudices can influence the theorizing as well as the practice of psychiatrists. This can be seen in a psychiatric report on the Mau Mau conflict in Kenya in the 1950s. The conflict was both a nationalist, anticolonial rebellion and a civil war within the Kikuyu tribe. It was linked to the Kikuyu claim that the "White Highlands" had been stolen from them by white settlers. Pressures, including evictions from land, had forced them to work as landless laborers, with a large loss of income.

Probably more than 20,000 of the rebels were killed in fighting. There were terrible religious-cum-sexual oaths and also terrible Mau Mau atrocities. Those they murdered included thirty-two European settlers and more than 1,800 Africans. Atrocities were not confined to the Mau Mau side of the conflict. Special Emergency Courts were set up, in which around 3,000 Africans were tried, often in mass trials, for Mau Mau offenses. 1,090 were hanged. Of these, 346 had been convicted of murder and the other 744 were hanged for other offenses, including possession of firearms, administering Mau Mau oaths or "consorting with terrorists."[17] 150,000 Kikuyu were put in camps, often by indiscriminate detention orders. Detainees included children. Overcrowding and too little food led to deaths from disease in the camps. There were brutal beatings. One culmination was at the Hola camp. When detainees refused to work, the African guards set on them with whips and clubs. Eleven were clubbed to death while European warders looked on.

Early in this grim conflict, Dr. J. C. Carothers was asked to produce a report for the colonial government on the psychology of the Mau Mau. Carothers was the psychiatrist in charge of Mathari Mental Hospital in Nairobi. He had previously published on frontal lobe function in the African. He suggested that Africans made little use of the frontal lobes, and likened their psychology to that of Europeans after prefrontal leucotomy. He had written more generally on "The African Mind in Health and Disease," work he drew on in his account of Mau Mau.

In his report "The Psychology of Mau Mau," Carothers did not mention political causes of the rebellion, such as the grievance over land, but gave an account purely in terms of individual psychology and its pathology. He did not rely on the neuropsychology of the frontal lobes, but attributed distinctive features of African psychology to differences of culture. The European "achieves a unique personal integration of his experience and a sense of continuing personal responsibility."[18] In African culture curiosity was stifled. Animism was a poor basis for explaining experience. So an African was "relatively unintegrate—an assemblage of memorized and disparate rules" without reflection, foresight, or responsibility.

Carothers thought colonization had undermined these traditional rules. Without them, Africans acted on the emotion of the moment: "The outsider has no rights and, if that outsider has inspired fear or hate, the vilest of behavior is appropriate." Without the evil spirits once blamed for misfortunes, they blamed Europeans. Many had taken the Mau Mau oaths, which had "all the depravity that is imaginable." But it should be possible to redeem many of them.

Carothers suggested forcibly isolating Kikuyu people in specially built villages, a policy previously used by the British in Malaya and later used by the Americans in Vietnam. He admitted that the Kikuyu would "not take kindly at first" to this. He thought they could be psychologically redeemed, partly by following the Catholic use of confession. As the African was not weighed down by past sins, "it should not be very difficult for him to cleanse his soul of any filth that has adhered to it." Carothers adds, "One has been much impressed by the activities of certain Screening Teams."

The pathologizing speculations about "the African," like Soviet theories about latent schizophrenia, hardly need refuting. But the references to confession and the Screening Teams have a sinister ring. Bad ideas can have bad consequences. One African man described being screened: "They put a rope round my neck, and the other end they put round Githinji. They said, 'If you don't say what we ask you, you will die.' Before being questioned we were beaten and the rope tightened. We were very frightened. I said we had killed nobody. We were beaten again, and they put to us that we had killed two persons. We denied this . . . The askaris beat us with open palms and with the butts of their rifles on my head and body . . . We stayed two days in the Screening Camp . . . What I told the first was true. Then I was beaten again and I said whatever they wanted me to say."[19]

Torture

> David Hicks: They pull you apart and put you back together, dismantling into smaller pieces each time, until you become something different, their creation, when eventually reassembled . . .
>
> Interviewer: Did you ever meet separately with a psychologist or psychiatrist when at Guantanamo, for ostensibly psychological reasons, either a psychological test or assessment, or for supposed treatment of any sort?
>
> David Hicks: No, but they did approach me occasionally during the last year or so I spent in GTMO to see if I would talk and cooperate. Apart from their contributions in interrogations they were always lurking in the background, waiting to "help a detainee," but to really act as another prong to interrogation. If a detainee even whispered for such medical intervention a "mental health expert" would appear with a pocket of unknown medication and a long list of probing questions. They were not there to help, but to harm.
>
> —David Hicks, interviewed by Jason Leopold, *Truthout*

Some American psychiatrists played a part in the more sophisticated torture set up in the camp in Guantanamo Bay.

"Major General Geoffrey Miller, who took command of Guantanamo in late 2002, approved the creation of a 'Behavioral Science Consultation Team' (BSCT, pronounced 'Biscuit') in order to develop new strategies and assess intelligence production. A principal BSCT function was to engineer the camp experiences of 'priority' detainees to make interrogation more productive. A psychiatrist and a psychologist staffed the Guantanamo BSCT."[20]

George Orwell would have been fascinated by the acronym to be pronounced like the comforting word "biscuit." Of course the Orwellian concept of "engineering the experiences" of prisoners in a concentration camp is not within accepted boundaries of medical ethics. To its credit, the American Psychiatric Association made a statement opposing participation in interrogation.

David Hicks, an Australian interviewed after his release from Guantanamo, had himself been physically beaten in Afghanistan. His abuse in Guantanamo included being forcibly injected at the base of his neck. The solitary and indefinite detention led to mental confusion, "huge mental blanks," and dependence on his captors. "They pull you apart and put you back together, dismantling into smaller pieces each time, until you become something different, their creation, when eventually reassembled." The effects lasted. "I have attended regular counselling since being released . . . Being exposed to such a consuming environment leaves a stain that cannot be removed overnight. It will take longer to reverse the consequences but even so, some experiences, especially one so prolonged, can never be entirely forgotten."

He described "teams of so-called experts" who advised on techniques to be used, such as sleep deprivation or loud noise: "A lot of effort went into these customized interrogations. Nothing was private. We were violated internally, psychologically, spiritually. They probed and tinkered in recesses so deep; parts of ourselves we are not conscious of or in touch with in our daily lives and may not even connect with and discover in our lifetimes."[21]

Patterns of Psychiatric Participation

Most of the human psychological flaws on display in these episodes are not peculiar to psychiatrists. These flaws include misplaced obedience, conformity, deference to those in power, and the cowardice that puts not losing a job or advancement before scruples about atrocities. They include the cruelty that can go with power over others, whether in Leningrad or in a Chinese Ankang, in an ECT unit in a British colonial hospital or in Guantanamo. Humanity can be distorted by hostility or by some uncritically accepted ideology. People can put on blinkers to evade seeing or caring about the consequences of their actions. And there is self-deception. Perhaps killing psychiatric patients really will improve the gene pool? Perhaps Soviet or Chinese communism is so good that people have to be crazy to oppose it? Perhaps "the African mind" is the explanation of rebellion? Might torturing people in Guantanamo save lives? And so on.

The horrors are obvious. Moral failures and self-deception are more likely than honest intellectual mistake. The failures of these psychiatrists and psychiatric nurses mirror the participation in atrocities of politicians, soldiers, policemen, professors, scientists, teachers, technologists, and many others.

But there are also indications of distinctively psychiatric moral vulnerabilities. One is the facilitation of atrocity by psychiatric stigma. Creeping psychiatric boundaries are dangerous. Rebels or dissenters are stigmatized through such elusive categories as latent schizophrenia, "bourgeois worldview," or "the African mind."

Carothers's thoughts on Africans also display the limitations of some kinds of psychiatric theorizing. Pathologizing whole groups can come from overconfidence in a set of current psychiatric categories, as in claims about the poor functioning of African frontal lobes and the supposed parallel with prefrontal leucotomy.

Jock McCulloch has suggested that, in the context of the loss of land and the impoverishment experienced by the Kikuyu, "it is significant that when the British government sought to explain the rebellion it turned not to an anthropologist or historian but to a psychiatrist," who would focus on culture, child-rearing, and personality rather than on the issue of land.[22] He says: "'The Psychology of Mau Mau' showed how well suited ethnopsychiatry was to the shaping and rationalization of conventional settler beliefs about Africans. It was the one science that was capable of providing a strictly hierarchical definition of human nature, and in that sense it was the one science whose shibboleths corresponded perfectly with the structures of colonial societies." Because it lacked the tensions raised in the fieldwork of social anthropologists, "for a psychiatrist such as Carothers, equipped with unambiguous definitions of normality and pathology, the understanding of Africans was far easier."[23]

Blinkered research is found in many disciplines. Sociologists may ignore biological factors, biologists may ignore cultural ones, and so on. Carothers's neglect of economic and political grievances may reflect something wider than a psychiatric phenomenon. And the racism of that period's ethnopsychiatry is hardly a charge against psychiatry as a whole.

But the other point goes beyond ethnopsychiatry and these dark moments in the history of psychiatry. The contrast between the anthropologist's awareness of how context complicates interpretation and the "unambiguous definitions of normality and pathology" found in the cruder versions of psychiatry is not confined to colonial Africa.

Medicalizing Social Disapproval

> There is no reason that all human existence should be constructed on some one or some small number of patterns.
>
> —John Stuart Mill: *On Liberty*

> (Her adoptive mother, disapproving of Jeanette Winterson having a girlfriend):
>
> *"Jeanette, will you tell me why?"* . . .
>
> "When I am with her I am happy. Just happy." . . .
>
> *"Why be happy when you could be normal?"*
>
> —Jeanette Winterson, memoir, *Why Be Happy When You Could Be Normal?*

Dubiously stretched diagnoses of mental disorder are not confined to big public atrocities. Another dark strand in the history of psychiatry is seeing psychiatric illness in the flouting of social norms. Public disgust may create pressure for those who do not conform to be "treated." Some psychiatrists have resisted this. Others have not. Victims have included unmarried mothers and gay people.

In the United Kingdom the Mental Deficiency Acts of 1913 and 1917 recognized four groups with mental deficiency. One was "moral defectives." It was said of this group that from an early age they had "some permanent mental defect coupled with strong vicious or criminal propensities on which punishment had little or no effect." In practice this was often taken to include unmarried mothers, who were sometimes locked away in asylums for years.

Being gay was classified as a sexual deviation and/or a personality disorder. It was included in the *DSM* as a disorder until campaigning forced its removal as late as 1973. In the 1960s homosexuality was sometimes "treated" by "aversion therapy"—same-sex erotic images were paired with electric shocks or drugs to cause vomiting.

One British victim in that period was Peter Price. Pressured by his mother to have his homosexuality "treated," he was admitted to a Chester psychiatric hospital. He was forced to listen to tapes saying he was a dirty queer, while lying for three days in his own excrement, urine, and vomit. While shown pictures of seminude men, he was forcibly injected with drugs. "The injection just made me violently ill. I just wanted to throw up." The doctors refused him a basin and made him vomit over himself. They gave him hourly injections. He escaped before the promised electric treatment. But the effects lasted: "If I hadn't had aversion therapy, I would live life as a normal gay person and I would have a partner . . . a long-lasting relationship. Aversion therapy changed my life totally. Three days has destroyed 25 years."[24]

Professor Hans Eysenck gave a lecture in London as late as 1972 advocating aversion therapy for homosexuality.[25] In the psychoanalytic tradition also, there was usually the same willingness to follow the conventional wisdom of the time. Though a striking exception was Freud himself. Thirty-seven years before Eysenck's lecture, Freud replied to a letter from an American woman who was obviously worried about her son's homosexuality. His letter started:

> Dear Mrs . . . ,
> I gather from your letter that your son is a homosexual. I am most impressed by the fact that you do not mention this term

> yourself in your information about him. May I question you, why you avoid it? Homosexuality is assuredly no advantage, but it is nothing to be ashamed of, no vice, no degradation, it cannot be classified as an illness; we consider it to be a variation of the sexual function produced by a certain arrest of sexual development . . . It is a great injustice to persecute homosexuality as a crime, and cruelty too.[26]

Freud lived long before the word "gay" was used as it is now. But I like to think he would have approved of its origin: G.A.Y. standing for "good as you." Regrettably, Freud's early followers concentrated, not on his rejection of the "illness" view, but on the "arrest of sexual development" theory. What might have gone wrong at the oedipal stage? How much could psychoanalysis correct this in the person? The questions showed a drift back to conventional prejudice. Anna Freud in 1956 advised Nancy Procter-Gregg not to quote Freud's letter in an *Observer* article. She said, "We can cure many more homosexuals than was thought possible in the beginning. The other reason is that readers may take this as a confirmation that all analysis can do is to convince patients that their defects or 'immoralities' do not matter and that they should be happy with them. That would be unfortunate."[27] This comment is sad in the context of what it aimed to suppress: Sigmund Freud's own clear, firm view that homosexuality is neither an illness nor a reason for shame.

Since 1973 the psychiatric and psychological professions have thoroughly distanced themselves from the medicalizing of sexual orientation. But there are still some freelance efforts to continue that approach. Some groups on the religious right in the United States practice "conversion therapy." In Britain as late as 2010 an investigation by Peter Strudwick found therapists who were willing to attempt to "cure" homosexuality by a mixture of therapy and prayer.[28]

As this history shows, psychiatrists were vulnerable to pressures to give such "treatment." It is linked to their role in relieving psychological distress. Social stigma can itself cause distress. The psychiatrist cannot eliminate society's attitudes, so it is not ill-intentioned to aim to alleviate the distress by changing the stigmatized person. Not an ill-intentioned aim, but one that often harms the person "treated" and also helps maintain the stigma.

Another vulnerability comes from the way stigmatized conditions can be powerfully but wrongly presented as being *in themselves* sources of unhappiness. It is now hard to grasp how strong this attitude to being gay once was.

Lord Devlin was a highly reflective judge. His decent instincts led him to produce a forthright report on atrocities under British colonial rule in Africa, a report most unwelcome to the government. But he was also a man of his time. In the context of proposals to end the criminalization of adult homosexual acts in private, he defended the right of a society to enforce its standards of morality. In a 1964 essay he wrote: "A man does not as a rule commit bigamy because he wants to experiment with two wives instead of one. He does not as a rule lie with his daughter or sister because he thinks that an incestuous relationship can be a good one but because he finds in it a way of satisfying his lust in the home. He does not keep a brothel so as to prove the value of promiscuity but so as to make money. There must be some homosexuals who believe theirs to be a good way of life but many more who would like to get free of it if only they could. Certainly no-one in his senses can think that habitual drunkenness or drugging leads to any good at all. Such are the vices that the law seeks to control."

Devlin also said, "I do not think that there is anyone who asserts vocally that homosexuality is a good way of life but there may be those who believe it to be so."[29] And in 1970 he wrote, "I agree with everyone who has written or spoken on the subject that homosexuality is usually a miserable way of life and that it is the duty of society, if it can, to save any youth from being led into it. I think that duty has to be discharged although it may mean much suffering by incurable perverts who seem unable to resist the corruption of boys."[30]

In their time these comments were not unusual in their confidence that most homosexuals would like to change and that their way of life was miserable. Psychiatry, as a discipline aiming to treat and cure malfunctioning minds, is likely always to be subject to such pressures. The history suggests a vulnerability to them. It matters to draw the boundaries of psychiatry in a way that gives a basis for resistance to the local prejudices of particular places and times.

15

Personality and Sexuality

> Before analysing, before classifying, before thinking, before trying to *do* anything—we should *listen*. Categories and classifications play a large role in the institutions of mental health care for veterans, in the education of mental health care professionals, and as tentative guides to perception. All too often, however, our mode of listening deteriorates into intellectual sorting, with the professional grabbing the veterans' words from the air and sticking them in mental bins . . . At its worst our educational system produces counselors, psychiatrists, psychologists, and therapists who resemble museum-goers whose whole experience consists of mentally saying "That's cubist! . . . That's El Greco!" and who never *see* anything they've looked at.
>
> —Jonathan Shay, *Achilles in Vietnam: Combat Trauma and the Undoing of Character*

Happily, psychiatric "treatment" of gay people or unmarried mothers is almost entirely a thing of the past. But even now the frontiers of psychiatric disorder are as fluid and disputed as those of eighteenth-century Poland. Notable attempts to map the boundaries are the two overlapping major systems of classification: The *Diagnostic and Statistical Manual of Mental Disorders (DSM),* now in its fifth edition *(DSM-5),* and the relevant section of the *International Classification of Diseases (ICD).* Among the most controversial psychiatric diagnoses are the "personality disorders" and some deviant sexual tastes or orientations, known as the "paraphilias."

"Personality Disorders"

What are the "personality disorders"? Lists vary, but both *DSM-5* and *ICD-10* include borderline personality disorder, obsessive-compulsive (or "anankastic") personality disorder, schizotypal (or schizoid) personality disorder, and antisocial (or dissocial) personality disorder.

How is "personality disorder" defined? *ICD-10* gives a number of criteria. "The individual's characteristic and enduring patterns of behaviour deviate markedly as a whole from the culturally expected range," as seen in their thinking, emotions, their control of impulses or their relations with other people. Their behaviour in different situations must be "inflexible, maladaptive, or otherwise dysfunctional." There must be personal distress or "adverse impact on the social environment."

This must be too broad. "Deviating markedly from the culturally expected range" at different times would have caught in its net dissidents in the Soviet Union or the Chinese Cultural Revolution, atheists in Saudi Arabia, and communists in 1950s America. Gays in the past (and in some of the more stifling societies now) would also be caught. In "the culturally expected range" we again glimpse William Blake's "mind-forged manacles."

"Inflexible, maladaptive, or otherwise dysfunctional" does not do much better. The word "maladaptive" sounds scientific, perhaps like an idea derived from Darwinian survival. But like "dysfunctional" it also has a worrying suggestion of not fitting well with prevailing social norms. "Maladaptive," even in the more literal Darwinian sense of not being conducive to survival in a particular environment, may still include too much. Bravery in a firefighter may reduce the firefighter's chances of survival. And Socrates held rather rigidly to the habit of asking questions that troubled people, a habit that eventually led to his death.

Definitions that include far too much may reflect on psychiatrists' philosophical skills rather than their diagnostic ones. Some of them say, "The definition may be no good, but you recognize it when you see it." There do seem to be people—not firefighters or Socrates—who seem messed up in ways that damage their relationships and their lives.

An anonymous person diagnosed with borderline personality disorder wrote: "Being a borderline feels like eternal hell. Nothing less. Pain, anger, confusion, hurt, never knowing how I'm gonna feel from one minute to the next. Hurting because I hurt those who I love. Feeling misunderstood. Analyzing everything. Nothing gives me pleasure. Once in a great while I will be 'too happy' and then anxious because of that. Then I self-medicate with alcohol. Then I physically hurt myself. Then I feel guilty because of that. Shame. Wanting to die but not being able to kill myself because I'd feel too much guilt for those I'd hurt, and then feeling angry about that so I cut myself or O.D. to make all the feelings go away. Stress!"[1]

Someone who feels like this does need help. The most urgent difficulties are practical. Are there effective ways to help? But behind the practical ones are theoretical issues, perhaps linked to helping people in future. If this a *disorder*, what makes it so? What kind of disorder is it, and how should we understand it?

Objections to the general definition of "personality disorder" are too easy. The substance is in the particular types. Is each of them a clear and unified condition? Leaving aside antisocial personality disorder, here are some of the key features given in the *DSM-5* accounts of three major categories:

> ***Borderline personality disorder includes:***
> Instability of self-image (often poor, with excessive self-criticism), of goals, values, or career plans, and of mood (with anxiety, depression, or feelings of emptiness);
> hostility, limited empathy, with hypersensitivity to possible slights;
> unstable personal relationships, marked by mistrust, neediness, alternating between extremes of idealization and devaluation, and between overinvolvement and withdrawal, anxiety about abandonment;
> impulsiveness and taking risks.
>
> ***Obsessive-compulsive personality disorder includes:***
> Sense of self derived mainly from work, constricted experience;
> perfectionism, rigid and unreasonably high standards of behavior; obsession with detail, organization, and order;
> thinking there is only one right way of doing things;
> persistence at tasks when this is no longer effective.
>
> ***Schizotypal personality disorder includes:***
> Confused boundaries between self and others, distorted self-concept;
> Unrealistic or incoherent goals;

> Difficulty in understanding the impact of own behavior on others, misinterpreting what others do;
> Suspicious, mistrustful, and poor at developing close relationships;
> Eccentric behavior, appearance, thought, or speech;
> Unusual beliefs or experiences;
> Withdrawal, coldness, limited emotional responses.

Lists of personality disorders invite an obvious party game, seeing which categories we and our friends fit. There is the risk of diagnosing personality disorders for what are simply unappealing personalities. Some of this looks very subjective. The person diagnosed with obsessive-compulsive personality disorder because of being perfectionist, rigid, obsessed with detail and order, with unreasonably high standards of behavior might reply that the psychiatrist who diagnosed her is slapdash, chaotic, and morally unprincipled. The person diagnosed with borderline personality partly on the basis of impulsiveness and risk-taking may see his psychiatrist as someone who has never been young or in love, and who probably started thinking about a pension at the age of 22.

Two different models lurk behind the diagnosis of personality disorder. One is based on the thought that some personalities dispose people to particular psychiatric illnesses: so "schizotypal personality disorder" is seen as incipient schizophrenia. The other model is based on dimensions of personality, with personality disorder being at an extreme of a continuum.

Each model has its difficulties. The incipient schizophrenia of one model has troubling echoes of the "latent" schizophrenia of Soviet psychiatry. The link between the personality disorder and the illness is unclear. On the other model, it is hard to see why a personality should count as disordered *merely* because it is at the extreme of some dimension. Why should extreme perfectionism or extreme solitariness count as symptoms of disorder while extreme honesty or extreme interest in mathematics do not? The choice of dimensions has a hint of "deviation from the culturally expected range." And what are unusual beliefs doing in this list of pathology?

Trying to think in terms of the current conceptual framework of personality disorder and its varieties is like walking over a bridge made of chewing gum. And yet, "Being a borderline feels like eternal hell.

Nothing less." The anonymous writer does need help and so do many like her. Effective help may depend on looking through the "borderline" category, to see more clearly what is going on in the person behind it.

The "Paraphilias"

The "paraphilias" are minority sexual tastes. To merit this diagnosis, certain kinds of intense sexual fantasies, urges, or behavior have to recur for at least six months. According to *DSM-5,* diagnosis is appropriate only where the urges have been acted on, or where they cause significant distress or impairment in important areas of the individual's functioning. Perhaps most people sometimes act on intense sexual fantasies and urges, and for quite a few people this causes problems in their lives. It is the kind of desire or act that leads to the diagnosis. Each "paraphilia" is specified by what triggers arousal:

Exhibitionistic disorder: the exposure of one's genitals to an unsuspecting stranger

Fetishistic disorder: the sexual use of nonliving objects or nongenital bodily parts

Frotteuristic disorder: touching or rubbing against a nonconsenting person

Pedophilic disorder: sexual desire for prepubescent or early pubescent children

Sexual masochism disorder: a desire for being humiliated, beaten, bound, or otherwise made to suffer

Sexual sadism disorder: a desire to cause the physical or psychological suffering of another person

Transvestic disorder: cross-dressing

Voyeuristic disorder: seeking sexual gratification from clandestinely observing another person who is naked, in the process of disrobing or engaging in sexual activity

Unspecified paraphilic disorder: erotic interest in activities including telephone scatalogia (obscene phone calls), necrophilia (corpses), zoophilia (animals), coprophilia (feces), klismaphilia (enemas), and urophilia (urine)

This extraordinary ragbag needs sorting out. Two lists are needed. One is of the conditions that, when acted on, invade or harm other people. The other contains the harmless, noninvasive ones.

The first list obviously includes pedophilia. Protecting children at risk of harm justifies making it illegal to act on these inclinations. (It is essential that the inclinations are contained. If nothing better can be found, then, sadly, by coercive means. But this doesn't mean stigmatizing, hating, or despising people for *having* the inclinations, which is probably outside their control.)

There are grounds for a legal ban where acting on some of the other conditions would be invasive of a person's private space and might cause pain, shock, or distress. People should be protected from nonconsenting exposure to sexual sadism, exhibitionism, frotteurism, voyeurism, and obscene phone calls. Dying people need protection from the perhaps remote risk of nonconsenting necrophilia.

The key is consent or its lack. For some of these activities, such as pedophilia and zoophilia, competent consent is out of the question. And for some others it is ruled out by definition: frotteurism is defined as needing a nonconsenting person, and exhibitionism and voyeurism need the "unsuspecting" person. For yet others, competent consent must be a very remote possibility. Who would sign the consent form to receive obscene phone calls or the advance directive for necrophilia? But for other conditions, it is important to keep the consent loophole open, because they can be competently consented to, as when masochists consent to sadistic acts.

The second list, of the harmless, noninvasive conditions, should include fetishism, sexual masochism, and transvestism. Of course any of these *can* involve harm to others. The large transvestite may ruin his girlfriend's clothes. But this is like the man whose obsession with stamp collecting leads to neglect of his family. The harm is contingent, not intrinsic to the activity. Perhaps, as once with homosexuality, the boundaries of psychiatry are being deformed by stigma and prejudice?

Whether or not people with conditions on either list should be candidates for psychiatric treatment (assuming, debatably, that effective psychiatric help is possible) depends on one of two reasons applying to their case.

One reason applies to conditions on the first list. The need to prevent harm to others might be argued to justify psychiatric treatment. If an effective treatment were available, there would be *a case for* requiring some people convicted of acts of pedophilia to accept it. I hope this case would be overridden by powerful opposing medical ethics and civil liberties arguments for the right of a competent person to refuse treatment. But prevention of harm to others could justify at least offering treatment.

The second reason could apply to conditions on either list. Some people, after serious consideration, might think their sexual preference constituted a disadvantage they would like to be rid of. Any legal or social penalties might be part of the disadvantage, although the wider social impact of further stigmatizing an otherwise harmless condition would be relevant here.

Where neither reason applies, there is no basis for psychiatric treatment. The idea that these conditions are in themselves disorders may come partly from a sloppy extrapolation from the fact that in some other cases the reasons do apply. Neither this blurred thinking, nor the kind of disgust once common as a response to homosexuality, has any standing as a reason for medicalizing these sexual tastes.

For sexual preferences not involving invasive or harmful acts with nonconsenting others, the approach should be very different from the stony-faced listing of "paraphilias." Sharon Olds caught the guiding spirit with humanity and humor in her poem "The Solution," which is about people saying what they want and then being paired up:

> You would stand under a sign saying *I Like To Be Touched And Held* and when someone came and stood under the sign saying *I Like To Touch And Hold* they would send the two of you off together.
>
> At first it went great. A steady stream of people under the sign *I Like To Give Pain* paired up with the steady stream of people from under *I Like To Receive Pain. Foreplay only—No Orgasm* found its adherents, and *Orgasm only—No Foreplay* matched up its believers. A loyal Berkeley, California policeman stood under the sign *Married Adults, Lights Out, Face To Face, Under A Sheet* because that's the only way it was legal in Berkeley—but he stood there a long time in his lonely blue law coat. And the man under *I Like To Be Sung to While Bread*

> *Is Kneaded on My Stomach* had been there weeks without a reply.
>
> From Sharon Olds, "The Solution."[2]

(Part of the Berkeley policeman's job was investigating obscene phone calls. Now he's retrained as a psychiatrist and calls them "telephone scatalogia." He enjoys his new work writing the *DSM* section on paraphilias.)

16

Dysfunction?

A "paradigm shift" is under way, which is carrying the speciality beyond the medical model, with its emphasis on the diagnosis and treatment of dubious disease entities, towards an entirely new conceptual framework which defines the basic components of human nature in terms of their evolutionary origins and their essential developmental needs.

—Anthony Stevens and John Price, *Evolutionary Psychiatry*

The flaw in the *DSM* approaches to emotional disorders is fundamental: the *DSM* fails to distinguish protective responses from diseases.

—Randolph M. Nesse and Eric D. Jackson,
Evolutionary Foundations for Psychiatric Diagnosis: Making DSM-V Valid

Jerome Wakefield and his colleagues have argued that mental disorder is "harmful dysfunction." This account has two parts. It is claimed to be a matter of scientific fact that a system honed by evolution has in some persons become dysfunctional. And then values come in: the dysfunction has to be harmful.[1] Harm will be discussed in Chapter 17. Here the question is whether psychiatric disorders should be seen in terms of dysfunctional systems.

Causal Models in Evolutionary Psychiatry

The gene that causes sickle-cell anemia also protects against malaria. One approach to evolutionary psychiatry explains the survival of some psychiatric disorders in terms of their possible genetic links to traits that have survival value. It has been suggested, for example, that schizophrenia might have a genetic link to the development of language,[2] or to the development of parts of the brain that underlie social relationships.[3]

Some of these conjectures may be right. But for now they are still speculative.

Other evolutionary models give explanations more closely tied to features of psychiatric disorders. Thoughts, feelings, or actions that are inappropriate to their context are taken to be signs that some chemical, physiological, or psychological system is not serving the function for which natural selection "designed" it. Hallucinations signal some fault in perceptual systems that evolved to give reliable information. The aim of correcting faulty systems justifies psychiatry as a branch of medicine.

How far do emotional and mood disorders fit this model? Are there emotional systems parallel to the cognitive ones? Darwin saw emotions as evolved from actions. They are the suppressed versions. Anger is suppressed physical aggression. Fear is the suppressed inclination to run away. Both fighting and flight can have survival value. So may the ability to suppress either of them. It is easy to see how the systems involved in Darwinian emotions might have evolved.

In particular, unpleasant emotions may, in parallel with physical pain, have evolved as defenses against threats or difficulties. On this view, feeling low after losing a job or being left by a partner is not pathology. The fundamental mistake is said to be treating protective responses as diseases.[4] These normal "protective" responses are different from cases where, in evolutionary terms, something is going wrong. There are two main models used to account for the pathological cases. On the "mismatch" model, some psychiatric disorders come from parts of our nature that adapted to an early human environment that is no longer part of the world of today. On the "over-reaction" model, some psychiatric disorders are exaggerated versions of responses that are still adaptive.

The Mismatch Model

There may be mismatches between our situation and our evolved human nature. We fear snakes but have no fear of cigarettes or of driving too fast. Some evolutionary psychiatrists see this mismatch in phobias and anxiety disorders. Once it may have been adaptive for some people to have stronger than average fears or anxieties. But these dispositions are no longer useful. Where they are also distressing or incapacitating, they are plausible candidates for treatment.[5]

The mismatch model faces questions about the supposed early environment when our nature was formed. John Bowlby coined the phrase "the environment of evolutionary adaptedness." But there might not have been one single environment. The view that the central characteristics of human nature were fixed in some early period, perhaps the Pleistocene, is too simple. Human evolution has continued, with varying adaptations in different cultural environments.[6]

The Over-Reaction Model

Tracy Thompson saw that some of her responses when she was depressed had been inappropriate. Her boyfriend suggested changing their weekend plans. This "sent me catapulting into hysteria, it was proof that Sam did not love me. I sobbed for hours." Sometimes it was anger: "Any minor inconvenience could set me off—misplacing a blouse, getting lost somewhere, missing a phone call from Sam, finding myself stalled in a traffic jam . . . I threw things; I beat helplessly on the floor with my hairbrush; I scratched and tore at my own skin. The provocations were always so minor that I had usually forgotten them by the next day; sometimes I would look at a bruise on my arm and think: What was that for?"[7]

What makes emotional responses inappropriate? Sometimes they reflect distorted interpretations. Usually they are disproportionate. Later Tracy Thompson saw hours of sobbing as an over-reaction to changed plans for the weekend.

Some psychiatric disorders may be exaggerated versions of responses that are otherwise still adaptive. Panic helps people escape from danger; panic disorder is panic without the danger. Suspicion helps people avoid survival-threatening traps. Low-key mood favors caution, avoiding the risks taken in a more euphoric state. Paranoia and clinical depression can each be seen as exaggerations of these adaptive traits, perhaps a failure in a system whose function is to regulate them.

The over-reaction model needs more clarity about the adaptive value of such traits as low mood. As well as the tendency to support caution, there are other suggestions about its adaptive value. Being depressed may be a way of signaling a need for help. Some have seen depression as a prompt to accept defeat in competition and to adjust to the resulting low rank. Some or all of these accounts may be right. It is not clear how we should decide. Critics of evolutionary psychology have asked the "just-so story" question: How do we tell evidence from plausible but ad hoc speculation?

The mismatch and over-reaction models pull in opposite directions. Perhaps each fits different disorders. How should we rate adaptive against maladaptive aspects of an emotional state? Gloomy and suspicious people may be cautious in a way that helps them survive. But how is this to be weighed against the fact that their gloom and suspicion can put other people off? How can we tell which traits are adaptive and which are not?

An Inappropriate Emotional Response

Richard Wollheim's horror of newsprint was a problem for friends when they had him over for a meal. "Every scrap of newspaper had to be either thrown away or thoroughly concealed (not just tucked away findably under a cushion): the mere sight of newsprint would make it impossible for him to eat his dinner."[8] In his autobiography Wollheim courageously called his disgust at the smell of newsprint "the most persistent thread in my life, stronger, more unchanging, than any taste or interest, more demanding than any intellectual challenge." He went on to say, "I have never seen any way in which the power of love could transform it. It was like a ghost in the house that could be expelled only by demolishing the house."[9]

Richard Wollheim could see that his horror was out of proportion. An Oxford colleague poured glasses of sherry for Wollheim and himself. Wollheim was overcome with nausea. The washed cupboard had been lined with newspaper. The rims of the upside-down glasses had touched the wet paper. His host washed the glass and gave him more sherry. This was not enough, as the other glass still smelled of wet newspaper. At first the response seems totally out of proportion. How can someone be so upset by wet newspaper? But this may be too hasty. Some judgments about appropriateness need complex interpretation.

Wollheim traced his revulsion to an early childhood event. He and his brother were with their nanny, who was reading a newspaper account of a royal death. His brother resented Richard being nearer the nanny. He did not want her to pin the paper on the wall for them to see. So he made pellets from the paper, wet them in his mouth, and flicked them at the page she was reading. "The juices that had risen up into my mouth in sheer horror at the scene seemed to duplicate the taste of the little pellets in my brother's mouth." Wollheim saw the page of newspaper slipping out of the nanny's hands onto the floor "like a great injured bird." As it fell, the dead Queen's picture was changed: her face, the emeralds, and the satin buttons "were now desecrated by spit, and smell, and the signs of disease."[10]

There is always a question about whether to accept a Freudian claim linking a childhood episode to an adult problem. First-person accounts are not infallible, but they have a degree of authority, particularly when so vivid. Wollheim's account is as claustrophobic as a Freudian case written up by Proust would be. And the causal link is given some support by the specific recurrence of wet newsprint.

If Wollheim's account is right, the revulsion seems more intelligible. But is it proportionate? Proportionate to what? At one level it is still an extreme reaction to sherry glasses' having touched wet newspaper. Wollheim himself saw this and tried unsuccessfully to eliminate it. But if it is a response to the residue of a childhood trauma, it is harder to say what is proportionate.

Doubts about Dysfunction

One concern about the "dysfunction" approach is that it could allow homosexuality to again be seen as a disorder. It is hard to avoid the view that the likely main evolutionary value of sexual desires is procreation. It is all too easy to see how the dysfunction view could be seized on.

Other doubts are conceptual and empirical. It can be hard to identify even cognitive systems and their functions. Where a feature of a species has lasted in the evolutionary struggle, it is likely to have contributed to gene survival or else be linked to other features that did. But evolution might not have honed it for a *single* function. This is obvious with large, complex features. Having a brain clearly contributes to survival, but it does so through many different functions. The brain is a hierarchy of systems: perceptual, cognitive, and so on. In turn perception is a hierarchy of systems: visual, auditory, and so on. And vision is a hierarchy of systems for recognizing color, shape, and such. The subdivision continues downward. It makes more sense to talk about *the* function of a system lower down than it does for a system higher up.

It is even more difficult to identify emotional systems and their evolutionary functions. There is the just-so-story question again. Maps of neurochemical pathways involved in emotions are starting to be unraveled. But now it is still optimistic to talk of clear emotional systems, each with an evolutionary function. Even the clusters of neurotransmitters, neural pathways, and so on that might make up an emotional "system" could serve many functions. This makes identifying emotional "dysfunction" problematic.

What is the evolved system that, functioning properly, might have kept Wollheim's revulsion within bounds? Revulsion against smells might have evolved to keep us away from poisonous plants, decaying meat, or dangerous animals. But must there be a faulty system when people dislike the harmless smell of cabbage being boiled? Is there a system to control reactions to childhood trauma?

These problems are not decisive against the "dysfunctional system" view. A functional system might exist even if we cannot say what it is. But it does not follow that all inappropriate emotional responses indicate a system failure. In Wollheim's case, we cannot identify a malfunctioning system, so we do not know whether there is one or not.

When is an inappropriate emotional response a sign of psychiatric disorder? The answer does not depend on speculating about systems. Whether a psychological condition impairs the good life is independent of what its causes are.

The Priority of Harm over Dysfunction

To call something a disorder or disability does not settle the issue of whether it should be treated. The treatment may be too painful or too expensive to be worthwhile. Or the disability may avoid something more dangerous, like wartime conscription into an army. Respect for autonomy is crucial. Under normal conditions a competent person has a right to refuse even beneficial treatment.

The person's relation to a disorder or disability can be a reason for not treating it. There are (disputed) reasons for thinking blindness is not just a difference but a disability. But even if this is right, curing blindness can still make things worse. One blind man, "S.B.," was cheerful, confident, and proud of his work as a carpenter and cobbler. After being given sight, he thought things looked drab and dull. Having changed from a blind man who coped well into a sighted man who coped poorly, he lost his self-respect. He died in the second year after the operation. Others given sight made the transition more successfully. But the case of S.B. suggests that treating a disability is not always the right thing to do.[11]

Despite these reasons for not always treating disorders or disabilities, disorder is still linked with treatment. If someone has a disorder, then, *other things equal* (which they may not be), it calls for the offer of treatment. The dysfunction may indicate the kind of treatment needed. But what calls for treatment is the harm: the way the condition makes someone's life worse. In the case of psychiatric treatment, it is a psychological condition that makes someone's life worse. Harm has priority. Whether or not a socially paralyzing horror of newsprint counts as a disorder depends, not on a conjectured mechanism going wrong, but on the kind and degree of harm it causes.

17

Harm

> Normality is not the point—harm is.
>
> —Derek Bolton, *What Is Mental Disorder? An Essay in Philosophy, Science, and Values*

Some moods or emotional states are so distressing or inhibiting that they call for psychiatric help. Severe depression can be so devastating that medication or therapy can save the person's life. But is the net drawn too widely? Critics say that feeling depressed over doing badly on an exam, or when left by someone you love, is not illness but normal response. They also say that extreme shyness is wrongly medicalized as "social anxiety disorder." These expanding boundaries of psychiatry may benefit pharmaceutical companies, but should the range of "normal" emotional life be narrowed in this way? If a line is to be drawn between variations of mood in normal emotional life and those harmful enough to call for psychiatric help, where should it come?

The Harm of Clinical Depression

> Depression is a disorder of mood, so mysteriously painful and elusive in the way it becomes known to the self—to the mediating intellect—as to verge close to being beyond description. It thus remains nearly incomprehensible to those who have not experienced it in its extreme mode, although the gloom, "the blues" which people go through occasionally and associate with the general hassle of everyday existence are of such prevalence that they do give many individuals a hint of the illness in its catastrophic form. But at the time of which I write I had descended far past those familiar, manageable doldrums.
>
> —William Styron, *Darkness Visible*

What should be the boundaries of "major depressive disorder"? In *DSM-5* this diagnosis is based on having had one or more "major depressive episodes." An episode is monitored over two weeks. For most of nearly every day the person must show five or more symptoms, in a way that differs from how the person was before. The symptoms must include at least one of two key symptoms: the person must be depressed and/or show loss of interest and pleasure.

The other symptoms are unusual weight change, disordered sleep, agitated or slowed movements, fatigue or loss of energy, feelings of worthlessness, inappropriate guilt, indecisiveness, impaired concentration, and either a planned or attempted suicide or else recurrent thoughts about death or suicide.

The diagnosis is not made where there are likely alternative causes, such as other medical or psychiatric conditions or medical or recreational drugs. The disorder is diagnosed only when the symptoms cause significant distress or impaired functioning.

Should "Normal" Grief Be Included?

> It is also worth notice that, although mourning involves grave departures from the normal attitude to life, it never occurs to us to regard it as a pathological condition and to refer it to medical treatment. We rely on its being overcome after a certain lapse of time, and we look on any interference with it as useless or even harmful.
>
> —Sigmund Freud, *Mourning and Melancholia*

> Is not grief simply a reaction to a life experience? How can one put it into the same category as the pathological states we call disease? To this we answer that it is "natural" or "normal" in the same sense that [wound or burns are] the natural or normal responses to physical trauma.
>
> —George Engel, "Is Grief a Disease?,"
> *Journal of Psychosomatic Medicine,* 1961

In different editions the *DSM* account of major depressive disorder has varied on whether or not to include grief on being bereaved. In *DSM-4* the symptoms did not count if they were part of normal grief when bereaved. (Sometimes bereavement causes mood disorders. To exclude these cases, normal or "uncomplicated" grief was contrasted with grief that lasted more than two months, or that had marked functional impairment, psychotic symptoms, or other symptoms such as preoccupation with worthlessness or suicide.) In *DSM-5* this exclusion has been given up. The previous exclusion and the current inclusion of grief have both been controversial.

Should "normal" grief be seen as a disorder, calling for psychiatric help if available? Or is this to wrongly medicalize an experience that is part of normal life?

The exclusion of normal grief has been challenged as arbitrary. Grief, like other sad or low emotional states, involves distress and can impair a person's functioning. It often involves depression and loss of interest and pleasure. Jerome Wakefield and others found that, for eight out of nine indicators of disorder, the profiles for "uncomplicated" grief are not significantly different from major depressive disorder.[1] Where normal grief also causes fatigue, insomnia, and weight change, only its specific exclusion would prevent it from being diagnosed as a major depressive episode.

George W. Brown and Tirril Harris, in their classic Camberwell study of female clinical depression, included bereaved women with major depressive symptoms. They thought that exclusion would let assumptions about causes distort their study.[2] They also brought out the role of previous bereavement in causing depression. Unsurprisingly, depression was often triggered by some bad event or major difficulty. Most women in the study had such problems, but of those only a fifth developed clinical depression. A deeper account had to look at the interaction between the triggering problem and other things in their lives. Factors influencing the development and severity of depression included weak or emotionally poor social ties, having more than two children living at home, and having no outside employment. By far the strongest factor affecting the severity of depression was previous bereavement, especially loss of a mother before the age of 11.

The clear parallels between grief and clinical depression, and the link with previous bereavement, make a case against excluding normal grief as a quite separate phenomenon.

Is "Normal" Grief Harmful? Interpretation, Context, and Meaning

But there is a case against including normal grief in "psychiatric" depression. Wakefield and his colleagues observed the similarities but ran the argument the other way. Perhaps "uncomplicated" depression following *other* losses should also not be seen as disorder. What matters is whether the grief is out of proportion. This is part of a strong case for moving from symptoms abstractly described ("loss of interest and pleasure," and so on) to states seen in context and evaluated for their appropriateness. This would allow finer discriminations. There is a hint of pathology in grieving for months for a great-uncle you hardly knew. But no pathology is needed to explain why grief for a loved lifetime partner, or for your only child, lasts long and may never quite go away.

George Engel's analogy with a burn suggests that grief is harmful. But the comparison was too hasty. Yes, a burn still needs treatment despite being a normal response to some physical traumas. But grief is not the same. We do anything to stop the pain and damage of a burn. But for grief, values and interpretation are central: "Before classifying, before thinking, before trying to *do* anything—we should *listen*." Jonathan Shay argued against defining as a breakdown the grief of the Vietnam veterans he worked with. Opposing "crudely medicating soldiers because they weep," he said the returning soldier needs "not a mental health professional but a living community to whom his experience matters."[3]

Is grief harmful? One response is that we would be poorer without it. Perhaps being fully alive means experiencing the deepest things, including painful ones. Intense sadness may be a valued alternative to the disturbing lightness of a person who feels no grief when someone close dies.

What matters is what it means to us. It can be seen as part of the seriousness and depth of the relationship. Julian Barnes, in his *Levels of Life*, describes his grief at the death of his wife, Pat Kavanagh. He did not want it evaded. He mentioned her name at a dinner with friends. They ignored it. He mentioned her twice more and they still ignored it. "Perhaps the third time I was deliberately trying to provoke, being pissed off at what struck me not as good manners but as cowardice. Afraid to touch her name, they denied her thrice, and I thought the worse of them for it."[4]

Another friend of Julian Barnes, who herself had lost her husband, wrote: "The thing is—nature is so exact, it hurts exactly as much as it is worth, so in a way one relishes the pain, I think. If it didn't matter, it wouldn't matter." At first the phrase about relishing the pain struck Barnes as unnecessarily masochistic. But later he realized, "I know that it contains truth. And if the pain is not exactly relished, it no longer seems futile. Pain shows that you have not forgotten; pain enhances the flavour of memory; pain is a proof of love. 'If it didn't matter, it wouldn't matter.'"[5]

To someone who interprets it in this way, grief is emphatically not harmful. Some people do accept medication to ease the pain of bereavement. Others would reject a pill to reduce or eliminate grief. Different people's grief is linked to the meanings they place on it. The questions of interpretation are of a different order from those raised by a burn.

What Is Harm? "Liberal" and "Human Flourishing" Versions

> So what is the proper domain of psychiatry; or rather, of multidisciplinary mental health services? The starting place is the matter of harm: the patient's distress and disability. Harm is agreed by (practically) all to be involved in our concept of mental disorder.
>
> —Derek Bolton, *What Is Mental Disorder? An Essay in Philosophy, Science and Values*

Harm is central. But what is harm? Derek Bolton is right to take distress and disability as the starting place. But their links to harm are not simple. Surgery may be distressing without being harmful. And disability is not always worse than the alternative, as when S.B. was given sight.

Of course some degrees of distress or disability are too acute to be problematic. William Styron's depression "in its catastrophic form," or the "eternal hell" of the anonymous person with borderline personality disorder, raise no subtle questions about whether help is needed.

Other cases are more problematic. Gays in the 1950s and later *were* harmed. They were imprisoned, stigmatized, and endured horrible "cures." They were assaulted or even murdered. In some places they still are. Of course these indirect harms do not make being gay a disorder. The intrinsic harm of major depression is not the same as the misery caused by prejudices about otherwise harmless conditions.

Even intrinsic harm is a plural and highly contested concept, charged with values. There are two main approaches to the assessment of harm. (Some see them as rivals, others as complementary.)

One view (linked to the idea of respecting autonomy) sees harm as something going against the person's own values. Following Bennett Foddy and Julian Savulescu, I will call this the "Liberal" approach.[6] The main issue raised by that view comes when people make choices that seem strongly against their best interests. Are such choices an authentic reflection of their values? This liberal approach, and its problem of authenticity, will be discussed in the last part of this book, especially in the context of eating disorders.

Here we will start with the main alternative view, to be called here the "Human Flourishing" approach. This takes an Aristotelian view of harm. It sees a condition as harmful when it is an impediment to the person's being able to live a good human life. This raises obvious questions about what a good human life is. One feature of this approach is that the assessment of harm is to some extent independent of whether or not the person concerned agrees with it. (This is linked to the appeal to a person's "best interests," which is generally thought appropriate when people lack the capacity to decide for themselves.)

Psychiatrists aim to help people whose thoughts, moods, emotions, desires, psychological abilities, or personalities are impaired. All this can be understood by contrast with the good life that is limited by the impairment. It is humans, not Martians, who seek psychiatric help. Aristotle rightly treats flourishing, or the good life, as overwhelmingly species-specific. Caging birds is cruel because it is their nature to fly. Solitary confinement of human beings is cruel because we are social animals. As with other species, what is a good life for us is linked to our human nature.

The View from Outside

Some ways of mapping the good life, and of mapping the human nature it has to fit, are from outside. One version looks at some social experiments that failed due to unrealistic ideas of what to aim for.

In the early Israeli kibbutzim there were hopes that collective child-rearing would create egalitarians who would cooperate, not compete. The children mostly did not absorb the ideals: "If anything, their experience of group life has turned them away from the group and encouraged them to value individual attainment. They find equality and cooperation boring; they are much more excited by personal achievement."[7]

Family homes were replaced by communal children's dormitories. The hope was to broaden parents' concern beyond their own children toward impartial concern for all the kibbutz children: "Parental love can be exaggerated . . . Just as we distanced the children from intimate parental relations, we must lessen and control love from parents to children. We do not approve of uninhibited hugging, kissing and caressing."[8]

Children's dormitories did not last. It was utopian to overlook the depth of parents' special love for their own children: "I thought our parents were crazy to abolish the communal sleeping for their children. Now that I am a parent myself, I can't understand how they ever permitted it."[9] The human needs of children were also overlooked: "There was no love . . . I needed love desperately, but I wasn't allowed to have it. My feminine side was repressed . . . I grew up like an orphan. My parents never kissed me until I was thirty!"[10]

Other, much larger, experiments also tested the boundaries of human nature. Immediately after the Russian revolution, some Russians hoped that an economy driven by people wanting to make money would be replaced by an equal society where people worked for the common good. This would mean a deep transformation of human psychology. Nikolai Bukharin wrote of "the manufacturing of Communist man out of the human material of the capitalist age."[11] This utopian project foundered partly due to human resistance to being reshaped. Efforts to impose the transformation by dictatorship, terror, torture, slave camps, and millions of deaths were a grim tribute to the stubbornness of the "human material," of people and their nature.

The Inner Exploration of Human Values

> We do not inquire into the human good by standing on the rim of heaven; and if we did, we would not find the right thing. Human ways of life, and the hopes, pleasures, and pains that are a part of these, cannot be left out of the inquiry without making it pointless and incoherent . . .
>
> It is no simple matter to find out what the deepest parts of ourselves are, or even to draw all the parts to the surface for

> self-scrutiny. Thus one can reasonably speak of a kind of discovery here: discovery of oneself, and of one's fellow citizens.
>
> —Martha Nussbaum, *The Therapy of Desire*

The external exploration of human nature often takes the form of looking across different cultures and historical periods for human universals. Finding them would not settle all questions about the good life. One plausible near-universal feature of human nature is war between different groups.[12] But this seems only to show a flaw in human nature, with a deep part of our psychology being a great obstacle to our own flourishing. Values cannot just be read off from behavior. We have to decide what to endorse.

Drawing the contours of a good human life has to go beyond how most human beings have lived, to an *inner* exploration of human values. "What exactly is it that you endorse or oppose, and why do you do so?" People are often inarticulate about their values. And Martha Nussbaum is right that it is no simple matter to discover the deepest parts of ourselves. Values may be developed, even partly created, by being articulated in the course of the conversation. The thought "I don't know what I think until we have had the conversation, and sometimes not even then" is not a silly one. In this virtually all of us are like the Broadmoor interviewees. Exploration is likely to be halting and tentative.

Different people and different societies have disagreements about a good life. This platitude is interpreted in two rival ways. Some say that behind surface differences there is deep agreement. Socratic questioning about values can suggest a degree of deep-level consensus about the good life. On the other view, our differences about the good life go all the way down.

How might the Socratic questioning go? A simple utilitarian version of the good life is that it consists of pleasurable experiences and no pain. The first reaction of many is to agree with this. But thought experiments showing the limitations of such a life often make them change their mind. One is Aldous Huxley's *Brave New World.* In that world, batches of genetically identical people are conditioned psychologically to want exactly what society provides. So there is no pain or misery. Life is all pleasure.

Teaching philosophy, I often ask people about *Brave New World.* As Huxley intended, most people are appalled. Reasons tend to be similar.

That world is stifling. People care about autonomy and want a richer conception of a good life. It raises the question of whether society should be shaped to fit people, not the other way around. These values and questions complicate the one-dimensional "pleasure and no pain" view of human values.

Another thought experiment with a similar upshot is Robert Nozick's "experience machine." This machine gives pleasurable experiences and eliminates bad ones by direct stimulation of the brain. If you want to be an Olympic athlete, the machine can give you the experiences of competing and winning. If you want to be a great scientist, you can be given the "Einstein" cassette. And so on. But the reality behind the experiences is that you are on a table with your head attached to the machine's electrodes. Nozick asked whether we would choose this for a lifetime.[13] As with Huxley's thought experiment, most people would not.

Some surface objections are practical. Suppose the machine breaks down? Or the operators turn malicious? You may end up in a nightmare. In a thought experiment we can wave practical objections away by stipulating benevolence and infallible technology. This moves discussion to deeper values. Even with permanent pleasure guaranteed, few would go on the machine for life.

People again tend toward the same reasons for refusing. They want to live in the real world, not a simulated one. They want relationships with real people, not fantasy relationships with imagined ones. They want to be active and in charge of their own lives, not passive consumers of the benevolent software program. And they want to make their own real contribution to the world, not to be given the Einstein cassette. This cluster of reasons, roughly Nozick's, is given by people who have not read his book.

Of course, the people I talk to about *Brave New World* and the experience machine may not represent the human species. Perhaps very different answers would have come from Chinese villagers or from medieval nuns. The conjecture, to some extent empirically testable, is that some of the reasons reflect near-universal deep-level agreement about the good life.

Wide Consensus about the Good Life Is Not Conclusive

Looking from the outside at what seems to work or not, or exploring values from the inside, are attempts to get clear about what things really matter to people. They give a rough account of a good human life, contrasting with psychological conditions that subvert it.

But this exploration may not be conclusive. It can give strong evidence, but still it is evidence that can be overridden. Even the discovery of wide and deep agreement about features of a good or a bad life would have its limits. People with body integrity identity disorder feel that some part of their body is not "them." What they want (often passionately) may be to have a functioning leg amputated. This conflicts with the views of many surgeons and most of society about what is in their interests. Near-universal agreement that amputation of a functioning limb impairs the good life does not show decisively that someone with BIID has "distorted" values. It could just bring the reply "Two legs are fine for them, but this second leg is wrong for me."

18

What Is Autism?

Jim Sinclair, campaigning for a new understanding of autism, has written against the hope of a "cure" for austim:

> Parents often report that learning their child is autistic was the most traumatic thing thaever happened to them. Non-autistic people see autism as a great tragedy . . . I invite you to look at our autism, and look at your grief, from our perspective. Autism isn't something a person *has,* or a "shell" a person is trapped inside. There's no normal child hidden behind the autism. Autism is a way of being. It's *pervasive;* it colours every experience, every sensation, perception, thought, emotion, and encounter, every aspect of existence. It is not possible to separate the autism from the person—and if it were possible, the person you'd have left would not be the same person you started with . . . Therefore, when parents say
>
> *I wish my child didn't have autism,*
>
> What they're really saying is
>
> *I wish the autistic child I have did not exist, and I had a different (non-autistic) child instead.*
>
> Read that again. This is what we hear when you mourn over our existence. This is what we hear when you pray for a cure.[1]

A parent of an autistic child has replied in a blog:

> Dear Jim,
>
> If I knew my son was going to turn out like you, intelligent, articulate, self-confident and alive, I wouldn't worry and grieve. I don't know that though. I can only speculate . . . And that future projection is based on what I see before me now . . . Simply on what it is I see autistic children struggling with, and I find it difficult to see how my child at this point in time

> might overcome such enormous obstacles . . . The observable reality of sensory overload, confusion, frustration and despair. It's hard for parents to overcome mourning when each year brings with it new obstacles for our children to navigate . . . In the same way non autistic people should not assume to understand what existence is like for autistics, those who are not parents of autistic children should not assume to understand what underpins our emotional responses. Parents will do well to listen to autistic adults such as yourself to hopefully better understand how the world might appear to their child . . . But likewise, autistic self-advocates may do well to listen to parents real concerns and challenges without presuming knowledge of what induces our turmoil.[2]

Some of the deepest problems in deciding whether a condition impairs a person's chances of a good human life come to the surface with autism. A humanly adequate way of thinking about it has to try to do justice to the thoughts expressed in both these impressive letters.

Disordered or Different?

> During my frustrating, miserable, helpless days, I've started imagining what it would be like if everyone was autistic. If autism was regarded simply as a personality type, things would be so much easier and happier for us than they are now.
>
> —Naoki Higashida, *The Reason I Jump*

People on the autistic landscape often have very successful careers, sometimes based on exceptional intellectual abilities. It is often said (at the same time both half jokingly and half seriously) that unusually many autistic people can be found among distinguished mathematicians, physicists, and philosophers. Others with autism can have outstanding computer skills. Some can read and remember pages of a book after rapidly glancing at them.

Autistic people who have no "compensating" ability are less likely to be able to speak for themselves. They may have different needs from those with "high functioning" autism who can articulate theirs. The very varied impact of autism on the lives of different people may partly explain the passionate disagreements it arouses.

Some who are "high functioning" argue strongly that autism is not a disorder but is part of a harmless and desirable neurodiversity. This can provoke outraged rejection among those close to a child who cannot talk and who is often anxious, screaming, and head-banging. To them it is just obvious that a cure would save both the autistic person and the family from great distress. The advocates of neurodiversity find it equally obvious that *they* have been caused much distress by the response to the way they are. As with the history of responses to gay sexual orientation, their distinctive features are not accepted and valued, but have been rejected amid talk of "cure" and "normality."

The issue is whether autism harms people by reducing their ability to have a good life. If it does, there is a case for psychiatric help, directed either at cure or at the containment and alleviation of the condition. In the dispute between the "disorder" and the "neurodiversity" views, the plurality of the autistic landscape may defeat any single answer. Perhaps the parents are right that the problems of their distressed autistic child does greatly impair the child's chance of a good life. *And* those who advocate the "harmless neurodiversity" view may themselves be instances of it.

The ideal might be to separate out autistic people who are "flourishing" from others and to offer treatment only to those in the second category. In what follows, the discussion will treat severe and high-functioning autism as separate cases. This is an obvious simplification, aimed at bringing out some issues more clearly before returning to the messier real world. Autism shows the difficulty of drawing a sharp frontier between flourishing and not doing so. Flourishing has many dimensions, and each is a matter of degree. Being "high functioning" is the same. Different dimensions, each with a blurred boundary, may still allow clear cases on each side to be separated from each other. But even some clear cases blur over time. People take off in unexpected ways.

Severe Autism

The autistic landscape is varied. There is no single "gene for autism." Many genes contribute to the autistic triad of social, communicative, and "imaginative" limitations. And, mainly, different genes contribute to different parts of the triad. Even so, there may one day be genetic predictors of the chances of developing autism. If so, familiar ethical dilemmas would follow. In choosing which embryo to implant, would it be ethical to select against autism? Would it be ethical to select *for* autism?

The idea of a good human life has been much debated in reproductive ethics. One lesbian couple wanted to have a child who would be deaf like them. Their choice of sperm donor fell on someone with hereditary deafness. Critics and supporters of this decision debate whether deafness is a disability and whether it makes for a less good life. In the reproductive debate, no final consensus has been reached. But one key question is, Will the person this embryo will develop into have a decent chance of a good life? ("Decent chance" and "good life" are intentionally vague. Rough-and-ready judgments are the best we can do here.)

The question in reproductive ethics has parallels in psychiatry. Obviously the psychiatric issue is not about bringing someone into the world. It is about whether a severely autistic person now in front of us has a disorder or is just different. A psychiatric disorder has to be harmful, so the question is whether the condition harms the person and, if so, how much. This comes down to, Will this person's autism significantly limit the extent to which he or she will be able to have a good life? Only if the answer looks more like yes than no is the offer of treatment for disorder appropriate.

There is a risk of answering the question wrongly. The view from outside can miss things. At a conference an articulate and obviously flourishing autistic woman described her inability to communicate as a young child. She said that her lack of communication had not worried her at the time. She had perhaps been happier then than she was later. Communication made her see she was disappointing people.

Then there is the danger of writing off people's expectations because we have not learned to read their language. A child with persistent head-banging may seem to have a nightmare life. But as noted in Chapter 11, Donna Williams has suggested that head-banging, seen from the inside, can have an intelligible purpose. This still may not stop the head-banging from making the person's life less good. But it is a warning about too readily making negative judgments about the autistic child's potential.

Other misjudgments can come from imaginative failures. If a condition such as severe autism greatly restricts the range of interests and enjoyments open to someone, the view from outside may underestimate the intensity of the delight the person gets from a hug, a meeting of the eyes, or a smile. The advantage of starting from what they say is that it links assessments of interventions more closely to the values of those they are supposed to help.

Starting from what they say will sometimes reveal an inner landscape that is less simple than the flattening view from outside. Naoki Higashida, asking what he would do if there was some way he could be normal, starts with the harm autism does him: "Living with special needs is so depressing and so relentless." This meant that "for ages and ages I badly wanted to be normal." Now he is not so sure: "But now, even if somebody developed a medicine to cure autism, I might well choose to stay as I am . . . For us, you see, having autism is normal—so we can't know for sure what your 'normal' is even like. But so long as we can learn to love ourselves, I'm not sure how much it matters whether we're normal or autistic."[3]

In so many ways the answer to the question "disorder or difference?" may be simplified or distorted. But this is not to write off the idea that severe autism calls for the offer of help. Sometimes a person's seriously impaired life can make talk of neurodiversity insensitive. Clear signs of severe and lasting distress can make criticisms of the mode of assessment seem pedantic. Where the harm is clear, if there is treatment that is likely to help, it should be offered. But even where there is clear harm, this may not be the whole story. There can be harms—contrasted with some Aristotelian view of the good life—that someone like Naoki Higashida might still choose to accept. Sometimes the Aristotelian and the autonomy views of harm pull apart.

High-Functioning Autism and the Core of the Person

> Out of the crooked timber of humanity no straight thing was ever made.
>
> —Immanuel Kant, in Isaiah Berlin's felicitous translation

High-functioning autistic people often echo Jim Sinclair's objection to hopes for treating and "curing" their condition: that there is no normal person behind the autism. The autistic person is who they are and so to wish away the autism is to wish them away.

Other high-functioning autistic people think autism is a disorder and bridle at being told it is part of their identity. Sandy Starr says that the benevolently intended use of the word "condition" rather than "disorder" may blur the distinction between medical and moral judgments. If autism stops the person from living independently, then there is something medically wrong but not morally wrong. It is not stigmatizing, or lacking in compassion, to say they have a disorder. He also resists the idea that autism is "an identity." He does not see his own having Asperger's syndrome as giving him credentials for discussing these issues. He does not think "the merits of your identity take logical priority over the merits of your ideas."[4]

It is right that saying someone has a disorder should not discredit the person (though, regrettably, there are those who see some disorders as a stigma). And it is important that we can to some extent choose which characteristics we endorse as part of our "identity."

Even if there is no "normal" person hidden behind the autism, an autistic mathematician may still choose mathematics but not autism as part of her identity. This is clearly true of some other psychological conditions or problems. Richard Wollheim saw his disgust at the smell of newsprint as too deeply rooted in him to eliminate. It was like a ghost in the house that could be expelled only by demolishing the house. He was "a newsprint-phobic philosopher." But he might have responded with justified irritation if someone introducing him at one of his lectures had so described him. Sandy Starr is equally entitled to have his ideas argued about on their merits and not as "the view from Asperger's syndrome."

But the core of Jim Sinclair's point is untouched. Some autistic people have good lives as they are, unless pressured to be "normal." If there is no "normal" person behind the autism, talk of "cure" can be a cruel pressure. This is so even if autism limits their relationships or other aspects of the good life. The human flourishing approach to psychiatry aims to remove obstacles to the good life. Sometimes, with consent, it may be legitimate to offer help in changing some core aspect of a person.

But cases where autism is inextricably bound up with the person's identity bring out a limit that should be placed on this human flourishing approach. Offers of help toward "normality" can be coercive. (As were offers of help for being gay half a century ago.) What a crude version of the good life tramples on is brought out by Clare Sainsbury: "'Normal' people may take it as a basic right to be accepted as they are; the rest of us are viewed only in terms of what will make us more acceptable to them. Far from seeming radical or positive, the philosophy of normalization seems painfully familiar to those of us whose very disability lies in our 'differentness.' Most of us have already spent years being taught that who we are is fundamentally wrong and in need of 'cure' and having others (whether parents or teachers or other professionals) try to force us again and again to do what we *cannot* do—that is be 'normal.'"[5]

19

Crossing the Medical Boundary?

On the human flourishing approach, it can be argued that psychiatrists need not confine themselves to offering treatment for the traditionally evolved psychiatric categories of illness or disorder. Psychological conditions that are not intrinsically harmful should not count as psychiatric disorders. But there are intrinsically harmful psychological conditions that do not fit the traditional disorders. The methods of psychiatry, whether psychotherapeutic or pharmacological, may also help someone escape a life-diminishing personality.

Altering Personality

Some thoughtful psychiatrists notice a shift in their own aims when prescribing antidepressants. Peter Kramer raised this issue in the context of his treatment of his patient "Tess." Her alcoholic father died when she was 12. Her mother went into permanent depression. Tess took over caring for her mother and the nine younger children until they grew up. At 17, partly to give her brothers and sisters a base, she married an older man, an abusive alcoholic. The marriage collapsed. Tess became a successful businesswoman and still also looked after her mother. She had a strong sense of guilt and responded, perhaps too much, to the claims of others. She thought she put off men, and she had unhappy involvements with abusive married men. She had all the symptoms of clinical depression.

Dr. Kramer prescribed medication that brought Tess out of clinical depression.[1] But she was still easily upset and cried when asked about her boyfriend. Wanting a more robust return to her personality before depression, Dr. Kramer suggested Prozac: "My goal was not to transform Tess but to restore her."

On Prozac Tess did seem transformed: relaxed, energetic, and with more self-esteem. She laughed more and had a new ease with people. She stopped crying over her old boyfriend and often dated other men. She felt less guilt about her mother and stopped living so close to her. She was less self-sacrificing. She felt relief at this "loss of seriousness." Her illness cured, she went off Prozac and continued to do well.

Yet, no longer depressed, Tess asked to go back on Prozac. She felt it had given her stability, ease, and confidence. Without it, she said, "I'm not myself." Dr. Kramer prescribed Prozac, and Tess recovered her ease and assurance, but he worried because that he was no longer treating an illness, but changing her underlying temperament and personality.

Psychiatrists are right to be concerned about crossing the normal medical boundary. On the Aristotelian approach, crossing the boundary could be justified in such a case. The aim was to overcome psychological obstacles to a good life. Peter Kramer's worries suggest a degree of commitment to the medical categories, but his policy here suggests the pull of the human flourishing model. If some or all of the "personality disorders" are not considered to be medical conditions, this approach could justify offering treatment aimed at eliminating the disorders or alleviating their harmful effects.

The conditions for crossing the medical boundary should be stringent. The aim must be to benefit the person concerned, not to promote the interests of the government, or the supposed interests of society, as in the Soviet, Chinese, and other political abuses of psychiatry. Also, of course, those treated must give their reflective and voluntary consent. They must be told about any risks and the element of nonmedical "enhancement" of their psychology. Under these conditions, psychiatry directed at enriching a person's life, not at curing illness, may sometimes be justified.

Psychological Obstacles? The Social Dimension

Tess, as Kramer describes her, had problems that seem to have arisen out of her childhood and family circumstances. But as thoughtful psychiatrists often notice, many of the psychological problems they are asked to treat have wider social origins.

The impact of poverty and unemployment on mental health and on suicide are well documented.[2] Soldiers in huge numbers return from combat with post-traumatic stress. Of the 1.3 million soldiers who have returned from the wars in Iraq and Afghanistan, 28.2 percent have sought mental health treatment.[3] In those wars, suicide has cost more American lives than death in combat.[4] An intelligent version of preventative psychiatry would focus on getting politicians and the public to see clearly the heavy psychological costs both of economic policies careless of the human dimension and of wars too easily embarked on.

Those choosing these uncaring or unintelligent policies prefer to see the associated psychiatric epidemics as mainly caused by individual psychology. This may also suit pharmaceutical companies, some of whose priorities are seen in their spending. About 35 percent of their revenues go to marketing and administration, "the largest single item in big pharma's budget, larger than manufacturing costs and much larger than R & D."[5] Peaceful foreign policies, or economic policies aimed at eliminating the stress of poverty and insecurity, could reduce the demand for their products.

Medical priorities are different. Education about smoking, carried out against the interests of the tobacco industry and the opposition of some uncaring politicians, has saved many lives. There is an obvious preventive medical case for equally vigorous public education about the social and political causes of psychiatric disorders.

Until public education succeeds, there remains a need for psychiatric help. The prime causes of suicidal thoughts in people who have lost a job or in soldiers back from war are to be found more in society than in individual psychology. But this is no help to the person who needs help for very real depression or post-traumatic stress. The dominant causes might not be medical, but the condition becomes psychiatric through being a psychological state that significantly impairs the person's chances of a good life. If there are helpful psychiatric interventions, of course they should be offered.

A Problem Case: Medication to Dampen "Sinful" Sexual Desire

It seems right for Dr. Kramer to have offered Tess help. What should be the limits of this boundary-crossing "human flourishing" version of psychiatry?

In the very conservative, ultra-orthodox Haredi community in Israel, antidepressants are said to have been given to yeshiva students, seminary girls, and married adults because these medications suppress sexual desire. An account, based on statements made by psychiatrists, patients, and family members, was given in the Israeli newspaper *Haaretz*.[6] Requests for these prescriptions are said to come from rabbis, yeshiva supervisors, and marriage counselors. There are claims that some rabbis pressured psychiatrists to prescribe particular drugs.

In 2011 the Israeli Psychiatric Association held a conference titled "The Haredi Community as a Consumer of Mental Health Services." Professor Omer Bonne, director of Hadassah University Hospital, Jerusalem, was reported as saying that antidepressants were sometimes prescribed to yeshiva students to dampen sexual desire. The aim was to reduce anxiety and depression. These were caused by the tension between their homosexuality, masturbation, or "compulsiveness in sex" and the religious teaching that these things were sinful.

Professor Bonne said that, when younger, he had been against prescribing the drugs: these sexual activities were not medical problems. But awareness that in that context they create terrible mental conflict changed his mind.

Professor Bonne's earlier view, opposing the use of psychiatric medication for nonmedical problems, gains support from the history of "treating" gays. But cases like Peter Kramer's "Tess" may support his later view, in licensing some uses of psychiatry against other obstacles to the good life, obstacles that do not fit the medical categories.

Further support for this use of antidepressants may come from the earlier discussion of whether the normal grief of a bereaved person calls for medical intervention. In grief the depression can be severe, but priority should be given to context and meaning. When the grief is meaningful to the person who is grieving, that person might not want to eliminate it. There is some parallel with the religious case. Sexual desires may have a different meaning to people when they conflict with deep religious convictions. In that context, wanting to dampen the desires could make sense. Should not context and meaning prevail here too?

Further support may seem to come from the discussion of severe and perhaps suicidal depression in people who have lost a job or who have postcombat trauma. The causes may not be medical, but the condition still calls for the offer of treatment as a severe psychological obstacle to the good life. Does not this also apply to the anxiety and depression of the yeshiva students?

This is a strong case. It would be decisive if it were the whole story. But it is not. Some religious communities may indeed see rejection of "sinful" homosexuality or masturbation as essential to the good life. Those who accept this may, in their own terms, be justified in requesting the medication. But what about the rest of us, who do not see these things as sinful and may distrust the indoctrination behind a student's acceptance of the medication? How should we, and especially psychiatrists who do not share these religious values, respond?

There are good reasons for opposing these interventions. Apart from any bad side effects of the medication, there are real doubts about the autonomy of the request, so influenced by external pressure from people who disapprove of the sexual desires. Even without immediate outside pressure, a request shaped by community-imposed indoctrination still might not be autonomous.

These are good reasons for rejecting the request. But psychiatrists who see this may still be pulled the other way by wanting to relieve the terrible mental conflict. Accepting that the desires are not sinful and that the request is not autonomous, they may see medication as the only way to rescue the person from cruel mental distress.

This is a decent motive. But that way lies the contentment of *Brave New World*. And the dark side of the history of psychiatry warns against it. If changing society is impossible, changing the person may seem to be the way out. This may be through trying to "cure" gay people to spare them the distress caused by society's prejudices. It may be through trying to help dissidents or colonial rebels escape conflict by curing their "latent schizophrenia" or the "inadequacies" of "the African mind." It may take the form of reducing normal sexual desires to help someone escape guilt about "sin." So, from good motives psychiatrists can become collaborators in oppression. The boundaries should be drawn to exclude this.

20

Strands in a Good Human Life

It is attractive to draw the boundaries of psychiatry in terms of trying to remove psychological obstacles to the good human life. One danger is seeing the good life too narrowly. The idea might have stifling consequences—some modern equivalent of imposing "treatment" on gays. Can we answer the question "What is a good life?" without forgetting that it takes all sorts to make a world?

There is an influential idea in the debate about choosing children with some sets of genes rather than others. If children are to have a decent chance of a good life, they should have "an open future." No one has a totally open future: we are all partly constrained by genetic, environmental, and other factors. But parents should not aim simply to reproduce their own version of a good life. They should leave children plenty of scope to shape lives of their own. A good life includes choices about how to live. We should not follow the *Brave New World* model of creating "happy" children living in a built-in prison. The idea of an open future applies to psychiatry too.

Aristotle needs to be combined with "experiments in living," John Stuart Mill's reminder of how open-ended the vision of the good life should be. What follows in this chapter is tentative: not a blueprint for "the" good human life, but suggestions about *some* strands in *a* good life. The account is shaped by obstacles found in psychiatric conditions. The strands selected here come in two groups. There are features of "me" that underpin a life a person is comfortable with. And there are things that help make a life add up to something, or have some meaning.

The Foundations: "Me"

A good life is supported by certain features of a person's psychology. One is being at peace with yourself. This is best understood by contrasts. It is what some of the artists in the Prinzhorn collection did not have. It is what John Clare missed: "I long for . . . / . . . sleep as I in childhood sweetly

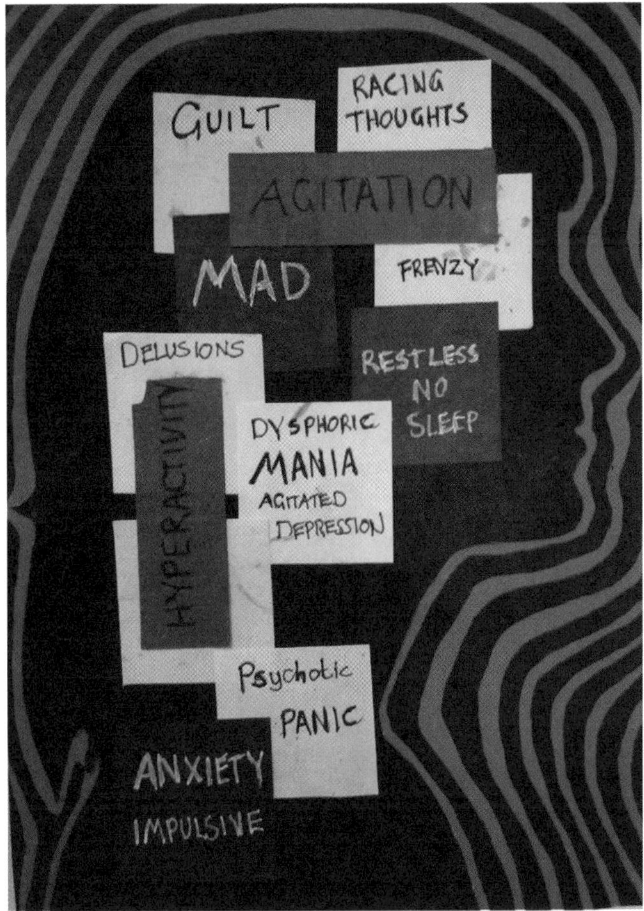

Figure 20.1: Laura Freeman, *Thoughts That Go Through My Head during a Mixed Affective Episode.* Courtesy of Laura Freeman.

slept, / Untroubling and untroubled where I lie / The grass below, above, the vaulted sky." Its lack is powerfully portrayed by Laura Freeman (Figure 20.1).

Another strand is having a good deal of control over your own life. No one is fully autonomous. We have been shaped by so many influences outside our control: genes, family, friends, the time and place we live in, the pervasive influence of a culture, our education, the media, and so on. But most of us are not fatalists and know we still make choices and that these choices make a great difference to our lives.

This sense of being in charge of our lives, at least to some extent, can be diminished—sometimes almost to a vanishing point. Lack of control can come from poverty, political oppression, hierarchical conditions of work, cultural pressures to conform, oppressive families, and the disabling limits of some physical or mental disorders. Our control over our lives is only relative, but it matters enormously. This is central to the widespread and deep rejection of both *Brave New World* and the experience machine. There is also evidence that, where people's work allows them little autonomy, the prospects for their physical health are poorer than for those whose position in the same profession gives them greater autonomy.[1]

A Life That Adds Up to Something

A sense of inner peace and a degree of control are important foundations. But ideas of a good life often go beyond the foundations to what we can build on them. People's hopes sometimes include the hope to have a life that adds up to something, that has some meaning. What does this come to?

The question "What is the meaning of life?" is sometimes asked seriously and sometimes ridiculed as pretentiously empty. What could possibly be the answer to such a question? It suggests that life is a puzzle to be decoded: the meaning of life to be interpreted like the meaning of a hieroglyphic. Like some hieroglyphics, life might elude our powers of interpretation. Or we might succeed in getting the answer. We might discover some plan of God's in which we have a part. Or scientific discoveries might suggest that humans have a crucial role in the scheme of things. There seems no reason to think life contains some secret message for us to decode. Yet many people do want their lives have some meaning. This hope is better interpreted as wanting to make something of their lives.

Some of the most powerful reflections on people's desire to give meaning to their lives came from a psychiatrist's observation of himself and other prisoners in Auschwitz. Viktor Frankl described the psychological impact of the imposed suffering and degradation. The impossibility of knowing whether it would end in death or release, or of knowing when it would end, made their existence "provisional." To some of the prisoners this made everything seem unreal, and so everything could seem pointless to them.[2]

Some prisoners suffered massive psychological collapse, others kept themselves intact. Frankl stresses that even there it *was* possible to retain human dignity. How a person accepts suffering and a terrible fate can still give a deeper meaning to his life: "Only the men who allowed their inner hold on their moral and spiritual selves to subside eventually fell victim to the camp's degenerating influences."[3] The values that had to be held on to varied from person to person. What persuaded a prisoner not to kill himself might be his irreplaceability for his waiting daughter, or the book to be finished. Frankl quotes Nietzsche: "He who has a *why* to live can bear almost any *how*."

One natural interpretation of making something of your life is giving it a pattern reflecting what you care about. For many people, this is part of the why that helps them bear almost any how. The natural expression of a pattern is a narrative that makes some sense of a life.

For many of us some kind of narrative is one of the threads holding our life together. But not everyone wants to give his life a pattern. Galen Strawson has drawn a distinction between two kinds of people: Narratives and Episodics. Narratives want to make something of their lives. Episodics do not; they include Galen Strawson himself: "I'm completely uninterested in the answer to the question 'What has GS made of his life?' or 'What have I made of my life?' I'm living it, and this sort of thinking is no part of it. This does not mean that I am in any way irresponsible. It is just that what I care about, in so far as I care about myself and my life, is how I am now."[4]

The point is a useful corrective to exaggerations about narrative. But perhaps Narrative/Episodic is less a sharp contrast than a continuum. Some neurological conditions reduce awareness to little more than the immediate present. Short of such impairments, can anyone be completely episodic? People at that end of the continuum may still feel a twinge of embarrassment at the memory of something they blurted out last month. In "What I care about is how I am now," a lot depends on the scope of "now." Perhaps it includes last month. But I wonder if Galen Strawson would be indifferent if the stimulating books he has written over the years were pulped, and all traces of them destroyed?

Clearly there are people at the episodic end of the continuum. Galen Strawson's list includes Virginia Woolf. It is true that what mattered most to her seem to have been what she called "moments of being." They were not part of any pattern but were moments of rich or intense experience. As a child, fighting her brother, she suddenly felt, "Why hurt another person?" She stopped and then felt hopeless sadness about her powerlessness as he continued to beat her. Another time, having overheard that someone she remembered had killed himself, she walked in the moonlight by the apple tree in the garden and felt with horror that the apple tree was somehow linked to the suicide. Many moments of being were less dark and less intense: responding to the willow trees "all plumy and soft green and purple" against the sky, reading an absorbing book, or starting to write one of her own. But these moments were always "embedded in a kind of nondescript cotton wool" of much of a day—contrasted with having a slight temperature or dealing with the broken vacuum cleaner.[5]

If Virginia Woolf was at the episodic end of the continuum, it would still be absurd to say her life did not add up to anything. Quite apart from the books she wrote, so many "moments of being" speak for themselves. A life that adds up to something does not have to be a life you *make* add up to something. Self-creative narrative is only one important thing among many that give meaning to a life.

This episodic version of meaning is important for people with severe autism and other conditions that make narrative difficult or impossible. On the other hand, finding different ways of telling a narrative may be crucial to helping people with post-traumatic stress disorder bring themselves together.

Upshot

I have argued in this part of the book that the core aim of psychiatry is to help people overcome psychological conditions that are harmful. On the human flourishing version, this harm consists in obstacles to their living a good human life. Most of the traditional psychiatric categories of disorder are such obstacles. But the medical conception of dysfunctional systems is too narrow to include all psychological obstacles calling for the offer of psychiatric help. In some cases there are problems in identifying psychological systems or their functions. Where dysfunctions can be identified, what calls for help is the harm rather than the dysfunction.

This in turn leads into questions about the kinds of harm that may justify offering psychiatric help, and the different accounts of the good life with which they are contrasted. Human flourishing and liberal accounts will sometimes diverge. And both may sometimes license nonmedical "treatment": help against harmful psychological conditions that do not fit traditional categories of disorder. This in turn raises acute ethical issues about the need for boundaries to block stifling versions of psychiatry based on narrow conceptions of the good life.

The rest of the book is based on strands of the good life that have been gestured at in this chapter. Relationships and work, from which people often derive a sense of meaning, are linked to having a degree of control over your life. Another source of meaning, at least for non-Episodics, can be the shaping of one's own identity. Control and the shaping of identity are both lost to external agents in *Brave New World* and the experience machine. The topics of the remainder of this book, Parts 5 and 6, are psychiatric issues affecting these two strands in the good life.

Some psychological conditions seriously limit people's control over their lives and their ability to shape their identity. This is a case for seeing such conditions as harms calling for the offer of psychiatric help. (It is only a prima facie case. There are the identity and neurodiversity issues raised by autism. And the obstacles to the good life may come less from the condition itself than—as with being gay or with having "sinful" sexual desires—from pressures coming from the reaction of others.)

Psychiatry is shot through with interpretation. Its goals are shaped and limited by values. The rest of this book will link these two central thrusts of the argument so far. Most current accounts of psychiatric geography are based on causal mechanisms, either conjectured or established. The aim here is not to replace this geography but to supplement it with a different map that takes seriously the person's own view from inside. This may bring out how different psychiatric problems subvert the values of control and identity. My hope is to open up new ways to interpret some conditions. Taking seriously the question of subversion of control in addiction or in some personality disorders means locating these conditions in a larger picture of agency and its distortions. And perhaps some versions of eating disorders and of post-traumatic stress disorder can be illuminated when they are seen as being, at their core, disorders of identity.

PART FIVE

Agency, Control, and Responsibility

I mean, I chose the route I've took, solely myself . . . I've chose it, so really my destiny as such was laid out by me. It wasn't laid out before and said, "Right, your destiny is to end up in Broadmoor in 30 years' time." I mean I actually walked the road that led me here. You know, no-one pushed me along.

I can't get it off my mind, for starters. Initially, obviously, it won't go away and I can't sleep. It makes me restless. It just plays on my mind . . . It worries me that eventually I will do these things and I don't want to particularly want to—difficult for me actually to say "no" to them . . . They involve kidnapping, rape and violence, and murder, so . . . *If you could choose not to have these thoughts?* I am trying to. That's a choice that I've already made, that I'm trying . . . At the moment I'm trying chemical castration, to work on the fantasies, which will do away with the sex and the murder/violence fantasies that I have, but I ain't having a great deal of success with it.

—Two voices from the "Socratic" Broadmoor interviews

21

Brain, Mind, and Agency

> I do not find the neurobiological theory of mental illness as helpful to my recovery because it deprives me of any sense of self-determination and responsibility. When I think I am a group of chemical reactions, each with its own scheme and plan, I feel dehumanized and powerless. I feel that I am thinking, feeling and acting at the whim of those chemicals, not through any effort or responsibility of my own.
>
> —Dan Fisher, "Humanity and Voice in Recovery from Mental Illness," in *From the Ashes of Experience: Reflections on Madness, Survival and Growth*, ed. Phil Barker et al.

> Doesn't his mind need help as well as his brain?
>
> —From a woman's letter about her brother's psychiatric treatment

Some psychiatrists, encouraged by scientific advances, may hope to avoid the philosophical issues discussed in this book. Pieter Geyl famously called history "an argument without end." Isn't philosophy even more so? For further progress do we need anything beyond the increasingly detailed causal accounts coming from epidemiology, genetics, pharmacology, and neuroimaging?

The pull of this antiphilosophical view is easy to feel. But it depends on not asking questions that matter. It is the vision held by people living in a city with buildings so solid that they forget they are in an earthquake region. Psychiatry's conceptual framework rests on the meeting point of two of the hardest and deepest problems in philosophy: the mind-brain problem and the problem of free will. The city is built at the intersection of two fault lines.

The challenge the mind-brain problem still poses to science and philosophy makes it a major fault line underneath our conceptual scheme. We are far from resolving the disputed issues about how conscious thoughts, feelings, and decisions relate to states of the brain, and about why consciousness evolved at all. Luckily psychiatrists can to some extent keep these problems about mind and brain at arm's length.

For psychiatry, by far the more serious fault line is the cluster of problems about agency and free will. These start to be noticeable when society has to respond to things done by people with psychiatric problems. When what someone does is partly the product of their mental disorder, psychiatrists, lawyers, and many others find it hard to draw the boundaries of responsibility. How far, when, and in what ways does having a psychiatric disorder absolve people from responsibility for what they do?

Here some comments will be made about the mind-brain problem before turning to issues of agency as they arise in psychiatry.

Mind and Brain

Thomas Nagel famously asked the question "What is it like to be a bat?" We do not have sonar, the "radar" that tells bats about nearby objects. If sonar fails and the bat can't locate food on the wing, we have some idea what this feels like. We do know perceptual failure. But we have never experienced the detection of objects by sonar. One day we may fully understand the brain mechanisms involved. But even then we will not know the subjective "feel" of it.[1] Even when all the neuroscience is understood, this subjectivity seems an unknown residue.

This applies to us as well as bats. When the mechanisms of human color vision are fully mapped out, a neuroscientist born blind could know all about them. If later the neuroscientist is given sight, the experience of color might still be a surprise: "This is amazing. I had no idea it was like this." If a complete neuroscientific account leaves this out, it seems not to be a complete account. If so, there is a huge question. What is this "extra" subjectivity, and how does it relate to the neuroscience?

How did consciousness evolve in a material universe? At one level the answer is not hard. Visual, auditory, and other experiences are useful, telling us things we need to know about the world. The experience of pain is a warning not to repeat harmful encounters. And so on. But this explanation may not go deep enough.

A person and a computer might carry out the same simple but long calculation: perhaps multiplying one immensely long number by another. A human might find the experience tedious, exhausting, or frustrating.

We might ensure that the person has a break during the task, or is not asked to do it often. We have no concern about the computer. This is not because computers calculate so quickly. It is because we think there is no answer to the question "What is it like to be a computer?" We do not think they have experiences.

This is why the easy explanation of the evolution of consciousness might not go deep enough. It is useful to be able to process visual and auditory information about the world and its opportunities and dangers. But computers can do all this without, we believe, having experiences. Perhaps we are wrong about computers. If not, the usefulness of all this information only explains why computer-like processing might have evolved. It fails to explain why in our version (or in some other species) subjective experiences are bundled up with these processes.

The problem is dramatized by the idea of "zombies"—beings that look and behave like us, and whose brains process information in ways neuroscientifically indistinguishable from ours, yet with the single but large difference that they have no subjective experiences.[2] Why has evolution thrown up humans rather than zombies?

Intuitively it seems conceivable that zombies could exist. If this is right, the materialist account of consciousness in terms of the brain and its functions seems incomplete. In this department, zombies have as much as we do. Something else has to explain why we have experiences they lack.

One materialist response is to challenge the intuitively plausible thought that zombies could exist. If zombies could do all that we can do, our states of consciousness would be unnecessary: mere by-products that do no work, feeding back no input to the brain. Each experience would be purely a product of its corresponding brain state. So experiences could not causally influence even each other. But we notice, compare, and think about our experiences. Noticing and comparing are also experiences. It has been suggested that a theory that makes experiences unable to interact with each other could not account for what we do here.[3] The claim is that, despite appearances, we can rule out the version of our consciousness needed to make zombies possible.

This is only one of the arguments against zombies. This one, like the others, has been challenged. The debate continues. No consensus has been reached on whether or not conscious states transcend the neuroscientific story. The problem for materialists is explaining why we and not zombies evolved, and how subjective experiences fit into a purely neuroscientific account. The problem for those who think conscious states involve something more than this is to explain what these nonphysical properties are, and how they can influence chemical and other events in the brain. Scientifically, isn't such interaction wildly implausible?

In our present state of knowledge, psychiatry needs the language of mind-brain interaction. But this need not involve any theoretical commitment to the implausibilities of dualism.

Everyday and Other Varieties of "Mind-Brain Interaction"

Although interactionist dualism may be a dubious theory, our lives are saturated with the body influencing the mind. A blow or an injury causes pain. Being tired or hungover can make us irritable. Drugs can relieve pain or cause euphoria. And so on. Equally platitudinous is everyday interaction the other way. Our mental state is one of noticing it is time to go somewhere, and our brain sends signals to the muscles needed for us to get up.

Other instances are more striking. Dr. Oliver Sacks described the physical response to stress of a patient in for a checkup: "On one of these return-visits I was dismayed to see a rather violent chorea, grimacing, and tics, which he had never shown previously. When I inquired if there was anything making him uneasy, he replied that he had taken a taxi to hospital, and that the taxi-meter was continually ticking away: 'It keeps ticking away,' he said, 'and it keeps *me* ticcing too!' On hearing this, I immediately dismissed the taxi, and promised Mr. E. we would get another one and pay all expenses. Within thirty seconds of my arranging all this, Mr. E.'s chorea, grimacing and ticcing had vanished."[4]

What in Freud's time was called "hysteria" involved apparent physical disorders such as paralysis, with no obvious organic cause. The Freudian view was that hysterical patients suffer largely from reminiscence: the memory of traumatic events was repressed and then burst out in the form of physical symptoms.[5] The diagnosis of hysteria is obsolete, but physical symptoms apparently caused by psychological problems are now classified as "conversion disorders." If genuine, these cases dramatically show the impact of the mental on the physical. But it is obviously difficult to be sure there is no organic cause. Malingering and other accounts have to be considered.[6] "Conversion" as a mental impact on the body is dramatic but debatable.

Less debatable are the adaptive capacities of "neuroplasticity." The brain responds to new demands made on it and to how we use it.[7] When brain injury damages a region used for a particular skill or process, the same region in the opposite hemisphere sometimes takes over. Or brain regions processing input from one sense might be reassigned to another. The visual cortex of people who have been blind for a long time may take over processing Braille and other input from touch.

The brain's plasticity includes the way a specialized region can enlarge with use. One case involves the hippocampus. We draw on "maps" laid down in the posterior hippocampus to find our way about. (The anterior hippocampus is involved in mapping somewhere new.) London taxi drivers need a huge mental map of the streets of London. To get their license, they have to pass "the Knowledge"—a test of their use of the mental map to choose the best routes. Later their daily work uses and maintains the map.

Scans detect the density of brain matter. Compared to controls, taxi drivers have greater density in the posterior hippocampus, the area used to access maps already laid down.[8] Could it be that people who already have this enlargement are those who choose to drive taxis? There is evidence against this. The density increases with years spent driving taxis. It does seem to grow with use.

On the other hand, the taxi drivers' anterior hippocampus, used for new mapping, had less dense gray matter than those of the controls. The two findings seem to reflect that the drivers make much greater use of a map already laid down and that they do not lay down new maps. It seems that growth that would have gone elsewhere can be hijacked by a more active region. How we use our brains can change their physical properties.

Mind-Brain Interaction and Dualism

These cases all show what is conventionally seen as the influence of mind on brain. This sounds like dualism: interaction between nonphysical (mental) states or events and physical ones. Perhaps the last systematic attempt at a general dualist account of mind and brain was by a neurophysiologist (J. C. Eccles) and a philosopher (Karl Popper) in 1977.[9] As Popper put it, the brain is owned by the self, rather than the other way round: "The active, psycho-physical self is the active programmer to the brain (which is the computer), it is the executant whose instrument is the brain. The mind is, as Plato said, the pilot."[10]

Eccles suggested how this might work. He saw the self-conscious mind as "an independent entity that is actively engaged in reading out from the multitude of active centres in the modules of the liaison areas of the dominant cerebral hemisphere." It "selects from these centres in accord with its attention and its interests and integrates its selection to give the unity of conscious experience from moment to moment. It also acts back on the neural centres. Thus it is proposed that the self-conscious mind exercises a superior interpretative and controlling role upon the neural events by virtue of a two-way interaction across the interface."[11] This interaction is described in terms of cortical modules "open to the self-conscious mind both for receiving from and for giving to . . . Each module may be likened to a radio transmitter-receiver unit."[12]

The puzzle in this theory is about the transmitting and receiving. Detail is given about areas of the cortex involved, neuronal modules, and so on. But what kind of "signal" is transmitted? Is it physical? Is it electrical or chemical, or of some other kind? Where does it go to? Because the mind is supposed not to be part of the brain, there is no physical place for the signal to go. Perhaps the signal is not physical but mental? But how should we think of physicochemical events in neurons being converted into a mental signal? And when the brain "receives" a mental signal, how does this cause changes in neurons? For Descartes, interaction involved "animal spirits" going between mind and brain at the pineal gland. The module account is the same story, updated for the age of radio or cell phones. The unanswered questions add up to a strong reason for skepticism about this kind of dualism.

Spinoza's View: Not Dualism, but Inner and Outer Perspectives

> The mind and body are one and the same thing, which is conceived now under the attribute of thought, now under the attribute of extension. The result is that the order, or connection, of things is one, whether Nature is conceived under this attribute or that; hence the order of actions and passions of our body is, by nature, at one with the order of actions and passions of the mind.
>
> —Spinoza, *Ethics*

Modern materialists believe that the reality of the mind is states and processes of the brain and nervous system, without any dualist residue. Some have adopted an "eliminative" version, according to which the "folk psychology" of subjective experiences can in principle (and, one day, in practice?) be replaced by talk only about brain states and processes. Others, equally skeptical of dualism, think this denies the problem of subjective experiences by fiat, and that the losses in the "elimination" of "folk psychology" are more obvious than the gains.

It seems that an adequate solution would bypass dualism without denying or downgrading subjective experience. One approach worth exploring can be seen as a kind of "noneliminative" materialism. Philosophers as different in outlook as Spinoza and Bertrand Russell have argued that the solution to the mind-body problem is to see subjective experiences and bodily or brain states as two aspects of the same thing. In itself this claim does not solve the mind-body problem. How do we know that we are dealing with two "aspects" of something, rather than with two things or processes? And can we sidestep asking "aspects of what?"? Despite these questions, the Spinozist approach seems worth exploring. A defensible version of it might mean we could escape the dubious metaphysical interactions of dualism and the procrustean "eliminations" of some versions of materialism.

Some have argued that modern physics gives an account of the physical world that might support this Spinozist approach. Michael Lockwood says that philosophers writing on the mind-brain problem have usually seen it as a task of trying to fit a problematic mind into an unproblematic physical world. For them all the "give" is on the side of the mind. Lockwood sees this as a prejudice. "Quantum mechanics has robbed matter of its conceptual quite as much as its literal solidity. Mind and matter are alike in being profoundly mysterious, philosophically speaking."[13]

The intuitively paradoxical aspects of quantum physics include "superposition": a particle exists in a way that includes its alternative possible states at the same time, until measurement pins it down to just one of the possibilities. Some particles interact in ways that result in their "entanglement" after they are separated: when measurement pins one particle to a particular state, measurement then pins the other particle down to a corresponding alternative state. This could allow information to be sent from one place to another without going through the space in between. David Deutsch has suggested that such phenomena create the possibility of "quantum computers." One version would allow vastly many simultaneous computations to influence each other and so produce a shared output: "In such computations, a quantum computer with only a few hundred qubits [quantum bits of information] could perform far more computations in parallel than there are atoms in the visible universe."[14]

Michael Lockwood has speculated that the physical basis of consciousness may be a brain whose interactions make a quantum computer possible.[15] I am nowhere near understanding quantum theory and take no view on whether this suggestion is true. The big models in neuroscience tend to follow current or predicted information technology. In the early twentieth century the brain was seen as a telephone exchange. In the mid-twentieth century it was a computer. The quantum computer model is in this tradition. Like its digital computer predecessor, it may create a fruitful research paradigm, even if it is at best a partial picture. If it does turn out that consciousness needs a brain that can support a quantum computer, we still may not have solved the mind-brain problem. A new question (Why only with quantum computing?) will be added to the question of why consciousness evolved at all.

There is a more general point. Lockwood pursues the thought that mind and matter are both mysterious. He suggests that physics might learn from introspective psychology: "If mental states are brain states, then introspection is already . . . telling us that there is more to the matter of the brain than there is currently room for in the physicist's philosophy." Developing an idea of Bertrand Russell's, itself similar to Spinoza's view, Lockwood says that consciousness "provides us with a kind of 'window' on to our brains, making possible a transparent grasp of a tiny corner of a material reality that is in general opaque to us." He suggests that the gulf, even in the brain, between mental and physical events is an illusion coming from two different kinds of access to the same reality. We know brain events from the outside, using our senses and instruments. We know mental events "from the inside, by living them, or one might almost say, by self-reflectively being them."[16] The epigraph to his book is an ancient Chinese aphorism: "We are that in which the earth comes to appreciate itself."

Whether the quantum computing suggestion about consciousness is right or wrong, we can reject the nineteenth-century view of matter as "inert." That view made the origin of life a puzzle, solved by an unnecessary nonmaterial "vitalism." Current models show how amino acids and more-complex molecules needed for life could emerge spontaneously on

Earth. Matter turned out to have the potential for the development of life. There is a parallel point about mind. It is a platitude that consciousness emerged from material brains and nervous systems. As matter has the potential for life, so life has the potential for consciousness.

How consciousness emerged is one of the great unsolved philosophical and scientific questions. We may hope that, as with the emergence of life, "interaction" with something nonphysical will be unnecessary. We do not know that interactionist dualism is impossible. But its unanswered questions make it implausible. In psychiatry it is desirable to be able to talk about neuroplasticity and other forms of everyday "interaction" of mind and brain without any theoretical commitment to dualism. In the rest of this book I will talk of mental states being "embodied" in neurophysiological or neurochemical states. My pragmatic hope is that this will be useful in thinking about psychiatry, without implying that the mind-body problem has been solved.

Mind-Brain "Interaction" without Dualism

A familiar central part of the program of neuroscience is mapping mental states, events, and functions onto the brain. Another way of describing this is as showing which brain states embody which mental states, events, or functions. For the philosophical mind-brain problem, this talk of "mapping" and "embodiment" is totally lacking in explanatory power. Is "embodiment" interaction or identity? How does a brain state "embody" a thought or a feeling? Could there be zombies who have the brain states without the embodiment? This language leaves all the deep questions unanswered.

But for thinking about neuroscience and psychiatry, this philosophically unilluminating language serves the purpose. We can talk about the taxi drivers' ability to navigate the London streets being embodied in the posterior hippocampus without denying a residual mind-brain problem. It allows us to talk easily of mental and brain events in the same sentence, facilitating the pluralist, rather than reductionist, explanatory models that psychiatry often needs.[17] It also allows room for the effectiveness of psychotherapy even if a materialist view of the mind is correct.

Some materialist account may be the whole truth. Even if so, in our present state of ignorance it is not wrong to talk in ways that sound like interactionist dualism. This choice of language carries no theoretical commitment to dualism. In principle the talk about mental states can be replaced by talk about whatever brain states turn out to "embody" them. Placebos are a paradigm of mind-brain "interaction." In some conditions the belief that you have been given medication often seems to contribute to improvement. The mechanisms include the release of opiates, action on the immune system, and so on.[18] "Mapping" beliefs onto the brain states embodying them will outline a neuroscientific account of this mind-brain "interaction." It will not solve the deep mind-body problem. But it does help neuropsychiatry dispense with mysterious transmissions to and from a nonphysical world.

Agency

Psychiatry cannot so easily bracket off the deep questions about agency and free will. How far do various degrees and kinds of psychiatric disorder impair free agency? The questions are partly empirical. What limitations do these disorders impose? They are partly philosophical. How do we decide what is a limitation? How is an irresistible impulse different from one that simply was not resisted? Which limitations are incompatible with free agency? If free agency is a matter of degree, how do we draw up the scale? At what point on the scale is a person's responsibility eliminated or diminished?

Quite apart from moral blame or legal punishment, these questions about freedom of mind and action are important from the person's own perspective. Part of human flourishing is being able to make decisions, to act on them, and so to have some control over your own life.

Thinking, Feeling, and Acting at the Whim of Those Chemicals?

> All these things indeed show clearly that both the decision of the mind and the appetite and determination of the body by nature exist together—or rather are one and the same thing; which we call a decision when it is considered under, and explained through, the attribute of thought, and which we call a determination when it is considered under the attribute of extension.
>
> —Spinoza, *Ethics*

Dan Fisher says that the neurobiological approach to psychiatry leaves him with the sense that he is thinking, feeling, and acting at the whim of those chemicals. Is he mistaken? How far do genetic and neuroscientific causal accounts leave room for input from the beliefs, desires, reasons, loves, hatreds, fears, and hopes at the heart of how we see ourselves and each other?

We have the experience of deciding to make a phone call and then doing so. Through such experiences we see ourselves as agents: we see our conscious decisions as causing our actions, or at least many of them. But neuroscience has thrown up some disconcerting questions about how far conscious decisions really control actions.

A classic study by Benjamin Libet and colleagues has been interpreted to show that a conscious decision comes after the action is initiated. An electrical change in the brain (the "readiness potential") takes place 550 milliseconds before a voluntary act. But people report first awareness of any urge to act only 200 milliseconds before the act itself.[19] Libet's own interpretation of this time lag was that the conscious experience of deciding or willing does not initiate the act, but that the 200 milliseconds left between awareness and action leave time for a conscious veto.[20]

The interpretation of the experiments is controversial. How accurate is the reported onset of awareness of the urge to act? And what is the "readiness potential"? Libet took it to be the initiation of action. But we know so little about the neural complexities of action that this is uncertain. In democratic countries the civil service makes plans corresponding to the programs of different political parties in readiness to implement the policies of the winning party. (The administrative "readiness potential"?) This does not mean that a new government has to rubber-stamp a decision already taken by the civil service, or that they at best have a hasty veto. Libet's interpretation might be right. But we will not know until neuroscience can tell whether the readiness potential embodies an unconscious decision or only preparation to implement a future decision.

Intuitively we think of our experience of the world as unmediated: that we simply see, hear, smell, or feel the world as it is. We now know that this picture leaves out the complex processes of interpretation that create our experience. These processes are unconscious, but neuroscience shows they are the real causal story of our perception. Something similar is clearly true of our actions. We do not know intuitively what goes on in the brain when we decide to call someone.

Daniel Wegner, invoking a wider range of evidence, follows Libet in suggesting that "the feeling of conscious will" is an illusion: we are wrong to think that what we experience as conscious decision causes our actions.[21] His case is partly based on our ignorance of the causal processes. He also cites cases where we are mistaken about our own involvement or lack of involvement in producing actions. (These include alien hand syndrome, automatic writing, and being "possessed by spirits.") Causation has to be established empirically, by finding conjunctions between events and then controlling for various factors to establish which are causal. The supposed causal link between conscious will and action is poorly based because it is assumed rather than investigated. Wegner suggests that the neural systems are the real causes. He thinks the experience of deciding or willing is probably a preview we are given so that we know, and can tell others, what we are about to do. It is a gauge on the control panel rather than part of the mechanism.

Wegner is clearly right that the full causal story of action includes brain mechanisms of which we are not conscious. It is more controversial that what we experience as a decision has no causal impact. Everything depends on how such experience is mapped onto the brain: in which brain states, events, and functions our experiences of agency are embodied. On this there is an intuitive appeal in the views of Spinoza and Michael Lockwood that conscious states are the brain states seen from "inside." (Though the metaphor—if it is a metaphor—of "inside" is a reminder of the still unsolved mind-brain problem.) If the brain processes embodying these experiences are a key part of the neuroscientific causal account of action, "conscious will" is not an illusion after all.

We know too little about the neuroscience of action to be certain one way or the other. But the "illusion" view seems less plausible than the standard one. Imagine designing an aircraft in a world without radar or satellites, so that the pilots have to radio other people about their flight path. On one proposed design, the plane is actually controlled by a robot rather than by the pilot. The robot also signals to the pilot's brain which levers to pull, and so forth. So pilots, who are in a cockpit that actually is disconnected from anything that would control the planes, believe they are flying planes. They can report their position and direction to others. If pilots are as efficient as robots, it is hard to see any reason why this absurd "disconnected cockpit" complication should be chosen rather than the simpler standard design. It is equally hard to see why the elaborate "disconnected consciousness" model of human decision, rather than the standard version, would have emerged in evolution.

So it is not unreasonable to think that our decisions do in general control our actions. Like Dan Fisher, we do not want to see ourselves as passive, just observing what happens as our brains do our thinking and deciding for us. Luckily the arguments and evidence thought to support the passive view are unconvincing. We need not give up on the idea that we are free agents. But there are still serious difficulties about the scope and limits of free agency. Does this freedom go "all the way down"? As Spinoza himself asked, to what extent are our decisions and the thinking behind them at the mercy of causal factors outside our control? There is the residual worry that, one level further down, we still may be "at the whim of those chemicals."

The Strategy of This Part of the Book

The account of agency and responsibility will be developed in three stages. First I will sketch the central framework of thought underpinning judgments of responsibility. Then I will relate this to how various disorders—addiction, for instance—create internal constraints, limiting or distorting motivation and action. Finally, I will turn the focus to people influenced by psychiatric conditions that are not easily described as internal constraints. Some conditions change people at their very core, in their basic desires and values. In contrast to the reluctant addict, some people diagnosed with "personality disorders" might not be constrained to do things against their will. Rather, the disorder shapes who they are, including shaping their will. How far should they be held responsible? Should we see the disorder as a piece of bad luck, for whose consequences they are not responsible? Or should we say that people who choose to do bad things because they have a bad will or a bad character, however this came about, are exactly those we should blame for what they do?

22

Psychiatric Conditions and the Framework of Responsibility

When should or should not people be held responsible for things they do under the influence of psychiatric disorder?

Questions about responsibility are often legal. Should this person be punished for an illegal act? Were there factors that diminish his responsibility or even absolve him altogether? The questions are often moral, often linked to praise or blame: If her terrible record of not meeting deadlines reflects her psychiatric problem, isn't it unfair to blame her?

Other questions about responsibility do not reflect the external standpoint of the law or the moral critic. People wonder about themselves. Should I feel bad about what I did? How far am I a free agent? How far am I in charge of my own life? For some people with psychiatric problems these questions can be even harder to answer than for the rest of us. And the answers often matter. When coping with some psychiatric disorders, it may be crucial not to take a fatalist view of your own life.

The Central Framework

It is extraordinary that, extended but otherwise almost unchanged, Aristotle's analysis of voluntary action still forms the central framework of thought about the conditions of moral and legal responsibility. The framework's persistence for more than two millennia suggests that it reflects something deeply rooted in our assessments of people and what they do.

Aristotle was giving an account of what makes actions voluntary, though he wisely approached it mainly by saying what makes an action involuntary. He said that voluntary actions attract praise and blame, while involuntary ones attract pardon and sometimes pity. So his account of involuntary actions is about how to decide when someone is not responsible for an action. The framework is simple. Involuntary actions are those done either in ignorance or under compulsion.[1]

To excuse an action, ignorance must be specific and relevant. Aristotle cites not knowing that the thing blurted out was a secret, mistaking a son for an enemy, or thinking the poison was lifesaving medicine. He rejects many kinds of ignorance as excuses. We do not excuse normal people because they do not know who they are, or because they do not know they are killing someone with a knife. Of these things "no one could be ignorant unless he were mad." Aristotle leaves dangling how we should respond to mad people who are deluded in these ways. But later development of the framework rightly allows these delusions as excuses.

Aristotle cites as central cases of compulsion being blown off course by a gale, or being carried off by men who have you in their power. He says that an act under compulsion is one "of which the moving principle is outside" and where "nothing is contributed by the person who is acting."

This account of the totally passive person has to be stretched a bit to fit being forced to do things. Being forced may be coercion (the tyrant who threatens to kill your family) or being forced by a storm to throw goods overboard in order to survive. A forced act is in one way voluntary: you chose to do it. But in another way it is not: "no one would choose any such act in itself." Aristotle thinks some acts are so terrible that no coercion excuses them: you should accept death or any other catastrophe rather than kill your mother. But according to how the circumstances and choices are assessed, being forced is a candidate for the compulsion that excuses from responsibility.

It is striking how external Aristotle's version of compulsion is. His view of madness seems limited to delusions (though his later discussion of weakness of will is highly relevant to addiction). His account of voluntariness leaves out the "inner" constraints of modern psychiatry: the addictive, the obsessive-compulsive, and so on. These are the main problem for his view that all acts whose "moving principle" comes from within are entirely voluntary.

He does consider the suggestion that we can be compulsively attracted, for instance to pleasure. But he rejects it, as pleasure is such a common motive that this could make all acts involuntary. And he objects that pleasure as a moving principle is internal: "It is absurd to make external circumstances responsible, and not oneself, as being easily caught by such attractions." He concludes that compelled actions are those "whose moving principle is outside, the person compelled contributing nothing."

The conflict between Aristotle and the modern view of drug addiction or compulsive handwashing is about whether inner constraints exist. The desire to take heroin or to repeatedly wash one's hands is internal to the person in a way that the gale at sea is not. We either have to hold the addict and the obsessive-compulsive fully responsible or else depart from Aristotle. The majority modern view departs from his view. It allows internal constraints to excuse people, either partly or entirely. But as Aristotle suggests, we need some limit to this loophole if it is not to excuse all actions.

Apart from the problem of internal constraints, Aristotle's broad outline is still the central framework of responsibility. The M'Naghten rules, drawn up to guide English law in the mid-nineteenth century, reflected the "ignorance" side of the framework, but not yet the "compulsion" side. In this, the jury in M'Naghten's case were ahead of the law.

Daniel M'Naghten was paranoid about the Tory party and the police. Sir Robert Peel, Tory prime minister and founder of the Metropolitan Police, was an obvious focus for him. In 1843 M'Naghten fatally shot in the back the prime minister's private secretary, probably in mistake for Peel. He said, "The Tories in my native city have compelled me to do this. They follow and persecute me wherever I go, and have entirely destroyed my peace of mind. They followed me to France, into Scotland, and all over England . . . They have accused me of crimes of which I am not guilty; in fact they wish to murder me. It can be proved by evidence. That's all I have to say."[2]

At his trial witnesses testified that M'Naghten was deluded. The defense argued that this took away "all power of self-control." The judge's summing-up centered not on self-control but on knowledge. Had M'Naghten at the time known that what he did was "a violation of the law of God or of man"? If he had been capable of distinguishing between right and wrong, he was a responsible agent and liable to all legal penalties. The jury, guided perhaps more by instincts of fairness and humanity than by the letter of the law, brought in a special verdict. M'Naghten went to Bethlem Royal Hospital and then to Broadmoor, where he spent the rest of his life.

The House of Lords, concerned about the lack of a "guilty" verdict, posed questions to the judges about the criteria to be applied in considering the responsibility of people acting under insane delusions. The resulting "M'Naghten rules" are essentially summed up in this passage from the majority response: "To establish a defence on the ground of insanity, it must be clearly proved that, at the time of committing the act, the party accused was labouring under such a defect of reason, from disease of the mind, as not to know the nature and quality of the act he was doing; or, if he did know it, he did not know he was doing what was wrong." Like Aristotle, the judges saw relevant ignorance as an excuse but, again like Aristotle, did not see the possibility of psychiatric conditions creating inner compulsions.

Some problems lurking in the M'Naghten rules were about "knowing" an act is wrong. Is wrongness the same as illegality, as some judges seemed hopefully to think? If not, there are also questions about resting the law on the debatable belief in objective truths about right and wrong. Are moral truths what "the reasonable man" believes? Or are they tied to religious belief, as the phrase "the law of God or of man" seems to suggest?

Another problem about "wrong" was raised in 1863 by the case of Townley, who killed his fiancée when she broke off their engagement. He was paranoid, saying six people were conspiring to kill him. He showed no remorse. He said he had as much right to deal with his fiancée as with any other property of his, and that he recognized no man's right to judge him. He seemed to know his act was illegal. The M'Naghten question about "knowing what he was doing was wrong" did not anticipate that someone might know it was both illegal and widely morally condemned, yet sincerely think he had a moral right to do it.

Extending the Framework: Psychiatric Constraints

The major defect of the M'Naghten rules was not seeing that mental disorder might make some things very hard or even impossible to resist. This was unfair to accused people who acted under the influence of such disorders. But allowing irresistible impulses raised a large problem, as James Fitzjames Stephen pointed out in 1855: "I fear there is a disposition to confound them with unresisted impulses." Over a century later the social scientist Barbara Wootton echoed this: "It must not be inferred that an impulse was irresistible merely because it was not resisted."[3]

One way of giving greater flexibility (though without solving the hard question anticipated by Aristotle and pressed by Stephen and Wootton) was the introduction in English law of the concept of "diminished responsibility." But this was not until the 1957 Homicide Act, more than a century after the M'Naghten rules. During that previous century there was pressure on both legislators and judges to find ways to mitigate the injustices coming from the rules' rigidity.

The rigidity was challenged by cases where a mother killed her baby under the influence of what would now in Britain be called postnatal psychosis (in the United States, postpartum psychosis). After childbirth women are at most risk of mental disorder. There are huge hormonal changes in pregnancy, some hormones increasing two-hundred-fold, followed by a rapid decline over the twenty-four hours after birth. According to modern studies, postnatal psychosis is characterized by agitation, huge mood shifts between mania and depression, a delirious state, delusions, confusion, and thought disorder. Dr. Margaret Spinelli points out that neuropsychiatric tests indicate cognitive impairments.[4] There is a 5 percent risk of suicide and a 4 percent risk of infanticide.[5]

In England the dark ages of the legal response to infanticide started to close after 1849, the year Rebecca Smith was hanged despite the jury having recommended mercy. She was the last mother to be executed in England for killing her baby. At that time, without epidemiological studies or neuroscience, many people already had quite a good idea of the pressures of postnatal psychiatric problems. Some personally knew women who had these problems, or heard what emerged in highly publicized trials. Where juries, with the support of the judge, recommended mercy toward a woman they convicted, she was not executed. Eventually all mothers committing infanticide were reprieved. Attempts were made to fit the law to this practice. For a long time they failed.

Success came (thirty years after most of the rest of Europe) with the passing in 1922 of the Infanticide Act. This allowed that a woman who had killed her newly born child before she had "fully recovered from the effect of giving birth to such child" could be convicted of the noncapital crime of infanticide rather than murder. This gave judges wide scope in sentencing. The punishment could be as little as a conditional discharge. Soon the standard sentence was either committal to a mental hospital or else probation on condition of accepting psychiatric treatment.

The Infanticide Act was recognition of diminished responsibility without the phrase. Yes, she did kill her baby and sometimes knew she was doing so. But her condition, with its delusions and desperation, was either an excuse or at the very least a strong mitigation. One kind of injustice and cruelty was starting to be defeated. The central framework of responsibility remained in place: only relevant ignorance or appropriately strong compulsion excuse someone from responsibility for an act. But the framework was extended to allow for degrees of inner compulsion. The boundary problems this change leaves us with are a price well worth paying for its humanity.

How Far from the Dark Ages Are We?

The Case of Caroline Beale

Caroline Beale was 30 in 1994, living in London with her boyfriend Paul and working in the Department of Health. She was very distressed by the death from cancer of her close friend Alison, the girlfriend of one of Paul's brothers. Alison had always wanted children and was devastated that she would not live to have them. At the same time Caroline found she was pregnant. Feeling it would be cruel to tell Alison, she kept her pregnancy secret from everyone.

After Alison's death, Paul found Caroline changed and their relationship was under strain. She had "visions" of Alison. After Alison's death she identified her own baby with Alison and believed the baby was dead too. Her great stress was noticed at work and she was offered compassionate leave. Having still told no one about her nearly nine-month pregnancy, she went to New York with Paul and his brothers. Later she said, "I couldn't tell anyone. It wasn't that Paul and I weren't speaking but we were going through a bit of a rocky patch . . . I didn't really want to go to New York . . . but I just went along with it. I didn't know what to do. And so I found myself sitting on the underground going to Heathrow and not being able to tell anybody what was happening."[6]

Caroline felt in a daze or a dream the whole time. On the last night in New York, she went to bed while the others went out. In the bath she gave birth. Since Alison's death, she had thought her baby was dead in the womb. In the bath, "I think I might have passed out. The baby's head was coming out. I knew she wasn't alive. Then I was awake again. I was so scared because I thought I was going to die as well. I just didn't know what to do. There were scissors on the sink so I just cut the cord with scissors and left her in the bath while I went to the loo . . . I was like on automatic pilot. I took her out of the bath and I didn't know what to do. I put her in a bag because I didn't know what else to do. I had to get her back to England, somehow."[7] The next day she carried the baby in the bag to the airport. A security guard found the baby and she was arrested.

The autopsy said the baby had taken a breath. Caroline was charged with murder. She was not granted bail, but was remanded to Rikers Island prison. In a diary she wrote, "The loneliness, the fear, the loss of self dignity, the hunger (and that really does exist). The worst thing of all is going to bed hungry and drinking water to fill yourself up. I think if a judge or DA was to spend a month here they would certainly be more hesitant about incarcerating people in this place. There must be some other way of doing things."[8] She had no access to treatment.

In England, Caroline's father had been put in touch with Dr. Channi Kumar at the Maudsley Hospital. Help was also offered by Professor Ian Brockington of Birmingham University, who went to New York to interview Caroline. Channi Kumar contacted a New York colleague, Dr. Meg Spinelli (the Margaret Spinelli whose paper "Maternal Infanticide Associated with Mental Illness" is cited in this chapter's notes). She was instrumental in helping Caroline obtain her defense lawyer, Michael Dowd, who negotiated terms with the district attorney, Marjorie Fisher, for release on bail. While on bail Caroline said she would kill herself rather than go back to Rikers Island.

Ian Brockington had found that leading experts were very skeptical about the autopsy claim that the hemorrhages proved suffocation rather than some injury during delivery. He, Channi Kumar, and Michael Dowd also assembled a powerful team of psychiatric experts for the defense.

On Caroline's condition, the psychiatrists were divided. Dr. Naomi Goldstein, interviewing Caroline for the prosecution, accepted that she had clinical depression and impaired judgment. But she did not think that at the time of the act Caroline had the psychosis needed for an insanity defense.

The defense psychiatrists, while differing on diagnosis, agreed she was not responsible. After spending time with her, Meg Spinelli had concluded that Caroline did not have postnatal depression but that she had had visual and auditory hallucinations and had been in denial about her pregnancy. Carrying the dead baby through the airport was a sign of acute psychosis. "In my judgement she lacked capacity to form intent by virtue of a defect in her ability to reason and should therefore be found innocent of charges under the insanity defense."[9] Channi Kumar interviewed Caroline twice, and diagnosed a major depressive disorder, linked to a pathological reaction to Alison's death. He believed that Caroline's disorder caused what she did. Criminal prosecution was inappropriate. He offered to treat her serious psychiatric illness at the Maudsley Hospital.

Michael Dowd was worried that in Queens a mainly Catholic jury might be prejudiced against anyone accused of harming a baby. He worried Caroline would not stand up well to a long trial. These concerns, and the risk of a very long sentence, made him support plea bargaining. At first, in exchange for a guilty plea, Marjorie Fisher would accept a sentence of from two to four and a half years. The final offer was that if Caroline pleaded guilty to manslaughter, she could receive a sentence that would not exceed the time she had already served in prison and so could return to England.

Because Caroline had believed her baby was dead, pleading guilty to manslaughter was a terrible and humiliating thing to have to do. She agreed to do it because the alternative risked so much. She was released and flew back to England. She had treatment and support from Channi Kumar and others at the Maudsley and after a storm of media attention started to get back to her life.

This tragedy has many layers. Caroline Beale was drawn into denial and concealment of the pregnancy by not wanting to hurt Alison. She found herself trapped in the deception, and invaded by a strange psychiatric condition triggered by the death of her friend. Then came the trauma of what she perhaps rightly thought was a stillbirth, with no one to turn to. It was followed by her "automatic pilot" state and the bizarre project of taking the dead baby to England. Then came the further trauma of arrest.

The next layers of the tragedy involve questionable decisions of others. Someone better trained might have produced a less overconfident autopsy report. A legal system that saw infanticide as the rest of the Western world does would not have brought a murder charge. In England people were shocked that the district attorney, Marjorie Fisher, made choices leading to Caroline's being confined in a hellhole of a prison and denied psychiatric treatment. The attorney became something of a hated figure. Though some of the criticism was justified, this response is too shallow.

Marjorie Fisher knew about the criticism in England. Asked about her decisions, she said, "In the United States you don't get extra points for killing babies." She also said, "A system that takes into account the life of a child is a very compassionate one. Sometimes I got the impression that people were more concerned about the defendant than about the victim . . . She hid it, she concealed it. To me that merited a murder charge." And she said, "I was satisfied with the sentence and I was most satisfied that she stood up and said what she did. She said that she knew that what she did at the time could end the child's life. She knew that and the people in Queens and the people in England knew that."[10]

Of these remarks, the most notorious was the suggestion that jurisdictions outside the United States give "extra points for killing babies." Perhaps a district attorney need not know about the development of law in other jurisdictions. Her ignorance that the special laws about infanticide come from concern about diminished responsibility, and not from a failure to "take into account the life of a child," is perhaps excusable. (Though the ignorance was aggressive: "extra points" suggests positive enthusiasm for a baby's death.) The other comments are weak. To the psychiatrically informed or the humanly imaginative, "She hid it, she concealed it" does not make murder more likely than that the concealment came from delusion, denial, and panic. And "she stood up and said what she did" is entirely undermined as evidence for her having committed murder by the system of plea bargaining.

The main issue goes deeper than the district attorney's decisions. It is about laws that, following the M'Naghten rules, are concerned only with whether a woman knew what she was doing, to the exclusion of issues about psychiatric conditions creating inner compulsions. This legal defect is the outer layer of the tragedy, making it very hard to avoid the kind of injustice and cruelty seen in this case.

The Case of Andrea Yates

This was demonstrated seven years later in Houston, Texas. In 2001 Andrea Yates drowned her five children in the bath. She was a devoted mother, whose first psychotic episode was after the birth of her first child. "She hid the episode in the hope that this would protect them from being harmed by Satan." After her fourth child was born, she attempted suicide twice while trying to resist "satanic commands" to kill her baby. When her fifth child was six months, she was "catatonic" and "like a caged animal." She was twice confined in a psychiatric hospital. When her medication was stopped, she obeyed Satan's command to save her children from hell by killing them. She said she was Satan.

Again, the story is a multiple tragedy. The horrifying tragedy of the five children killed, and by their own mother. And the tragedy of Andrea Yates herself: of her tormenting insanity and the indelibly horrible thing it made her do.

The tragedy has another dimension. Andrea Yates was charged with capital murder. Her plea was innocent by reason of insanity. The State of Texas still used the M'Naghten tests. Did she know the nature and quality of her act? Did she know it was wrong? The prosecution argued that she knew right from wrong because she called 911 and her husband after the killings. The jury found her guilty of capital murder but substituted life imprisonment for the death sentence the prosecution demanded.[11]

The cases of Caroline Beale and Andrea Yates show that the modern version of the central framework of responsibility has not percolated everywhere. In some places, more than a century and a half after the hanging of Rebecca Smith, legal failure to recognize internal compulsions still multiplies their cruel consequences.

Including internal compulsions was a great advance. Backward jurisdictions still need to be persuaded of this, and there is still intellectual work to be done. There is a need for a finer-grained analysis of what counts as excusing internal constraint. This needs to be seen in the context of particular psychiatric conditions.

Excuses as a Defense of Character

The continuing dominance of the central framework of Aristotle's two excuses, ignorance and compulsion (in modified form), reflects the way actions are guided by beliefs and motivated by desires.

It also reflects links between judgments of responsibility and how we view motives, values, and character. If someone knowingly steals money, this reflects on his honesty. This is not so if he just picks up a pile of documents, without seeing the paper money among them. If a bank clerk hands over the key to the safe because the robber demanding it is armed and dangerous, this reflects fear, not complicity in the crime. What matters is motivation, which tells us something about the person's values and character. Pleas of ignorance ("He did not see the money") or of compulsion ("She was forced to hand over the key") defend a person's character. They defeat accusations of being a thief or an abbettor.

The psychiatric versions of the two pleas—ignorance and compulsion—raise problems of their own. A delusion may stop someone from knowing what he is doing. But it is often hard to tell how far someone really is deluded. And the strangeness of delusions can make them hard to understand. Psychiatric states may involve compulsion, but the "inner" compulsion of addiction is harder to assess than the external kind used by the armed robber.

The Reactive Attitudes

Morally blaming people is bound up with the belief that what they did reflects badly on them. The excuses of the central framework, ignorance and compulsion, sever the link between action and character, and so prevent the person's character being stained by the action.

These excuses, with complications, apply in many psychiatric cases. (Though where the person's character itself has defects caused by the psychiatric disorder, the problems are much more acute.)

Blaming someone, judging their character, can have the unemotional detachment of the recording angel. But there is another view of blame that makes it less detached by locating it among people's relationships and attitudes.

In his classic paper "Freedom and Resentment," P. F. Strawson argued against those who see determinism as undermining blame. He suggested that they overlook the way blame is embedded in a network of "interpersonal reactive attitudes" such as gratitude and resentment. He argued that blame cannot be separated from these other attitudes—that they stand or fall together. And, he argued, determinism could not justify giving up this whole network of attitudes. It would be psychologically impossible for us to give them up. Even if it were possible, it would not be rational to do so. These attitudes are at the core of human relationships. Giving them up would impoverish us. It would replace our present emotionally involved reactions to each other with the clinical objectivity of a psychiatrist or a social worker.[12]

This line of thought might not succeed in defusing the issue of determinism. (Is it too hasty to see the reactive attitudes as an indivisible web? Will undermining blame really make all relationships so cold and detached?) But one merit of this approach is that it makes questions about blame less abstract, shifting the focus to our reactions and attitudes to the person.

Attitude Spirals

Relationships are shaped by people's attitudes toward each other. Some attitudes pervade a whole relationship: liking, disliking, love, hatred, friendship, and enmity. These attitudes are often responses to what the other person does. But not always. I may not deserve the dislike of one person or the love of another, yet have both.

Some attitudes are less free-floating because they are based on evaluation. Respect, admiration, and contempt claim to reflect someone's good or bad qualities. Some attitudes reflect people's good or bad luck. If I break a leg trying to windsurf, I may trigger sympathy, gloating, or amusement. Other attitudes are reflexive. Jealousy, envy, and condescension all compare the other person with oneself. All of these are "interpersonal reactive attitudes." Each may be, and some must be, a reaction to what other people are like. But without further layers, they are limited.

Relationships include interplay between attitudes to each other. We have attitude spirals. I have attitudes to your attitude to me. You have attitudes to my attitudes to your attitudes. Lovers or friends respond to each other's attractiveness or wit. But the relationship is thin without reactions to each other's love or trust. Enemies may dislike each other's faces or voices, but the enmity is shallow unless they mind each other's contempt or gloating.

Relationships go deeper as we develop attitude spirals. Some attitudes are centrally responsive to the attitudes of others. At this level are gratitude, indignation, vengefulness, blame, and forgiveness. (These need not be in response to attitudes to ourselves. We might be indignant on someone else's behalf, or blame a person for generalized malevolence.) At least mainly, we see in actions the attitudes that shine through them. These attitudes to attitudes are at the core of human relationships. For those who know people whose psychiatric conditions contribute to objectionable behavior, there is a possibly insoluble dilemma. Blaming them may be unfair. But just as the reactive responses are at the core of relationships, exclusion from these responses is exclusion from part of that core.

23

What Is Addiction?

> Addiction is a chronic, often relapsing brain disease that causes compulsive drug seeking and use, despite harmful consequences to the addicted individual and to those around him or her. Although the initial decision is voluntary for most people, the brain changes that occur over time challenge a person's self-control and ability to resist intense impulses urging them to take drugs.
>
> —U.S. National Institute on Drug Abuse, *Drug Facts: Understanding Drug Abuse and Addiction,* 2011

> The Liberal View is not so minimal that it cannot say what addictions are. They are strong appetites towards pleasure . . . Addiction is an illiberal term invented to describe those who seek pleasure in a way that expresses our social disapproval.
>
> —Bennett Foddy and Julian Savulescu, "A Liberal Account of Addiction"

Distortions of motivation occur in people who can and do carry out intentional actions. At the moment of acting, they intend what they do, but the intention may express an overwhelming desire they would not choose to have.

Choices motivated by addiction seem less free than many other choices. Why is this so? This raises the question of what an addiction is. Most people think they have a clear intuitive idea of addiction, but the clarity fades when questions are asked. Here these questions will be raised by contrasting medical models of addiction with what Bennett Foddy and Julian Savulescu have called a "Liberal" account.[1]

Neurochemical Systems and Hijacking

When is a habit an addiction? The "chemical addictions" form the inner circle. Why is it so hard to give up alcohol, nicotine, heroin, Ecstasy, and so on? The bad experience of withdrawal has been seen as the key. But it is rare for withdrawal symptoms to be as terrible as their reputation. And "recovered" addicts sometimes relapse long enough after withdrawal for it not to be an issue.

There is evidence that addictive drugs mimic neurotransmitters. Different addictions involve different kinds of neurochemical disruption, but the dopamine system is often involved. Release of dopamine at the relevant sites in the brain used to be thought of as the chemical correlate of pleasure. But when monkeys have been trained to recognize a signal that apple juice will soon come, the relevant dopamine neurons fire as soon as the signal comes.[2] The dopamine system seems to be part of a more complex process of learning to seek and repeat pleasure. The dopamine release might embody, not pleasure, but enthusiastic anticipation: what in humans might be expressed as "Wow! Yes, please!"

William James, writing before modern understanding of neurotransmitters, said of many drunkards that "their nervous centers have become a sluiceway pathologically unlocked by every passing conception of a bottle and a glass. They do not thirst for the beverage; the taste of it may even appear repugnant; and they perfectly foresee the morrow's remorse. But when they think of the liquor or see it, they find themselves preparing to drink, and do not stop themselves: more than this they cannot say."[3] Drinking even when the taste is horrible shows that wanting and liking do not have to go together, something that fits the evidence about the anticipatory acceptance system.[4]

In one route into addiction, drugs mimic "natural" anticipatory signals of pleasure by releasing dopamine directly at the key points in the brain. The high levels of dopamine release may trump conflicting signals. In this way, as Steven Hyman puts it, addictive drugs hijack ordinary systems of motivation and learning.[5]

The hijacking metaphor has been criticized for implying that addicts are compelled to act in a way that allows no possibility of choice.[6] I want to retain the vivid word "hijacking," but without this implication. The word is striking, but also ambiguous. When pirates hijack a ship, they can either force the captured sailors to sail the ship under orders or lock them away. If forced to work, the captives still may have a chance to disobey the orders. Locked away, they have no power to change anything. In the addict with the hijacked dopamine system, it may be exceptionally hard, but still possible, to override the anticipatory acceptance. Or it may be literally irresistible. There may be no sharp boundary between the two, only a difference of degree. But in responding to addiction, the distinction matters.

Advocates of the Liberal view of addiction are skeptical about appealing to chemical changes in addicts' brains to support a conclusion that addictive desires are irresistible. Foddy and Savulescu point out that brain changes are not peculiar to addictive drugs but are also found in other desires. They remind us of neuroplasticity: "Living our lives changes our brains." They argue that these "supposedly compulsive adaptations" are caused by dopamine release in the brain's reward pathways, not only as a result of drugs but also in regular pleasures of other kinds. They reject any sharp line between drug addiction and other habits.[7]

It seems likely that the systems of learning and reward will be active in nonaddictive pleasures ranging from sex to what Hume called "calm passions." Even birdwatching may have its share of dopamine release. And it may be true that, for strength of desires, there is no sharp boundary between drug addiction and other desires for pleasure. These are important points, but they do not end the debate. The milder version of the hijacking claim is that the level of dopamine release may still make it very much harder to resist the associated desire. There might be no sharp distinction between the motivational force of drug addiction and of other strong desires. But there is still an empirical question whether there are differences of degree great enough to justify the intuitive view that addiction is a trap from which it can be either impossible or at least extraordinarily difficult to escape.

Chemical accounts of addiction bring out the importance of drawing on each of the two sides of Spinoza's picture of mental states as embodied in states of the brain. Without the neurobiology, we would never know the underlying mechanisms. We would also miss the clues suggesting that the key to addiction might not be pleasure itself but anticipated pleasure. Equally, without being able to talk about the psychology, we would have little chance of seeing the human significance of the various patterns of neural firing in the dopamine system and so on. Whether or not the "two perspectives" model is ultimately right, at least it is a corrective to views where only one is taken seriously.

The Disputed Boundaries

What about what are sometimes called "behavioral addictions"—addictions that seem to lack the obvious chemical basis of direct stimulation of neurotransmitters? Can there be behavioral addictions to the Internet or to gambling?

Or is this to wrongly medicalize strong ordinary desires? Foddy and Savulescu, making this objection, quote an 1851 case from the *New Orleans Medical and Surgical Journal.* Dr. Samuel Cartwright reported a new disease among local slaves. "Drapetomania" was an addiction to running away from their owners. The currently claimed behavioral addictions are not so ludicrous. But the question remains: Does this way of thinking medicalize ordinary unhijacked motivation?

There are people who spend so much time on the Internet that they disrupt other important things in their lives.[8] Are they addicts? Grounds for skepticism can come from another case. In 1796 a German writer was alarmed by what he saw as the addictiveness of books: "Readers of books . . . rise and retire to bed with a book in their hand, sit down at table with one, have one lying close by when working, carry one around with them when walking, and . . . once they have begun reading a book are unable to stop until they are finished. But they have scarcely finished the last page of a book before they begin looking around greedily for somewhere to acquire another one . . . they take it away and devour it with a kind of ravenous hunger. No lover of tobacco or coffee, no wine drinker or lover of games, can be as addicted to their pipe, bottle, games or coffee table as those many hungry readers are to their reading habit."[9]

But skepticism may be too easy. Perhaps repeated use of the Internet could be linked to changes in brain chemistry of strong motivational force. Could the "nonchemical addictions" just be those whose chemical basis has not yet been discovered?

If the brains of London taxi drivers are changed by learning "the Knowledge," why should not habitual gambling or use of the Internet have as great an impact? Perhaps everything we do both influences and is influenced by chemical states of the brain, so that it may be more fruitful to replace the question about chemistry with a question at the psychological level. Intuitively, gambling seems a more plausible addiction than reading. One way of thinking about this intuition is to ask whether the psychology of gambling has anything special about it.

Addictive Gambling? Possessed by Frenzy

> Another win! That meant I now had altogether eighty friedrichs d'or! I moved all eighty to the dozen middle numbers . . . the wheel turned and twenty-four came up . . . now I had altogether 200 friedrichs d'or . . .
>
> Feeling as though I were delirious with fever, I moved the whole pile of money to the red—and suddenly came to my senses! For the only time in the course of the whole evening, fear laid its icy finger on me and my arms and legs began to shake. With horror I saw and for an instant fully realized what it would mean to me to lose now! My whole life depended on that stake!
>
> "Rouge!" cried the croupier, and I drew a deep breath, while my whole body tingled with fire . . .
>
> Possessed by frenzy, I seized the 2,000 florins I had left and staked them on the twelve first numbers—haphazard, at random, without stopping to think! . . .
>
> I no longer feared anything, whatever it might be, and I flung down 4,000 florins on black . . .
>
> Black turned up. After that I remember neither the amount nor the order of my stakes. I only recall, as if it was a dream, that I had already won, I think, about sixteen thousand florins . . .
>
> But I, with strange perversity, deliberately went on staking on red after noticing that it had turned up seven times running . . . I really was overcome by a terrible craving for risk. Perhaps the soul passing through such a wide range of sensations is not satisfied but only exacerbated by them, and demands more and more of them, growing more and more powerful, until it reaches final exhaustion.
>
> —Fyodor Dostoyevsky, *The Gambler*

This is lightly disguised personal experience. While writing *Crime and Punishment* Dostoyevsky took a month off to alleviate his acute money problems. He dictated the whole of *The Gambler* for publication. Describing the casinos of Wiesbaden, he knew what he was writing about. As a desperate money-raising strategy, he invented a system for roulette. At first he won 10,000 francs. "The next morning I got excited, abandoned the system and immediately lost. In the evening I returned to the system, observed it strictly, and quickly and without difficulty won back 3,000 francs. Tell me, after that how could I help being tempted, how could I fail to believe that I had only to follow my system strictly and luck would be with me? And I need the money, for myself, for you, for my wife, for writing my novel . . . Suddenly I began to lose, could no longer keep my head and lost every farthing."[10]

The sense of loss of control comes over strongly: "feeling as though I were delirious," "possessed by frenzy," and "could no longer keep my head." Of course one case, even when the person is Dostoyevsky, does not prove that all passionate repeat gamblers are the same. But Dostoyevsky's gambling seems far more possessed than the enthusiastic German readers who so worried their critic in the 1790s.

Dostoyevsky's frenzy suggests a view of the boundaries of addiction. He knew he needed the money for himself and for his wife, and for writing his novel. In the fictionalized version, with icy fear he came to his senses: his whole life depended on that stake. But in real life he did not act on these thoughts. The frenzy was dominant. He lost his head and lost all his money too. Full-blown addiction is the pull that often trumps even total awareness of how much more is at stake. Chemical tests can sometimes be decisive evidence, but what they are evidence for is this motivational force.

Loss of Control: The Liberal Critique

In the fictionalized version, Dostoyevsky describes being overcome by a terrible craving for risk. On the Liberal view, the word "overcome" misdescribes his state: He did not lose control, he simply acted on a very strong desire to take the risk. His choices were against his best interests, but this is not decisive proof of loss of control. He might just have cared more about taking the risk than about needing the money for himself, his wife, and his novel. And this is extended to addicts in general. The reason the view is called "Liberal" is its reluctance to discredit people's own choices in the name of an outside view of their best interests.

It is admirable to respect other people's different values. Still, the picture is too simple. The conflict is not usually between the happily unconventional hedonist and intrusively advice-giving outsiders. More typically it is within the addict's own mind, often between conflicting priorities at different times.

The apparently cheerful addict, single-mindedly pursuing pleasure, needs interpretation. The Liberal view is right that, when people act in ways that seem to go against a good life, this does not prove they have lost control. But most people do feel the pull of many of the "normal" ingredients of the good life. So going against that pull may still suggest diminished control. Few people would not care at all about needing money for themselves, for those they love, or for writing their novel. At the moment of betting, Dostoyevsky's craving for risk trumped everything else. But some internal conflict is still a reasonable expectation. And at other moments he did come to his senses, shaking with horror on seeing "My whole life depended on that stake!"

There are also different inner stories behind addictions. "Primary" addiction is driven by the love of a drug or of an activity such as gambling for its own sake. "Secondary" addiction is a means of dealing with other problems, such as escaping from worries and stress. Mark Griffiths says that secondary addicts lose control more than primary addicts do, though sometimes secondary addiction can be overcome by dealing with the other problems.[11] He quotes cases of adolescent boys whose slot machine addiction was an escape from feelings of having no control over their lives at home. Their gambling problems stopped when they moved away from their homes.[12]

The Liberal view fits willing addicts. Whatever may be true of heroin addiction or frenzied gambling, some other addicts are very much in control. Foddy and Savulescu cite the willing coffee addict who becomes irritable and slightly unwell without it. They claim that the neurological changes in coffee addiction are weaker versions of those in heroin addiction. "You are obviously addicted. Nevertheless, you endorse your desire for coffee; when you satisfy your cravings each day you do not regret it; and you do not yearn for the power to abstain. You are a willing addict."[13]

Willing coffee addicts do not call on psychiatrists. The addicts needing help are the unwilling ones. They do care about their damaged relationships, lost money, lost jobs, bad reputation, impaired health, or risk to life. That they do care about them yet still give way to the addiction is evidence (though not decisive proof) that their "guidance control"—their responsiveness to reasons for acting differently—is impaired.[14] Control is a matter of degree. Paradoxically, while it is the control they do not have that calls for psychiatric help, the effectiveness of the help usually depends on the control they do have.

24

Unwilling Addiction as Diminished Control

The modern debate between liberal views of addiction and the medical model reflects a moral debate with a long history. Are "unwilling" addicts to blame for their condition, because they just do not choose to change? Or are they victims because they are not able to give up their addiction?

If Plato's account is accurate, the "blaming" view goes back at least as far as Socrates:

> Socrates: You mean they'll live like people who are ill, but lack the discipline to give up a way of life that is bad for them.
>
> Adeimantus: That's it.
>
> Socrates: And what a nice time they have! All their treatments get them nowhere . . . and they're constantly expecting every medicine they are recommended to make them better . . . The thing they can abide least of all is someone telling them the truth—that until they stop getting drunk, stuffing themselves, whoring, and doing no work, no medicine or cautery or surgery, and no spell or amulet or anything like that either, is going to do them the slightest good.[1]

The "victim" riposte to Socrates is given vividly in Coleridge's account of his addiction to laudanum:

> For my Case is a species of madness, only that it is a derangement, an utter impotence of the Volition, & not of the intellectual Faculties—You bid me rouse myself—go, bid a man paralytic in both arms rub them briskly together, & that will cure him. Alas! (he would reply) that I cannot move my arms is my Complaint & my misery.[2]

At the core of understanding unwilling addiction is the question of loss of control, of irresistibility. Was Socrates right in implying that of course addicts can give up drunkenness, gluttony, sex, and laziness: they just need to decide to do so? Or was Coleridge right that his addiction involved a paralysis of will, no easier to overcome than paralysis of the limbs?

An "irresistible impulse" may go against what the person strongly wants at nearly all other times—the moment of weakness after two years' effort to give up smoking. The good question asked by Fitzjames Stephen and Barbara Wootton about how an irresistible impulse differs from one that just wasn't resisted is hard to answer. Part of the difficulty comes from resistibility being a matter of degree.

Degrees of Irresistibility and of Weakness

What Is Irresistible? The Two Sentries

Soldiers have been punished, even shot, for falling asleep on sentry duty. A sentry may say that he really tried but could not resist going to sleep. A common response is that he should have tried even harder. Obviously there is no sharp line such as "Everyone can keep awake for five hours but not longer." Circumstances vary: some sentries are fresh; others have marched for hours. People's ability varies. But even when the soldier starts fresh, and on earlier spells of duty has kept awake far longer, the boundary is still blurred. Did he fall asleep because he did not care enough or because his tiredness was too great to resist? How do we tell? The blurred boundary is real, but it does not follow that irresistible tiredness is unreal. There is no sharp boundary between sentry duty lasting five minutes and lasting five days. But it is absurd to blame someone who falls asleep after several days awake. Some things really are irresistible.

The case of the sleeping sentry shows how difficult it is to separate defects of character from limited ability. There are two extremes. One soldier has no commitment to sentry duty. As soon as he is alone he makes himself comfortable and goes to sleep. The other has real commitment and stays awake. After very many hours he feels sleepy. He conscientiously struggles against sleep but finally is overcome. If anyone deserves blame, the first sentry does. The second sentry obviously does not. The problems come from the real cases somewhere on the continuum between the two.

It is usually hard to see where on the continuum a particular case falls. Evidence can be about motivation. What did he say to his friends about sentry duty? Or it can relate to ability. How much sleep had he earlier? Had he easily managed sentry duty before? Is there medical evidence? Even detailed answers are often inconclusive. Ability is not all or none but on an ascending scale.

Sometimes unwilling addicts do respond to reasons. They may give up smoking in pregnancy, give up heroin to care better for a child, or just stop buying drugs when they get more expensive. Others do not respond to reasons but a lot of the time wish they did. On the Liberal view, this is just the weakness of will we all know so well, and not because they are powerless. The weakness-of-will model seems right. But how easy it is to overcome weakness of will varies with the strength of the desire to be resisted. Resisting the temptation to spend longer in bed is likely to be incomparably easier than resisting a deep-rooted addiction.

Weakness of Will as the Core of Unwilling Addiction

> I was—all the empirical evidence suggested—in a pathetic losing battle with the economy of my desires run amok, sometimes fighting off overwhelming craving for my drug, other times knowing, in some sense of "know," that my relationships with genuinely good people, my work, my life could, indeed would, be lost if I chose to use. And I'd still choose to use. Well, I'd use. That much was clear.
>
> —Owen Flanagan, "What Is It Like to Be an Addict?"

Philosophers from Plato onward have seen in choices like these a paradox needing resolution. People know that marriage, relationships, work, and health matter much more to them than satisfying the craving. They see that they will lose them all if they give way. Socrates (on Plato's testimony) thought it impossible to make what is seen to be the wrong choice. So he believed people act against what is best only because they do not see what the right choice is. Aristotle saw that some other account is needed, as Socrates's view "plainly contradicts the observed facts."[3] Lack of self-control does lead people to act against what they think is best.

Denying this comes partly from a seeming paradox: How can someone opt for what is seen to be the less good choice? The paradox comes partly from blurring different things together. There is what I think will be best for me, what I think is morally right, what most of the time I most want, and what at this moment I most want. Dostoyevsky could truthfully say that a decision not to gamble the money would be in his own best interest. He could agree that the decision would be morally right and would fit what most of the time he would want to do. But it can still be true that, in that moment of frenzy, taking the gamble was what he most wanted to do. How can the relative strength at a particular moment of different desires be measured except by seeing which one wins?[4]

What someone chooses shows what they then most want. But this truth can suggest two pictures, each too simple. One is that, given that the addict chooses what she most wants, the choice reflects a bad desire, not lack of ability. So there is no excuse and she should be held fully responsible for taking the addictive drug. At the other extreme is the view that, because no one chooses what at that moment they do not most want, it was utterly impossible for Dostoyevsky to resist the gamble: he was fated to do what he did and so was not responsible.

These pictures simplify by treating control as being all or none when it is a matter of degree. Yes, the relapsing alcoholic chose what at that moment she most wanted. But that desire went against other things that nearly all the time she cares about much more. She struggled against the desire but was defeated. It is true that Dostoyevsky could not have gone against his strongest desire at the time of acting. But fatalism about his act does not follow. Perhaps he could have thought in advance about approaching his money problems in less risky ways and so have avoided the casino that triggered his frenzy?

In the psychological dimension that runs from being fully in control to total collapse of will, few cases are at the extremes. Most of us, most of the time, are somewhere along the continuum. The blur about drawing a line gives rise to the saying that an alcoholic is someone who drinks more than the doctor.

And abilities are patchy. Ability to resist depends on context. When someone is in the grip of gambling frenzy or of one of the clearly chemical addictions, desire may be too strong to deflect. At that moment the belief that resisting is better may be powerless. But the desire need not be utterly irresistible. Facing a gunman's threat to shoot if he gambles, the addict may resist. At other times good reasons may still lose out to the brute strength of the desire.

In court cases involving diminished responsibility, the question is sometimes raised: "Would he have done it with a policeman at his elbow?" The answer "no" tends to undermine the defense. But this is too crude. The sentry struggles to keep awake, but after an extremely long time he falls asleep. He should not be blamed. But the answer to the question "Would he have fallen asleep if at that moment his commanding officer had arrived?" might also be no. All the same, without the stimulus or goad of this visitation, sleep may still have been irresistible. Context is crucial.

There was a lot of heroin use among American soldiers in Vietnam, partly because it was easily available. Of the army enlisted men there, 34 percent tried it and 20 percent reported having been addicted to it at some stage. Once back in the United States, 95 percent of those who had been addicted had not relapsed in their first year and 88 percent had not relapsed in their first three years.[5] For this large majority, their addiction was reversible. But this does not show that under the stress of war they had the same ability to give it up. The fact that context can increase or limit ability casts doubt on the view that all addictions are either utterly voluntary or utterly inescapable.

Because abilities vary in degree and are patchy, often there is no simple yes or no answer to the question of whether someone can help their gambling or their drug taking. In court cases that hang on issues of responsibility, the law often needs a yes or no answer. Psychiatrists, aware of degrees of capability, can find this difficult. Nigel Walker once said, "The psychiatrist in the witness box is like a wrestler who is compelled to box."[6]

Weakness of will is the core of unwilling addiction, but this tells us too little. How much control has an unwilling addict at the time of giving way to a desire? Here another question will be taken first. At an earlier stage, how far could the person have avoided becoming addicted?

Can People Help Becoming Addicts?

> And we punish those who are ignorant of anything in the laws that they ought to know and that is not difficult . . . we assume that it is in their power not to be ignorant, since they have the power of taking care. But perhaps a man is the kind of man not to take care. Still they are themselves by their slack lives responsible for becoming men of that kind, and men make themselves responsible for being unjust or self-indulgent, in the case of one by cheating and in the other by spending time in drinking-bouts and the like; for it is activities exercised on particular objects that make the corresponding character.
>
> —Aristotle, *Nichomachean Ethics*

Aristotle thought becoming an addict was voluntary: We create our character by what we freely choose to do. Repeating the same actions changes them into habits, which in turn harden into our character. People are responsible for becoming addicts, by choosing lives of drinking or drug taking. What does this picture of self-creation leave out? Not all decisions leading to addiction are equally free. Degrees of constraint vary in two ways of walking into addiction: the primrose path and walking the tightrope. More important, addiction can be an attempt to escape from sometimes daunting problems.

"The typical addict goes down the primrose path believing that there is little danger of losing control."[7] This seems to make such people's addiction voluntary. But they were mistaken about the risks. Should their ignorance excuse them from responsibility?

Ignorance excuses, unless it is culpable. Was it possible to find out the risks? Should they have taken the trouble to do so? Answers vary in different cases. Distressed parents and friends may say he always brushed aside their many warnings. At the other extreme is a child of 8, with no idea of any risk, liking the smell of glue and becoming addicted. Or someone may not know about her own rare genetic susceptibility to an addiction. Degrees of knowledge and control can vary in ways hard to trace.

The more obviously voluntary route is "walking the tightrope"—seeing the danger but not caring, or even being drawn to the risk. But even here there may be a hint of compulsion. Some people are "sensation seeking," looking for intense experiences, often through risk in sports, driving, unsafe sex, or drugs. This is correlated with addiction to Internet dependence and with online gaming.[8] Evidence suggests that genetic polymorphisms linked to the dopamine system play a role in sensation seeking.[9] It is not known how difficult this makes it to resist walking the tightrope. Even this route may be less voluntary than it seems.

These different pathways into addiction are like weather. Larger social and psychiatric problems are climate. Addicts are disproportionately poor people, victims of abuse in childhood, or have other psychiatric problems. In one British study, people diagnosed with personality disorders made up 4.4 percent of the general population.[10] A Dutch study found they were 78 percent of drug users and 91 percent of alcoholics.[11]

"Secondary" addiction comes from these problems and pressures. People choose to take an addictive substance to escape them and become trapped: "Both alcohol and benzos did produce some sort of safe feeling . . . It was more of an existential anxiety involving not feeling safe in my own skin . . . I found some substance that alleviated a certain kind of inchoate fear . . . I used it. Eventually it produced a much worse dreadfulness than the fear it initially provided relief from. But by then I couldn't find my way to stop."[12]

One woman describes some of what she escaped from into alcohol: "A basic fragility; a feeling of hypersensitivity to other people's reactions, as though some piece of my soul might crumble if you looked at me the wrong way; a sense of being essentially inferior and unproductive and scared. Feelings of fraudulence are familiar to scores of people in and out of the working world—the highly effective, well-defended exterior cloaking the small, insecure person inside—but they're epidemic among alcoholics. You hide behind the professional persona all day; then you leave the office and hide behind the drink."[13]

Many addicts describe trying to escape the pressures of these feelings of fear, inadequacy, or worthlessness.[14] They are like Aristotle's sailor blown off course by a strong wind, except that here the wind is internal. This is where Aristotle's view conflicts with modern psychiatry.

The thought that addiction is voluntary comes from the way it normally stems from choices made and then repeated. But the thought is too simple. It ignores inner pressures. People's inner history is usually elusive when someone else wonders if they could help becoming addicts. Even where the history seems fairly clear, there is usually no single question with an all-or-none answer. There are complex questions about how far ignorance was culpable or how far a genetic predisposition could be resisted. And about how strong the pressures were on the small, insecure person inside the well-defended exterior. To most of these questions, the brisk answer is too brisk.

We are not all addicts, but we all know weakness of will. Benefits of a healthy lifestyle are long-term, but at this moment coffee and conversation easily trump a brisk walk. Reluctant addicts are extreme cases of weakness of will. There is the moment of the weak-willed decision to have another drink or to gamble one more time. And there are further motivational problems obstructing attempts to escape addiction. Chemical hijacking may often have a role, but so can other psychological vulnerabilities.

Being in control is being able to take and implement decisions. The processes underlying decision and action are complex, so in unwilling addiction, control can fail in different ways. In current psychology there is an influential two-track model of decision making. One track is planning: consciously investigating and evaluating different possibilities. Planning gives relatively reliable results because its response to new information is flexible. But it is slow. An alternative is to act intuitively. The intuitions may come from stored memory of what has worked before. Intuitive decisions are rapid but their rigidity makes them less reliable.[15]

This is linked to the contrast between computer and human chess. The "brute force" of computer chess-playing, scanning millions of results, is a vastly accelerated and more thorough version of planning. By contrast, the intuitive human strategies are often rooted in the "feel" memory gives for which moves have promise and which are nonstarters. Often the best strategies combine computer scans with human intuition. Something similar seems to hold for good decision making in general. It calls on both. The skill is seeing when to switch backward and forward between slow, thorough planning and rapid but less reliable intuition.

This two-track model has been used to map how patterns of addiction reflect different vulnerabilities in decision making.[16] Intuitions can be fooled by the hijacking of neurotransmitter systems into overvaluing a drug not really liked. Planning is vulnerable to distortions in beliefs about the situation: in slot machine games a gambler may see patterns not really there. Planning is also liable to "judgment shift," where the pressure of the addictive urge leads the person to downgrade the importance of the values it threatens.[17] Or the switching between the two tracks can fail: chemical hijacking can make it hard for the planning system to override a misguided habit.

Efforts to escape addiction are hindered by further problems. Some of these affect willpower and stamina. Others are subtle cognitive distortions affecting the sense of agency.

Motivating Resistance: Problems of Willpower and Stamina

According to one influential picture of free will, found in Immanuel Kant and many others, desires are the products of causes but the will somehow transcends them. The strength of different desires is caused by levels of sex hormones, or by the person's degree of hunger, thirst, or tiredness, and so on. But this leaves the person free to choose which desires to act on and which to override. This freedom is seen in terms of the will being outside the causal realm. Philosophers going back at least to Thomas Hobbes have doubted that the will is in this way outside the world of causes. Modern psychology is starting to colonize the will on behalf of the causal realm.

Strength can be exhausted by heavy physical tasks. There is evidence that willpower too can be depleted by repeated demands on it.[18] In some experiments people were asked to do stressful things. They had to control their emotions while watching a distressing clip, to list their thoughts while trying not to think of a white bear, or to eat only radishes while next to delicious-smelling freshly baked food. People need willpower for these tasks. Afterward they showed less physical or mental stamina in second tasks. In these they were asked to trace impossible geometrical figures, to solve anagrams, or to keep a painful grip on a handle. They gave up more quickly than control groups.

These unenticing second tasks may not have inspired much commitment. But even when people are committed, stamina seems to fade. In one study people already making a serious effort to diet were less able than nondieters to resist eating ice cream placed temptingly near them.[19]

Neil Levy has argued that this depletion of willpower helps explain why addictions can be so much easier to resist for a short time than for long periods. People oscillate in what they most want: to escape addiction or to give way to it. However, different strengths of the addictive desire may not be the whole explanation. Varying strengths of the willpower opposing the desire may also be part of the story.[20]

Perseverance with dreary and frustrating tasks can reduce willpower. But as Janet Treasure has pointed out, "motivational interviews" may increase it. Interviewers show people conflicts between their actions and what they care about, and help give them hope they can change. There is evidence that this procedure helps build stamina in resisting addiction.[21] Other evidence suggests that willpower is less depleted when the earlier task is more autonomous. People in one study were asked not to eat something tempting. Those who refrained because they had chosen to diet showed less depletion than those who were simply obeying the instruction.[22] In general, there is support for the comparison likening willpower to a muscle. In the short term either physical exercise or exercising willpower can lead to exhaustion. But the habit of such exercise develops strength.[23]

Fostering Awareness of Agency

Fostering the sense of agency is central. As Hannah Pickard and Steve Pearce have argued, if something seems impossible, it is hard to see how a person can form the intention to do it.[24] ("Just decide to sprout wings and fly away.") This is part of something more general. The difficulty of escaping addiction is compounded by the self-fulfilling belief that it is too difficult. And this paralyzing belief is supported by a crude view of decision making, one too readily seen as obviously correct.

Part of building awareness of agency is helping addicts escape from the crude view: from what Jay Wallace has called "the hydraulic model." This portrays desires as being just like physical forces, with the strongest simply winning.[25] As Wallace has pointed out, some decisions are like this, but many others are not so simple.

Some conflicts are settled by brute strength of desire. A runner, thirsty and exhausted after a race, can either collapse into a chair or walk for five minutes to get water. His choice depends only on which he wants more. He is almost passive, letting the desires fight it out. He discovers he wants rest more than water by finding that he slumps into the chair. It wasn't just collapse, but had an element of decision. Told he would die without water, he would have gone to drink. Such marginal cases of decision fit the hydraulic model.

When pressures are weaker, there is room for active decisions. The strongest desire at the moment of decision does win, but it is possible to influence which desire that is. At one point someone's strongest desire may be to get rich. By the time of deciding what job to try for, that desire may have been weakened. Active questioning can contribute. Why do I want to be rich? What would I do with the money? How will getting rich change me? And so on. The more active decision goes deeper and expresses more of ourselves.

There are ways of fostering these more active decisions. Hanna Pickard and Steve Pearce, drawing on their work in the Oxford Complex Needs Service, picture a therapeutic community in which people are encouraged both to support each other and to look for deeper understanding of themselves.[26] At the core of this is the hope of being able to change. For this, the person needs to see that change may be possible: "We do not help patients by thinking that, at a certain point, they are in a sense beyond help. If we do not explicitly treat them as responsible agents, capable of choosing to make changes for the better in their lives, then it is less likely that they will find a way to treat themselves as such."[27]

Active decision making may include thinking about how one choice will affect other choices. This suggests that things you want, like avoiding alcoholism, are to a surprising extent at risk from a single choice.

People discount future benefits and harms compared to present ones. Given this, how do people stop addictive drinking? Liver disease may be years away. A drink now may be tempting, and just one will hardly make a noticeable difference. It can seem surprising that people ever resist.

There are strategies against the weakening effects of this discounting. George Ainslie argues that the calculations should include our own psychology.[28] If this time we give in, why suppose we will act differently another time? Each defeat lowers the expectation of future success. And expecting failure makes success even harder. Knowing all this pushes us further into a downward spiral. It turns out that, when deciding about one more drink, the whole fight against ill health is at stake. So we have much more incentive to resist. Resisting this time helps us expect we can do so again and so may start an upward spiral. Because choices influence each other, they should be considered together in bundles. This helps us make and follow supportive rules.

This self-awareness opposes weakness of will. Thoughts about spirals help control the wayward desire. When someone is in the grip of addiction, winning is much harder. Reminders given early of psychological spirals may help more than those given later.

The core of unwilling addiction is weakness of will. Unwilling addicts need to develop willpower to escape. This supports the view of Socrates quoted at the start of this chapter: The thing they can abide least of all is someone telling them the truth—that until they stop getting drunk, stuffing themselves, whoring, and doing no work, no medicine or cautery or surgery, and no spell or amulet or anything like that either, is going to do them the slightest good. The view is often expressed, as in this passage, in terms heavy with blame and disapproval.

But Coleridge's plea, also quoted above, brings out how unfair the blame may be: You bid me rouse myself—"go, bid a man paralytic in both arms rub them briskly together, & that will cure him." It may be unfair because, as we have seen, the question of how far a person could have prevented themselves from becoming an addict is often very difficult to answer. It may be unfair because in some cases the escape from addiction can be, as Coleridge suggests, too difficult. Coleridge, like some other addicts, may have been wrong about his own case. But as with the sentry falling asleep after struggling long to keep awake, there are irresistible desires. It is extremely hard to know where the blurred boundary comes between what is resistible and what is irresistible.

It is psychologically difficult to hold simultaneously the two perspectives we need. We should be reluctant to blame, because we are unsure how much freedom of action a particular addict has. On the other hand, the key to helping addicts is fostering their sense that they may be able to resist.

Often a lot of willpower is needed to overcome the intense desires that sometimes are produced by hijacked neurotransmitter systems. Perhaps disconcertingly, willpower itself no longer seems a fully autonomous force. Its strength may vary according to different causal histories. But a causal account of the will does not destroy agency. Causal explanation does not obliterate the distinction between active decisions and those that fit the hydraulic model. Causation is not an argument for fatalism. Agency with a causal story behind it is still agency.

In supporting someone's escape from addiction, the default assumption should be that resistance may be possible: that willpower, like a muscle, can grow with exercise. Challenging crude models of decision making can be important in fostering the hope of escape. Sometimes that hope can be self-fulfilling.

25

Character, Personality Disorder, and Responsibility

> As in our own society a scientific theory of causation, if not excluded, is deemed irrelevant in questions of moral and legal responsibility, so in Zande society the doctrine of witchcraft, if not excluded, is deemed irrelevant in the same situations. We accept scientific explanations of the causes of disease, and even of the causes of insanity, but we deny them in crime and sin because here they militate against law and morals which are axiomatic.
>
> —E. E. Evans-Prichard, *Witchcraft, Oracles and Magic among the Azande*

Some psychiatric conditions can take over a person's character and change it. They include some dementias and also schizophrenia. They come on after the person's original character and personality have developed. We can (to some extent) oppose the person to the character-distorting illness.

Some other conditions go deeper, to shape a person's original core. These "foundational" conditions, including autism and some personality disorders, are more fully present much earlier. They do not appear to strike people from outside. Even where early environment plays an important role, there is no alternative "real" person, remembered by friends and family but now submerged by the disorder.

Antisocial Personality Disorder and the Case of Mr. H

As we saw in Part 1, some of the Broadmoor interviewees suggested that their childhoods may have strongly influenced the people they became. They did not choose that kind of childhood. Does this then mean that it is unfair to blame them for how they turned out and for what they did as adults? I want to look at this line of thought applied to a particular person,

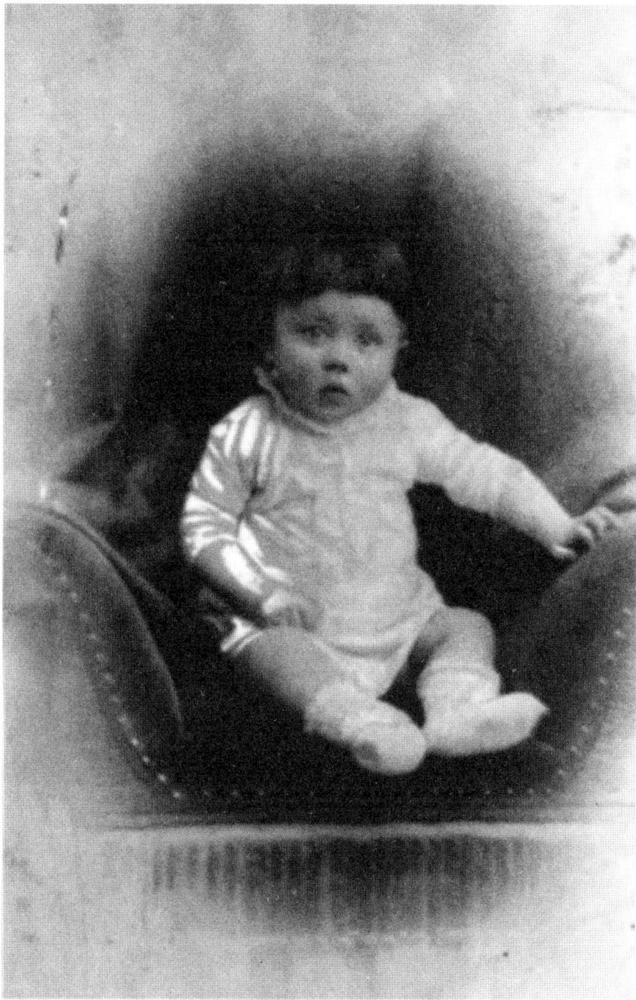

Figure 25.1: Mr. H as a young child. Bundesarchiv Bild 183-1989-0322-506.

without describing a possibly identifiable Broadmoor patient. The person to be considered, although he never had a psychiatric diagnosis, clearly illustrates the combination of a cruel childhood with a distorted adult psychology.

Mr. H, pictured as a baby in Figure 25.1, had an unhappy childhood. His father was strict and had a terrible temper. He was a "demon" about punctuality. He insisted on silence in the family. The children never dared speak in his presence unless spoken to and were not allowed to call him anything less formal than "Father." When the father summoned his son, he never called him by name but always whistled for him in the way he called the dog. The father often beat the dog, his wife, and each of the children. The adult Mr. H remembered having once been given 230 strokes of the cane by his father. He also said he remembered seeing his drunken father rape his mother.

Mr. H grew up with a very rigid personality. As an adult he was obsessed with cleanliness, passionately hating any untidiness or dirt. He was also obsessed with wolves, sometimes thinking of himself as a wolf, and calling his Alsatian dog "Wolf." He took the dog for exactly the same walk every day, throwing a stick for it at exactly the same place. Any suggestion of varying these routines made him agitated and angry. He hated being left alone at night, and hated the moon because he thought it was dead. He was obsessed with his own possible death from cancer, which his mother had died from.

Mr. H had difficulties in his love life. As a boy he had been terrified of being kissed. His first love affair came when he was 37. It was with a teenage girl, who tried to kill herself when he abruptly broke off the relationship. He then fell in love with his niece, who did not reciprocate his feelings. She killed herself with his pistol. At age 41 he had another affair, with an 18-year-old girl who made an unsuccessful suicide attempt early in their relationship. Mr. H seems to have been disgusted by normal sexual intercourse, saying he did not want it because he would become infected. His niece said his main sexual pleasure was getting her to urinate on his face.

Much of his emotional life seems to have been diverted to patriotism and politics. He fought in a war, with great patriotic enthusiasm. He was temporarily blinded in a gas attack, which left him with great resentment against those who did not fight in the war. He took up extreme right-wing politics and was passionately anti-Semitic. He was highly successful at appealing to the public. He became leader of his country. He started a world war. He ordered the systematic murder of millions of his fellow citizens. He killed himself when his country lost the war.

Now that Mr. H's identity has emerged, there are questions about how, if at all, his childhood and its effects on his character and personality are relevant to our reaction to him and to what he did.[1]

Rigidity, sexual problems, neurotic health worries, obsessive racial hatred, extreme anger and resentment, fixations about dogs and the moon: these are things people are better off without. They perhaps suggest he was a candidate for being diagnosed with a personality disorder. But there is not much mileage in the idea that the real Mr. H is not reflected in all this. There is no reason to believe he had a quite different unexpressed personality. The anger and the anti-Semitism were characteristics as genuinely his as it is possible to find.

Mr. H raises in acute form the problem of personality disorder. The excuses that normally defend someone's character from criticism all fail. There is no conflict in which a set of higher-order desires or deeper values is defeated. There is no alternative obscured "real" self. If blame is a negative evaluation of character on the basis of actions, it is hard to see how Mr. H can escape it.

And yet, as with the Broadmoor interviewees, this seems not quite the whole story. In the interviews, although I did not ask the interviewees about their early life, they often talked about childhoods of pain, rejection, and humiliation. It was natural to see them too as victims, to glimpse their life from the inside and to feel sympathy. The emotional responses to what they have suffered and to the terrible things they have done are hard to reconcile. Sometimes, going back from the hospital after hearing about both, I struggled to get the two perspectives into one coherent picture.

When a terrible childhood is offered as an excuse, people often reply with what can be called "the dismissive response": most children treated in this way do not grow up to commit the rapes and murders that lead to Broadmoor, or crimes like those of Mr. H. The suggestion is that even people given a desperately bad start have a choice about how to respond to it. So those making worse choices than others with similar childhoods can be blamed for this. Environmental determinism is too crude.

The Effects of Combining Genetic Risk with an Adverse Childhood

The story certainly is more complex. Some of it is starting to be unraveled. One study followed the development of 442 males born in 1972–1973 in the New Zealand city of Dunedin. Terrie Moffitt, Avshalom Caspi, and others investigated how far either a particular genetic polymorphism or childhood ill-treatment are linked with later antisocial tendencies.[2]

Several measures were made of "antisocial" outcome: an adolescent diagnosis of conduct disorder; convictions in adulthood for violent crime, a personality assessment of aggression, or reports (by people who know them well) of symptoms of antisocial personality disorder.

The genetic variant they studied affected the gene that encodes monoamine oxidase A (MAOA). Low levels of MAOA are plausibly linked to aggression. It is the enzyme that metabolizes some neurotransmitters, including norepinephrine, serotonin, and dopamine. Early ill-treatment affects all these transmitter systems.

Of the male cohort studied, 37 percent had the "risk" variant linked with low MAOA activity. In childhood, 36 percent of the cohort were ill-treated—8 percent had maltreatment graded as severe, and 28 percent had maltreatment graded as probable. The study found that severe ill-treatment on its own increased the likelihood of the antisocial outcome, as did the "risk" genetic variant on its own. Neither increase was dramatic.

But there was a much higher increase in the probability of antisocial outcome when boys with the genetic risk were also rated as "probable or severe" cases of maltreatment. They were 12 percent of the population and had 44 percent of the convictions for violent crime. Moffitt and Caspi claim that, of those with the genetic risk who were also severely maltreated, 85 percent developed some sort of antisocial outcome.

It might be wondered if attempts to repeat the study would bring the very high figures down a bit. Terrie Moffitt quotes another study as supporting the impact on antisocial tendencies of combining genetic risk with maltreatment.[3] This was a Virginia twin study, which showed the impact of the combination, but at less dramatic levels.[4] In this study, combining the genetic risk with childhood adversity raised the level of diagnoses of conduct disorder (from 15 percent with childhood adversity only) to 35 percent. The contrast between the two results may be explained partly by differences between conduct disorder and the Dunedin measures of antisocial outcome. The Virginia study also used a different assessment of childhood adversity, based on parental neglect, violence between parents, and inconsistent discipline.

The considerable difference between the two studies' methods and results makes it hard to assess the extent of the multiplying effect of combining genetic risk with adverse childhoods. But even if the figure were the much lower one of the Virginia study, the general conclusion would remain striking. Adding genetic risk to an adverse childhood would still more than double the level of conduct disorder.

Part of the complex emotional response to hearing about the childhoods of Broadmoor interviewees or of Mr. H. can be some secular version of "there but for the grace of God go I." This looks less of a worry if the dismissive response is right: most people override bad childhoods.

If the claimed excuse is not a bad childhood alone but one combined with a genetic risk, though, the dismissive response looks less impressive. It is not so clear that most people can override this combination. Depending on how the figures finally settle down, it seems that the number who do not manage to override it may be somewhere between 35 percent and 85 percent. We do not know the full causal story that led to the crimes of the Broadmoor interviewees or to the crimes of Mr. H. So we cannot be confident that we would have responded differently to the upbringing they had. Of course we all hope that, given that terrible childhood, we would not have been like Hitler. No doubt many of us would not. But certainty here is overconfidence. This adds a disquieting perspective to our attitudes to Mr. H and to other possibly personality-disordered people who have done terrible things.

Decision and Action: Determinism without Fatalism

> Suppose, for example, one's values or "higher order" desires have been instilled in one in an unreflective, coercive way. Even if one is able to make one's "lower order" desires march in step, there is a sense in which one's whole harmonious will is an expression of enslavement . . . he is not free from his environment, for he has not engaged in a process of separation and individuation. His will cannot be free because it is not his will.
>
> —Jonathan Lear, *Love and Its Place in Nature*

Despite skepticism discussed earlier, what most people intuitively believe seems likely: our deliberations shape our decisions, and our decisions cause our actions. But what is the full causal story behind our deliberations and decisions? Despite the growing contributions of genetics, epigenetics, perhaps quantum physics, neuroscience, psychology, and the social sciences, we still have large areas of ignorance about the springs of action. But scientific progress is reducing our ignorance. There seems no reason to expect this stop.

This suggests the thought that one day we could have a full causal account of decision and action. Some deny this. Those of us who accept the possibility divide over whether it is welcome. "At the whim of those chemicals" may be too simple. As I said at the end of Chapter 24, agency with a causal story is still agency. But the studies just discussed suggest a considerable narrowing of possibilities when an adverse childhood is combined with just one genetic risk factor. If just these two factors change the picture in this way, how may things look when we know about many more?

Might not a full causal account mean that we are, after all, at the whim of a combination of our DNA, epigenetic factors influencing its expression, our mother's anxiety during pregnancy, other influences in the womb, our brain chemistry, early parenting, our degree of secure attachment, and thousands of other interacting biological and social factors? If one day this is all understood, will we not be looking at a totally determinist picture? And will that picture really leave room for genuine agency?

Some of those worried by this would like determinism not to be true. They hope that there will, in principle, be some gaps in the causal story, so that not everything about our decisions and actions is even in principle predictable. But indeterminism does not give much help to free agency. How can we tell the difference between an uncaused event—say at the level of neurochemistry—and one whose cause just has not yet been discovered?

Perhaps an answer to this question might emerge from quantum physics. Even if a decision could be shown to be partly uncaused, though, there is the problem identified in the eighteenth century by David Hume. How does lack of a complete causal story make a decision free rather than just random?[5] On a pessimistic view, free agency is incompatible with indeterminist randomness and with determinism. As these seem to exhaust the possibilities, free agency appears impossible. Perhaps this is too pessimistic. But looking for uncaused events is less promising than aiming for an account of agency compatible with determinism.

The first step toward this is to recognize that determinism does not entail the fatalist view that things will be as they will be, regardless of what people do. Fatalism has absurd implications. If it were true, a person's decision to drive when drunk makes no difference to anything: the accident would have happened whatever he decided. This view need not detain us.

There is a slightly more subtle picture. Our decisions issue in actions that do make a difference to the world, but our genes, neurochemistry, and so on in turn are causal influences on our deliberation and our decisions. As we have seen, it is implausible in most cases to think of our deliberation as passive or ineffective. Through it, we can change what we most want. We can look at the possibly coercive environmental influences that shaped our values, and decide whether or not to make those values truly ours. We actively decide many things on the basis of weighing reasons, and what we decide leads to one kind of action, or toward becoming one kind of person rather than another. This may well be a fully causal process, but that does not make it less ours.

It is self-defeating to give determinism as a reason for deciding never to make decisions based on reasons. In a determinist world, our reasoning can be (and usually will be) part of the causal process influencing decision and action.

Two Perspectives on Agency, Two Perspectives on People

There is a tension between two views expressed in comments already quoted from different Broadmoor interviewees.

The first is: "I mean, I chose the route I've took, solely myself . . . I've chose it, so really my destiny as such was laid out by me. It wasn't laid out before and said, 'Right, your destiny is to end up in Broadmoor in 30 years' time.' I mean I actually walked the road that led me here. You know, no one pushed me along."

These thoughts are completely right. But in psychiatry, as in much of life, they are often only one side of the story. Sometimes even where a person does decide on an action and carries it out, it would have been difficult or impossible to have chosen an alterative. This comes out in the second comment, from another interviewee: "It worries me that eventually I will do these things and I don't want to particularly want to—difficult for me actually to say no to them . . . They involve kidnapping, rape and violence, and murder, so . . . *If you could choose not to have these thoughts?* I am trying to. That's a choice that I've already made, that I'm trying . . . At the moment I'm trying chemical castration, to work on the fantasies, which will do away with the sex and the murder/violence fantasies that I have, but I ain't having a great deal of success with it."

Understanding these issues needs both these viewpoints on agency. This is a central dilemma for anyone thinking about the responsibility of people acting under the influence of some psychiatric disorders. These two quoted thoughts do not sit comfortably together, but each expresses an important truth applying far outside the walls of Broadmoor. Acts influenced by addiction are not "fated" but really are the person's choice. Accepting agency rather than fatalism can be crucial in escaping addiction and other conditions. But it is also true that such psychiatric problems can greatly impair the power to choose.

Are the reactive attitudes appropriate as responses to antisocial acts of people who have been diagnosed with antisocial personality disorder?

What counts against this is that the condition is still at least partly, and perhaps largely, a piece of bad luck. There are constraints on self-creation. If the condition was caused by having particular genes, or by what happened in the womb, none of this was under the person's control. If it was caused by parental rejection, cruelty, or abuse, none of this was the person's own fault. Such people are themselves victims. So blame and resentment seem unfair.

On the other hand, to withhold the reactive attitudes is to exclude those individuals from a central part of human relationships. This also seems unfair. And it may be that participating in human relationships, including the spirals of reactive attitudes, is the only chance those individuals have to transcend the limits of their original personality.

The reactive attitudes are not totally under our control. We cannot just switch them on and off at will to bring about the best consequences. But we have a degree of choice about how far we do or do not inhibit them. To the extent that we have a choice of response (say, to aggressive violence stemming from antisocial personality disorder), something complex seems called for. This includes retaining the reactive attitudes to the person's own appalling attitudes toward his victims. But it also includes remembering that he is a victim too, that his character has been badly shaped by causes largely outside his control. This dual response is not easy, as I found in the interviews in Broadmoor.

It is probably right that we cannot entirely, or even largely, abandon the reactive attitudes. It is also probably right that, even if we could, life would be impoverished if we did. But there is also a determinist thought that should make us uncomfortable about these attitudes. It is about those of us who do not have personality disorders. As Aristotle saw, we shape our characters by our own voluntary actions. Yet there is likely to be some causal explanation of how we came to choose some actions rather than others. And these causal explanations may often go back to factors beyond our control: to early childhood, or further back to the womb or to genes.

For us, as for those diagnosed with antisocial personality disorder, some important parts of our psychology certainly belong to us yet are not mainly of our own making. In the long run, the dual response we develop to people with some psychiatric disorders may turn out to be appropriate to the rest of us as well.

PART SIX

Identity

Dear Doctor: I am feeling very sick. I have a heart in my stomach which throbs and mocks. Suddenly the simple rituals of the day balk like a stubborn horse. It gets impossible to look people in the eye: corruption may break out again? Who knows. Small talk becomes desperate.

Hostility grows, too. That dangerous, deadly venom which comes from a sick heart. Sick mind, too. The image of identity we must daily fight to impress on the neutral, or hostile world, collapses inward; we feel crushed.

—Sylvia Plath, *Journals*, February 20, 1956

Aware of how little I was able to show my true self, I insisted that my name was not Donna any more and that I was to be called Lee . . . At home I would still spend hours in front of the mirror, staring into my own eyes and whispering my name over and over, sometimes trying to call myself back, at other times becoming frightened at losing my ability to feel myself.

—Donna Williams, *Nobody Nowhere: The Remarkable Autobiography of an Autistic Girl*

They had warned me that I was likely to fall into a depression: a high and then a low. The inevitable sequence of the cyclothyme, which was what I appeared to be. What they had not told me was that I would end up at such a distance from myself, such a hopeless distance.

—Roger Garfitt, *The Horseman's Word*

26

The Sense of Self

As features of the good life, agency and identity are in mutual support. Awareness of one's own agency is an important part of having a sense of self, and psychiatric conditions disrupting one often disrupt the other. In this chapter psychiatric disruptions will be used briefly to indicate some contours of the sense of self. People care about feeling at home in their own body, "being comfortable in their own skin." They need recognition by others to create a secure awareness of being the person they are. Without this, efforts to create an identity may be shallow and self-defeating. People can also care about their moral identity, wanting to shape the *kind* of person they are.

The Bodily Expression of the Self

Bodily shape may not fit a person's idea of the shape they should be. It may not fit the person they feel they are. The feeling of such conflict in gender identity disorder has been succinctly expressed by Jan Morris: "But it all seemed plain enough to me. I was born with the wrong body, being feminine by gender but male by sex, and I could achieve completeness only when the one was adjusted to the other."[1]

There is a something similar in body integrity identity disorder. People with this disorder feel that some bit of their body is not part of them, and so want it amputated. This can involve great distress, suicidal feelings, and even attempts at self-amputation.[2] They may feel it when the offending arm or a leg is touched, but the appendage does not become part of their body image.[3]

Evidence links this to poor functioning of mechanisms in the right parietal lobe that map actual bodily boundaries on to the person's body-image. One response might be that it is the body image, rather than the body, that needs adjusting. But we have no means of adjusting the body image, so it is amputation or nothing. Obviously, help offered should reflect the facts of each person's case. But refusing an informed and considered request for amputation would need reasons strong enough to outweigh the distress of the felt mismatch: "BIID seems weird and alien at first, but it is a very real condition that affects a lot of people. I have needed to be paraplegic as far back as I can remember . . . 'First do no harm.' But the surgeons' refusal to help us is actually what is doing harm. You cannot begin to understand the amount of anguish and emotional pain we live with. Day after day. Refusing us surgery, the only thing that actually helps with BIID symptoms, is condemning us to a life of utter misery."[4]

The Deep or Shallow Sense of Self, and the Empty Jar

> I'm horrible, I told the man at the other end of the phone. I hate myself. I'm crazy. It would really surprise him that once upon a time I used to be somebody, I used to accomplish things.
>
> —Rachel Reiland, *Get Me Out of Here: My Recovery from Borderline Personality Disorder*

Some of the men interviewed in Broadmoor wanted recognition and had been denied it. As children they felt hardly noticed—not picked up from school, or for years not visited in the hospital. They would have been pleased just to be seen, wanted, accepted, and loved for who they were. These are likely foundations of the deeper sense of self: the secure and untroubled awareness of the distinct person you are.

One conjecture put forward earlier about the Broadmoor patients was that denial of recognition aroused in them a hunger for it. Some of them tried to satisfy this hunger in shallow ways—wanting to impress other people, and themselves, that they were really "somebody." This shallow way of being "somebody" evades the deeper sense of self. Gwen Adshead's comment that some of the Broadmoor patients were "not very real to themselves" touched on this. Having not been recognized or not been respected themselves, they might not have learned through the usual reciprocity to recognize and respect others. If this is right, they may have a weak sense both of other people and of themselves.

There are other causes of the failure to develop a deep sense of self. Gunilla Gerland has described her autism partly in terms of a sense of personal emptiness. This also was linked to lack of recognition. She was different from nonautistic people. She felt that their mental maps had no space for the person she was: "I was trying to be someone, but *I* didn't seem to exist among all the possibilities available, so it had to be someone else." This left her feeling she had no character of her own: "I felt I was empty. I had peeled away the unafraid person, those individual characteristics, the special tastes I had as a child. I hardly knew what I liked at all now. I didn't know if I was hungry or satisfied. I didn't know what kind of music I liked, or whether I liked music at all. I didn't know whether I liked the books I was reading or whether I just read them anyway. I didn't know if I preferred doing one thing or another."

Having lost her own individuality, she borrowed from other people, but this left her with no sense of any self of her own: "People asked me what I wanted, what I thought. I took features from people I met and added them to me. I often took features from people who seemed very self-confident. I did this immensely skilfully. I became a chameleon—if I adopted Karin's way of sighing as she spoke, I could use it with everyone except Karin, and if I adopted Maria's taste in music, then I didn't talk about music with Maria. I was an empty jar that could be filled with anything. People's behavior simply fell into the jar and I used it to try to feel myself someone, like a real person. I developed this strategy in order to be able to relate to people. If you were no one, you couldn't relate—you had to be someone."

But this borrowing to relate actually hollowed out relationships: "I sensed that Dirk liked the features I had adopted from other people. He didn't know he was having a relationship not with me but with a woman I had invented. It couldn't work. How could it have done? The invented woman wasn't real. She was empty, and I who was playing her was not real either. No one, not even I myself, had ever seen me as I really was. Things got worse when more intimacy was called for. Imitation couldn't rise to it—I didn't know who I should be. I started screening myself off . . . Dirk was annoyed when, as he put it, I disappeared into the wall. I just wasn't present, he said."[5] Helping people escape this emptiness raises difficult questions about what makes characteristics, tastes, and desires authentically one's own.

Moral Identity

As well as caring about being "somebody," people care about the kind of somebody they are. Many—though perhaps not all—care about the pattern that emerges, wanting their life to add up to something. This can be reflected in what they contribute to the world or to a few people close to them. Or it can be about achievements that may not reverberate into the lives of others. (One obituary of an Oxford academic, with the fine discrimination examiners show between alpha and alpha minus, said he was a great, perhaps even a very great, collector of books.) It can be a sense of moral identity, to care about the kind of person you are—wanting to be a person whose life is shaped by *these* values, not those. Moral identity also can be damaged in ways that call for help.

27

Moral Identity and Moral Injury: Combat Trauma

> My conscience seems to become little by little sooted . . . [H., accused of being the local Gestapo agent] was an old man of seventy. His wife and he looked frightened and old and miserable. I was quite harsh to him and remember threatening him with an investigation . . Day before yesterday word came that he and his wife had committed suicide . . . At the bedside was a card on which he had scrawled: "We must perish miserably. God forgive us. We have done no one any harm." The incident affected me strongly and still does. I was directly or indirectly the cause of their death . . . I hope it does not rest too hard on my conscience, and yet if it does not I shall be disturbed also.
>
> —J. Glenn Gray, *The Warriors: Reflections on Men in Battle,* quoting his own 1945 wartime journal

In the 1982 Falklands War, 256 British combatants were killed. Twenty years later, in 2002, the South Atlantic Medal Association said that those killed during the war were outnumbered by the 264 former combatants who had committed suicide.[1] In both 2009 and 2010, more active-duty U.S. troops committed suicide than were killed fighting in Iraq and Afghanistan. In 2010 there were 468 suicides compared to 462 killed in combat.[2] By 2011 there were 197,074 soldiers (about 15 percent of the total number back from Iraq and Afghanistan) being treated for post-traumatic stress disorder.[3] These psychiatric conditions are a major feature of modern war. In some of them, but not in others, the soldier's sense of moral identity has taken a battering.

Trauma and Unhealed Wounds

Agent-Reaction

> In my opinion, the person who went to the Falklands and the person who returned are two different people. I feel I lost my boy in the war, only he didn't die. I fear it is only a matter of time before he takes his own life and finally gets some peace.
>
> —Tony McNally's father, in Tony McNally, *Watching Men Burn: A Soldier's Story*

In the Falklands War, Tony McNally was a rapier missile operator. His job was to shoot down Argentinean aircraft attacking British targets. Because of a technical fault, when he aimed at Argentinean planes attacking the British ship *Sir Galahad,* pressing the fire button did nothing. The bombs exploded on the ship, which was laden with fuel and ammunition. Forty-eight men were killed, with many more were badly burned and wounded: "Soldiers were jumping into the water, their clothes on fire, as others ran around on the deck trying to get off. As the carnage unfolded in front of me, I could do nothing but stand there, watching men burn . . . The Paras turned their anger on us, screaming and shouting obscenities . . . How do you explain that it wasn't our fault? That a fuse had blown, or the computer had crashed?"[4]

The aftermath of this experience was felt much later. "As night fell, we switched to our normal routine—food, sentry duty and sleep. It sounds harsh, but life had to go on. It's no use crying over burnt Guardsmen, and we didn't. Though it would eventually hit me hard, very hard—terrible feelings of guilt, sobbing tears, horrific flashbacks, wishing I'd died out there myself—my mind had shut down those emotions for the time being. All that lay a good ten years in the future."[5]

Back in England, the problems started. "I went totally berserk with my family a week or so into the leave. We had a row about something irrelevant and I smashed up the house and stormed out. That night I dug a trench in the garden and slept in there, wearing my combat gear . . . It was obviously very odd behaviour—though I didn't realise it at the time—and I slid further and further out of control . . . I'd wake up, often in a cold sweat, at 2 a.m. or 3 a.m., and find myself replaying the events of the attack on the *Galahad* over and over again in my head."[6]

Some years later the factory where Tony McNally worked was closed down. He had no hope of finding work. He felt low and the nightmares of death and horror started again. "I thought a lot about the *Sir Galahad,* and would find myself in tears, wondering why the fucking Rapier hadn't fired, feeling a mountain of guilt on my shoulders for all those deaths and the awful injuries of many of the survivors."[7] Later he had terrible flashbacks and night terrors, and became violent and destructive. His wife tried hard to cope, but "I'd put her through hell" and she left him, as did his second wife.

No one could reasonably hold Tony McNally responsible for the deaths of the troops on the *Sir Galahad.* The technical failure was out of his control. But the terrible feelings of guilt, however unjustified, are part of a cluster of natural human reactions. A suicidal person jumps in front of a train. The train driver is in no way to blame, but he is still likely to feel terrible. Before backing out of the parking space, the driver takes all reasonable precautions, including checking in the mirror to see that no one is behind his car. But he runs over a small child, too low to be seen, who had crawled into his path. The car driver's role is more active than that of the train driver, but he still cannot reasonably be held responsible. He will still feel terrible, though, because "It was me who ran over her"—what Bernard Williams called "agent regret."[8]

Nancy Sherman has rightly said that in military contexts the phrase is inadequate: "'Regret' for these kinds of tragedies is, in fact, too light a word, not close enough to remorse and too close to the kind of regret we feel about inclement weather."[9] So, although the term "agent regret" is well entrenched in philosophy, here "agent reaction" may be a better phrase. Tony McNally's agent reaction to its being his gun that failed was long-lasting. It shows how much a matter of bad luck, how unfair, and yet how devastating, feelings of guilt and self-blame can be.

Killing Believed Justified

Karl Marlantes grew up in Oregon. Aged 19 and with Marine training, he was in the Marine Corps reserve. After studying at Yale, he was a Rhodes Scholar at Oxford. But in 1968, after one term, he left to fight in Vietnam. He commanded a platoon and was awarded fifteen medals, including the Navy Cross, two Navy Commendations for Valor, and two Purple Hearts. After a year he returned to Oxford and completed his degree in philosophy, politics, and economics. Thirty years after Vietnam he asked Veterans' Affairs for help with his post-traumatic stress disorder.

Once, Marlantes went to shoot two enemy soldiers who were attacking his platoon with grenades. There was "one particular NVA soldier whose desperate fearful eyes I still vividly recall, standing out like black pools in an exploding landscape of mud and dying vegetation . . . I can still see him rising from his hole to throw a hand grenade at me. The wild desperation, the animal cornered . . . His friend crumpled over next to him, dead. He was a teenager, like my radio operator."[10]

Some would believe what Karl Marlantes did was wrong. Absolute pacifists would think so, as would those of us who think the Vietnam War was immoral and that killing in such a war cannot be justified. But Karl Marlantes did not hold either of these views. He believed he was justified in fighting. Given that, it is hard to see he had any rational basis for guilt. Killing an enemy soldier who is attacking your unit, and who is about to throw a grenade at you, is surely one of the easiest acts of wartime killing to justify. And Marlantes clearly did not feel guilt. Asked about it, he said, "Well, it's hard to say that it's guilt. Because I've killed people, more than one. And I feel sadness about it, a great deal of sadness. That's different than guilt."[11]

At the time he felt only exhilaration that the grenade threat was over. But ten years later, in a therapy group, he was asked to imagine saying sorry to the mother and sister of someone he had killed: "Within a minute of starting the apology I broke down wailing like a frightened child. Out came a torrent of terrible memories and remorse. This was the first time I felt any emotion about having killed . . . The crying started again the next day, and would start again days and even weeks afterward and go on for hours at a time. Even at work the faces of dead friends and mutilated bodies on both sides would come unbidden to mind. I'd have to make excuses to go outside where no one could see me shaking, throat aching to hold back the sobs . . . It went on like this for months, until I quit my job. I got into something new and everything went away, until next time. This pattern went on for nearly three decades."[12]

Going Berserk

Jonathan Shay, a Veterans Affairs psychiatrist who has treated the war-induced problems of many returned American soldiers, says that soldiers who rout the enemy single-handedly often have episodes of going berserk. A Marine veteran described one: "He fired and I felt this burning on my cheek . . . I emptied everything I had into him. Then I saw blood dripping on the back of my hand and I just went crazy. I pulled him out into the paddy and carved him up with my knife. When I was done with him he looked like a rag doll that a dog had been playing with . . . I felt betrayed by trying to give the guy a chance and I got blasted. . . . I felt a drastic change after that. I just couldn't get enough. I built up such hate, I couldn't do enough damage . . . Got worse as time went by. I really loved fucking killing, couldn't get enough. For every one I killed I felt better. Made some of the hurt went away [*sic*]. Every time you lost a friend it seemed like part of you was gone. Get one of them to compensate what they had done to me. I got very hard, cold, merciless. I lost all my mercy."[13]

Among the triggers of going berserk, Jonathan Shay lists being wounded, surrounded, overrun, or trapped. He also cites grief at the death of close comrades, compounded as a trigger by the sight of seeing their bodies mutilated by the enemy. This grief can swing between rage and emotional deadness. It can also involve guilt, and sometimes the thought "I should have been the one who died," a thought that can lead to suicide.

Dishonoring the Enemy

Tony McNally describes a group of British troops looking into a hole at the headless torso of an Argentinean soldier. Two were prodding the remains with sticks, trying to open the rib cage. "We were all giggling like adolescents as the two with the sticks started to flick bits of rotting flesh at each other. One of the lads ended the game by throwing a small Argie grenade into the hole . . . This act was to haunt me to this day. It was a shameful thing to do, impossible to justify or even to explain, and I have asked the dead soldier for forgiveness for being part of it. Although I wasn't physically involved, I should have intervened. In our defence, all I can say is that we weren't ourselves that day . . . The war had dehumanised us and we didn't give too much of a toss about anything."[14] Years later the eyes of the abused Argentinean soldier looked at him accusingly in a dream.

Sometimes, whether about dishonoring the enemy or simply killing them, human responses can break through. A psychiatrist was told by a veteran that killing the enemy was fine until he looked in one dead man's wallet and saw pictures of the man's family, very like those in his own wallet. The sudden empathy triggered a lot of guilt.[15]

It is also possible for an officer to succeed in creating such breakthroughs in his men, and thereby help keep their humanity alive, despite their dishonoring the enemy dead:

> I mean we had been fighting for days. And their friends had been killed. And the dead bodies laying around the hole. So they cut some ears off . . . the corpses of the enemy. And they stuck them to their helmets. And like I said, these are 18-year-olds. So it's like a high school letter. "Hey, look, I shot these two guys" . . . And I said . . . "You can't do this . . . You're going to bury those two bodies" . . . That restored their humanity. They realized they were burying another person. And they felt sadness. Again, I don't think the word is guilt. Those people were trying to kill us. But the sadness that those people were there just like we were. They were 18. We were 19, 18. And there we are killing each other. That broke through for that moment . . . you kill them when they are animals. And then you have to try to come back. If you don't, then the atrocities can start.[16]

The Light and the Dark in Human Nature

> It is the darkest pit of therapy for the common soldier. It is where my vets least want to take me but most need my help. It is where I am least able to help them. All I can do initially with them is listen and hold their hands, if they want, praying silently that they can get through this. When I first started this work I couldn't go there with them. I was afraid. I eventually learned what I was afraid of: they never told me anything so awful that I could not imagine doing it myself.
>
> —Larry Dewey, *War and Redemption: Treatment and Recovery in Combat-Related Posttraumatic Stress Disorder*

The psychology of soldiers going berserk or dishonoring their enemies has elements that come close to being human universals. Of course very many soldiers do not do these things. But the pattern cuts across cultures and historical periods. Jonathan Shay, whose books compare the narratives of his patients with *The Iliad* and *The Odyssey*, has shown many striking parallels between the psychology of combat in Homeric times and now.[17]

These are dark parts of our psychology, as Karl Marlantes sees: "There is a dark side that can come out instantly if the bonds are removed . . . And when you get in combat, you're going to die if you don't do it. And believe me, the old civilizing things that's saying, 'Well, let's be nice. Let's see if we can be good to the guy and stuff.' It's like when it's your organism at stake, all that stuff finally disappears. And that's why I think there's a deep genetic component to us. That we just don't want to admit. It comes out. Carl Jung talks a lot about shadow, how we have a violent side of us that we don't like to talk about."[18]

Returning soldiers notice how people are in denial about this. Jonathan Shay quotes what one said about a dinner given for his return: "Her father said, 'So, tell us what it was like.' And I started to tell them. And I told them. And do you know within five minutes the room was empty. They was all gone, except my wife. After that I didn't tell anybody I had been in Vietnam."[19] Before being in combat, those who become soldiers may be as much in denial as anyone else about the dark side of human nature. Part of the trauma of such things as having gone berserk may be the sudden breakthrough of awareness of the dark side, compounded by the horror that the discovery is in themselves: that *they* have done these things.

"I *Became* That": Moral Identity

One veteran had started in Vietnam at 18 with strong religious beliefs:

> I was no angel either . . . But evil didn't enter it 'till Vietnam. I mean real evil, I wasn't prepared for it at all. Why I became like that? It was all evil. All evil. Where before, I wasn't . . . I look back today, and I'm horrified at what I turned into. What I was. What I did. I just look at it like it was somebody else. Somebody had control of me. War changes you, changes you. Strips you, strips you of all your beliefs, your religion, takes your dignity away, you become an animal . . . You know, it's

> unbelievable what humans can do to each other. I never in a million years thought I would be capable of that. Never, never, never.

Another was similarly changed: "When I just come there, I couldn't believe what I was seeing. I couldn't believe Americans could do things like that to another human being . . . but then I *became* that. We went through villages and killed everything, I mean *everything*, and that was all right with me."[20]

Torture is also something that can traumatize soldiers who obey orders to take part in it. Daniel Keller had blasted loud music in victims' ears and had poured gallons of water into their mouths and noses as they gasped for breath. Afterward he had therapy, which partly wiped the memories. But he still had to deal with it, as these impressively honest comments show: "None of us were like this before. No-one thought about dragging people through concertina wire or beating them or sandbagging them or strangling them or anything like that . . . before this . . . I don't think I'll ever be done coming to terms with it for the rest of my life. I am just going to learn how to be a better person and live with what I have done."[21]

Responding to Moral Injury

> I shall argue what I've come to strongly believe through my work with Vietnam veterans: that moral injury is an essential part of any combat trauma that leads to lifelong psychological injury. Veterans can usually recover from horror, fear, and grief once they return to civilian life, so long as "what's right" has not also been violated.
>
> —Jonathan Shay, *Achilles in Vietnam: Combat Trauma and the Undoing of Character*

Some psychiatrists object to the term "post-traumatic stress disorder" to describe the condition they treat. Jonathan Shay says it is better seen as an injury: it is more like losing a limb in battle than like a psychiatric disorder. Edward Tick quotes one veteran saying that PTSD is "a name drained of both poetry and blame" and that a name is needed for "a disorder of warriors, not men and women who were weak or cowardly but . . . who followed orders and who at a young age put their feelings aside and performed unimaginable tasks."[22]

The Post-Traumatic Landscape: Flattening the Contours

It was only after large numbers of affected soldiers returned from Vietnam to the United States that post-traumatic stress disorder (PTSD) was included in the *DSM*. The criteria in *DSM-5* for identifying the disorder still do not distinguish combat-related trauma from other kinds. The first criterion (A) says the origin must be exposure (personal, or through witnessing the exposure of others) to actual or threatened death, serious injury, or sexual violation.

The resulting disturbance is identified by four further criteria:

> (B) Intrusion symptoms (such as recurrent intrusive memories, dreams, flashbacks, etc.);
> (C) Avoidance of memories, thoughts, feelings, or other reminders of the traumatic events;
> (D) Negative changes in cognitions and mood (such as not remembering aspects of the trauma, persistent, distorted negative emotions or beliefs about oneself and others, feeling detached or estranged from others, or inability to have positive emotions);
> (E) Marked alterations in arousal and reactivity associated with the traumatic events (such as being irritable, aggressive, excessively vigilant or startled, or having problems concentrating or sleeping).

PTSD is usually seen as a unitary condition that happens to have various origins. There are some good reasons for this context-neutral view. Rachel Ychuda points out that "the demonstration of a distinct set of biological alterations that correlates with symptoms of PTSD has served as an important validation of the concept of PTSD."[23] Some medications and kinds of psychotherapy seem helpful in treating PTSD in general. And "traumatic events able to cause PTSD vary considerably, but the core symptom domains remain remarkably consistent across populations." The context-neutral view is reflected in the goals of treatment: to "reduce the frequency and intensity of intrusive trauma memories, restore social and occupational functioning, and enhance resilience against future traumatic life events."[24]

But there are also limitations to the context-neutral account of PTSD. The view is from the outside. It ignores differences between being a passenger in an air crash and the experiences described by Karl Marlantes or Daniel Keller. The air crash is unlikely to lead to guilt, agent reaction, or to damage to the sense of moral identity. When symptoms are seen as floating free from context, this flattens the contours of the returned soldier's inner landscape. The goals of treatment make no reference to moral identity or to healing moral injury.

Although all post-traumatic stress involves inner turmoil, there are different ways of not being at peace with yourself. The air crash may come up in terrible flashbacks, but without self-accusation. Even where there is agency, there are different reactions. Tony McNally was changed, but he knew he was not responsible for the gun breaking down and so there was no violation of his moral identity. And Karl Marlantes, who was responsible for his acts, felt no guilt. He saw his act as a necessary defense of himself and his comrades in a war he believed in. His tears at the therapy session, the torrent of terrible memories and the unbidden images of mutilated bodies, were a breakthrough of previously rejected human responses. But they were not signs of damage to his moral identity. He believed what he had done was horrible but justified.

Perhaps the most important boundary is between those cases and ones where moral identity has been damaged. As Jonathan Shay says, there may be a different prognosis if "what's right" has been violated. This is most likely where someone has gone berserk, dishonored the dead, or tortured someone. From the outside Tony McNally, Karl Marlantes, and Daniel Keller may all show similar *DSM* symptoms of flashbacks, negative emotions, and feelings of estrangement. But inside there is a world of difference between Karl Marlantes's sadness without guilt and Daniel Keller's thought, "I don't think I'll ever be done coming to terms with it for the rest of my life. I am just going to learn how to be a better person and live with what I have done." It is hard to believe that these differences are irrelevant to the kind of help needed.

Home from the War: Needing Recognition and to Be Listened To

Many people, for good reasons and bad, avoid discussing the war with returned soldiers. Some suspect they would be disturbed by what they might hear and so shy away. There is also a decent concern not to cause distress by opening psychological wounds. So veterans are often met by silence on the topic. Some, like Karl Marlantes, say they would like to talk about it and be listened to. "You know, you come back and there is this code of silence . . . And it's all done out of trying to be kind. But you know, it's like, 'Well, I don't want to say something that upsets him . . .'—and the fact of the matter is if someone would genuinely ask, 'Well, you know, can you talk about it?' I think most guys would be delighted, you know? And sure there are those who are going to say, 'I don't want to talk about it' . . . So then you wait a year or two and ask him again. And believe me, at some point, they're going to want to talk about it."

Awareness of the silence also goes with a sense of alienation. Karl Marlantes accepts that some things, which to a soldier in combat seem a terrible but necessary duty, will to most people seem horrific: "'Thou shalt not kill,' even for the atheists in our culture is a tenet you just do not violate unless you're, you know, crazy or a sociopath or something. And so all your young life, that's drilled into your head. And then suddenly, you know, you're 18 or 19 and they're saying, 'Go get 'em and kill for your country.' And then you do that. And then you come back. And then it's like, 'Well, thou shalt not kill' again. Well, believe me, that is a difficult thing to deal with."

But Marlantes thinks talking could lead other people to make the effort to understand. "And then you say, 'Hm, maybe I should feel bad that I feel good about this.' And so you get these moral reverberations going around in your head that you're sure no-one else is going to understand. I think that's probably not true. I think people with a certain amount of wisdom can certainly try to understand it. But you do have a sense of alienation."

The alienation comes partly from the sense that only soldiers are held responsible for terrible acts of war whose origins reach back into the whole society. Karl Marlantes: "It's the sense that you're carrying the entire burden. And no-one is aware of it, no-one wants to cop to it." He points out that people pay taxes that support the war and scientists build bombs in factories that society funds. "Everyone in this country is involved in that war. What the soldier did is at the end of an enormous long chain, he pulled the trigger. That was his part. But we all like to believe that he did it. We didn't do it . . . people come back, and they realize that nobody really cared. And they don't even want to take responsibility for the fact that they were part of the enormous machinery that had all this take place."

Marlantes thinks an ideal response to the returning soldier would not be silence. But it would not be cheering either. "What they need is recognition that what they've just done is something that should be thanked not cheered."[25]

What often is not recognized is the help the returning soldier needs to cope with trauma. When Tony McNally was diagnosed with post-traumatic stress disorder, he took part in a class action of 1,900 people against the Ministry of Defence for compensation. They claimed the MOD had known of the likelihood of post-traumatic stress disorder and had failed to give the help they could. It was "mainly because I wanted someone, somewhere, to recognise what had happened to me . . . it was never, for me really about money. I wanted someone to put their hands up and say, 'Sorry, we could have done more.'" The judgment went against them. Although effective treatment was available, it was ruled that the MOD had no duty to identify sufferers to get them help. "War and warlike operations inevitably take their toll, both physical and psychological." Tony McNally commented, "That didn't mean, apparently, that those in charge needed to give much of a toss about the people at the sharp end."[26]

The Need to Heal That Split

Returned soldiers with these psychological injuries, whether or not they think their traumatic experiences involved acts against their own moral identity, need healing. Karl Marlantes eventually came to identify the healing he needed: "I killed him or Ohio did and we moved on. I doubt I could have killed him realizing he was like my own son. I'd have fallen apart. This very likely would have led to my own death or the deaths of those I was leading. But a split occurred then that now cries out to be healed. My problem was that for years I was unaware of the need to heal that split, and there was no-one, after I returned, to point this out to me."[27]

What are the prospects of healing such a split? What of other psychological damage—the sense of being already dead, the uncommunicated grief that turns into rage? How far is cure possible?

The answers vary with different people and their different histories, and also with what is meant by "cure." Jonathan Shay says clearly, "If recovery means return to trusting innocence, recovery is *not* possible." But he says partial recovery can take place, although by *DSM* standards the people who have partially recovered "remain highly symptomatic." Even if they have persistent problems like difficulty being in public spaces, many of them have flourishing lives. The best treatment puts the survivor in control: "Healing is done *by* survivors, not *to* survivors."[28]

How can psychiatry help them to heal themselves? Different wounds may need different help. It is possible that, even for those who did not violate their own ethical beliefs, some kind of expression of sadness and process of purification might be appropriate. Penances were often imposed on returning warriors in the early Middle Ages. The eighth-century Penitential of Theodore said, "One who slays a man in public war shall do penance for forty days." Wisdom about the horror and burden of killing, even killing that was believed to be justified, may have been reflected in the early ninth-century Penitential of Pseudo-Theodore; it said that the man who is blameless in committing homicide in war should still seek purification because of shedding blood.[29]

There are many ways to help the healing. Those who were not responsible for any horror, but who feel agent reaction because of their close involvement, might benefit from questions about agent reaction in other kinds of case. "Do you blame the driver of the train that kills the person who jumps into its path?" "Should he go on feeling bad about what happened if it is possible to stop doing so?" "Are you really so different from the train driver?"

Jonathan Shay says that "narrative enables the survivor to rebuild the ruins of character," but "only if the survivor finds or creates a trustworthy community of listeners," people willing to experience something of the same terror, grief, and rage. His suggestion for this "communalization of the trauma" is, like taking Shakespeare to Broadmoor, an Aristotelian appeal to what tragic theater can do: "Combat veterans and American citizenry should meet together face to face in daylight, and listen, and watch, and weep, just as citizen-soldiers of ancient Athens did in the theater at the foot of the Acropolis. We need a modern equivalent of Athenian tragedy."[30]

For Bill Ridley, the healing started on a journey of reconciliation back to Vietnam. He had been in the battle that destroyed much of the city of Hué. Returning thirty-five years later, he worried about his likely reception. A Vietnamese guard, "wearing the uniform [Ridley] had fought against," recognized him as an American. The guard smiled and said, "Let me be the first to welcome you back. You are our honored guest." After two days, Bill Ridley said, "The VA hospital has given me dozens of different pills in every combination for sleep, nightmares, nerves, stress, depression, and every damned PTSD symptom you could name. Tell me why none of it ever worked. Then tell me why it only took two nights back in this country to get my first full night's rest in thirty-five years!"[31]

The split Karl Marlantes saw in himself was between what he did, justified according to his beliefs, and what he needed to blank out: "I doubt I could have killed him realizing he was like my own son." One of the deepest debates in ethics is about how far what is right or wrong can be detached from which acts we do or do not find humanly possible. Perhaps most combat is possible only with this blanking out. If so, the issues raised by Karl Marlantes have near-universal military significance.

His own healing started with facing up to this conflict between doing what he thought right and its human horror. "I forced these images back, away, for years. I began to reintegrate that split-off part of my experience only after I actually began to imagine that kid as a kid, my kid perhaps. Then out came this overwhelming sadness—and healing. Integrating the feelings of sadness, rage or all of the above with the action should be standard operating procedure for all soldiers who have killed face-to-face. It requires no sophisticated psychological training. Just form groups under a fellow squad or platoon member who has had a few days of group leadership training and encourage people to talk."[32]

Forgiving Oneself

Those who did some of the clearly horrible things like torturing people, or killing when berserk, may need to forgive themselves. There are complications to this. Torture may wreck the lives of victim and torturer. It is right to help rebuild the life of the guilt-ridden torturer, but the victim should not be forgotten. Any pretense that the act was not all that bad is a failure of moral seriousness. (The issues of combat trauma have some parallels with those raised by the Broadmoor interviews.)

The seriousness should go with gentleness. We who have not experienced combat should remember the huge pressures on fighting soldiers. Would we have returned with less to forgive? And the person with flashbacks about torturing or bestial killing, while rightly being held responsible, is often far less culpable than the politicians who too lightly declared war or who authorized torture, or than the many other people who too easily accepted these things.

Another complication is found in Glenn Gray's journal: "I hope it does not rest too hard on my conscience, and yet if it does not I shall be disturbed also." This too is a matter of moral identity. His impact on the old couple was far more than he intended or had reason to predict. Even so, he did not want to become a person who took such things lightly. It mattered to him that forgiveness should not come too easily. And this should go for those who have done more terrible things. Daniel Keller avoided paralyzing guilt while facing what he did with seriousness: "I don't think I'll ever be done coming to terms with it for the rest of my life. I am just going to learn how to be a better person and live with what I have done."

When I talked at a meeting about the need of people who have done some of these things to forgive themselves, Thomas Nagel raised a deep skeptical question about whether this is intelligible. What does forgiving oneself *mean?* First I thought the difficulty was about *self*-forgiveness. But perhaps it is about any forgiveness. What is it to forgive those who have harmed you? It is not to forget what they did, nor is it to stop thinking it was wrong. It is to stop holding it against them. But what does this mean? If they sincerely express regret and resolve to act differently in future, you can decide not to judge their reformed character in the light of their repudiated past. The result can be the fading of resentment, and an easy relationship may develop. *Self*-forgiveness can be like that too. It is neither forgetting what you did nor denying its wrongness. It is not holding it against yourself: not tormenting yourself about it but starting afresh. Daniel Keller put it well: learning how to be a better person and living with what you have done.

Psychiatrists should aim to help those burdened with a damaged moral identity to forgive themselves. The forgiveness should obliterate neither the memory nor the wrongness. Larry Dewey sees denial as an obstacle to healing: "The beginning of this last phase of spiritual or moral healing always seems to start with having the courage to face the truth no matter how painful and shameful it may seem to be. Once the truth is faced, we can start looking for further understanding and resolution. At this point have we left the realm of psychiatry? I am not sure what the realm of psychiatry is any more. I have been changed by this work."[33] Psychiatry should be changed by it too.

28

Psychotherapy, Autonomy, and Self-Creation

> . . . he merely told
> The unhappy Present to recite the Past
> Like a poetry lesson till sooner
> Or later it faltered at the line where
> Long ago the accusations had begun,
> And suddenly knew by whom it had been judged,
> How rich life had been and how silly,
> And was life-forgiven and more humble.
>
> —W. H. Auden, *In Memory of Sigmund Freud*

The aims of psychotherapy vary with who is being helped: a child, an adult, or a family. The aims vary with different problems: depression, post-traumatic stress, anxiety, compulsions, and so forth. Further variety comes from the different schools and theories behind the approach. Underneath all this is a common aim: release from distress by removing psychological obstacles to a good life.

This vague aim usually takes three more specific forms. One is helping people see and escape from cognitive and emotional traps. Another is helping people see how their relationships with each other may be working badly, and to find ways of untangling them. A third is trying to help people discover things about themselves and—if they so decide—to help them turn self-understanding into self-creation.

Release from Cognitive and Emotional Traps

Stressful situations, including such life events as divorce or losing a job, are powerful triggers of depression. Clinically depressed people often underrate the causal role of these triggers. Instead they may blame their own supposed inadequacies. In depression this is one way that interacting beliefs and emotions cause a downward spiral. Being depressed supports a pessimistic bias in thinking about the future. This also gives people a very poor view of themselves, making them feel hopeless. In this circular trap, depression distorts beliefs, which in turn maintain depression.[1]

Evidence supports therapy as one of the more effective treatments. A UK Department of Health report found that both cognitive behavioral therapy and interpersonal therapy are effective, and that there are indications of possible benefit in some other types, including psychodynamic therapy.[2] Paul Biegler has made a strong case for the view that cognitive and emotional traps found in depression give good reasons to expect this. Spinoza's two perspectives on the same state are important here. Only medication directly attacks the chemical side of depression. Only therapy directly attacks the cognitive side. Seeing depression simply as a chemical problem obscures the role of stress. Therapy can help people escape the trap through seeing both the causal role of stress and the distorting effects of depression.

Relationships, Families, and Therapy

Family therapists could reasonably sigh at Tolstoy's famously confident assertion that all happy families are alike, while an unhappy family is unhappy in its own way. Questions can be asked about both claims, but family therapists have a stake in challenging the second claim. Part of their expertise rests on experience of what has been useful in understanding other families' problems. Lack of any common structure would make their experience useless.

Therapists look for particular patterns. Families may be trapped in vicious circles. They may communicate poorly. They may have unrealistic mutual expectations, or stereotype each other. There may be too much criticism and intolerance. They may blame problems too much on certain members. Some of them may have low self-esteem.

How real are the claimed patterns? Are they present in the families or only in the belief systems of therapists? They are obviously plausible causes of family stress and disruption. But what evidence is needed to justify overriding how families see their own problems? What are the causal theories family therapists draw on? How good is the evidence for them? And how is it decided which one fits a particular family? When these patterns are involved, how should therapists respond? Some answers are shaped by therapists' theories, notably about families as systems.

Families Seen as "Systems"

The historical origins of the systems approach are important. It started in the mid-twentieth century with the general systems theory of Ludwig von Bertalanffy and with the "frames and paradoxes" of the anthropologist Gregory Bateson. Both of these influenced Mara Selvini Palazzoli and the still-influential Milan school of family therapy.[3]

Bertalanffy's general systems theory was "a theory, not of systems of a more or less special kind, but of universal principles applying to systems in general."[4] A "system" can be anything with interacting components: the central heating, cells in a living organism, a family, an army, the international financial system. It is hard to see that a general theory of systems can have much specific content. Is it more useful than a "general theory of events," meant to fit anything from the melting of an ice cap to the French Revolution or a child patting a dog?

Bertalanffy applied his approach to psychology: "Any system as an entity which can be investigated in its own right must have boundaries . . . Psychopathology shows the paradox that the ego boundary is at once too fluid and too rigid. Syncretic perception, animistic feeling, delusions and hallucinations, and so on, make for insecurity of the ego boundary; but within his self-created universe the schizophrenic lives 'in a shell,' much in the way animals live in the 'soap bubbles' of their organization-bound worlds." This account of "the schizophrenic" does not suggest Bertalanffy has much familiarity with people with schizophrenia, but he concludes: "Psychiatric disturbances can be neatly defined in terms of system functions."[5]

Gregory Bateson's view of psychotherapy centered on frames and paradoxes. A psychological frame "is (or delimits) a class or set of messages (or meaningful actions)." Frames are "metacommunicative," by which he meant that "the subject of the discourse is the relationship between the speakers." He explained these abstractions with an illustration. When young monkeys nip each other in play, they signal that the aggression is not real. Humans do this too. We frame what we are saying as playing or joking.

Bateson thought that in delusions, people with schizophrenia take fantasies that are metaphors and wrongly frame them as literal truth.[6] He drew on Russell's paradox: "Is the class of classes that are not members of themselves, a member of itself?" Either answer, yes or no, seems self-defeating. One way out, the theory of types, postulates a hierarchy of levels of language. The class of classes is on a higher level than the class of houses or the class of dogs. So the (level two) class of (level one) classes that are not members of themselves cannot be a member of itself. Finding this paradoxical is said to come from confusing different levels of discourse.

Bateson saw the monkey's nip and the signal "only playing" as being on different levels. He thought that schizophrenic conflation of the metaphorical and the literal called for reframing. Therapy could help a person with schizophrenia to see that what appeared to be literal truth is really metaphor. Like the "different levels" approach to Russell's paradox, it dissolves the problem by reframing it.[7] There are limits to this view of schizophrenia. It is purely cognitive, focusing only on delusions, and only on the view that schizophrenics confuse metaphor and reality. (What is hearing hostile voices a metaphor *for?* How can we tell?)

Bateson used framing problems in developing his "double bind" theory. An example of a double bind is a child's being given conflicting commands, one verbal and the other by gesture or tone of voice. This might cause schizophrenia through a failure to discriminate between frames. This interesting theory influenced R. D. Laing and others in the 1960s. But it is backed by little evidence and is ignored in current discussions.[8]

The theoretical approach of the Milan school started from Bertalanffy's ideas about self-maintaining systems, and those of Bateson about paradox and the hidden rules governing mutual interpretation and interaction. Its classic exposition is Mara Selvini Palazzoli's *Paradox and Counter-Paradox*, the stated aim of which is to test the hypothesis that "the family is a self-regulating mechanism which controls itself according to rules formed over a period of time through a process of trial and error."[9]

The hypothesis is hardly controversial. In hundreds of ways families avoid chaos by regular patterns of behavior. On days when she goes to work, he does the shopping. At meals some families have regular places to sit; others sit randomly. They do not hang up on calls for each other, but take messages. For these patterns the family therapist John Byng-Hall has drawn on the apt theatrical metaphor of "family scripts."[10] Families were not born with all this, so the rules must have evolved over time. And errors are corrected: "There was no towel, so I dried my hands on her dress. Her response wasn't good, so I haven't done it again."

The interest comes from applying to schizophrenia this emphasis on unconscious or barely conscious family rules. The central claim is: "Families in which one or more members present behaviors traditionally diagnosed as 'pathological' are held together by transactions and, *therefore,* by rules peculiar to the pathology" (italics mine).[11]

It is claimed that this points to a cure: "Since the symptomatic behavior is part of the transactional pattern peculiar to the system in which it occurs, the way to eliminate it is to change the rules . . . when we are able to discover and change one fundamental rule, pathological behavior quickly disappears."[12] Given the evidence about genetic, early environmental, and other factors in schizophrenia,[13] it is perhaps optimistic to hope that it can be cured by a family rule change.

The claim is that a pattern of pathological family rule systems causes schizophrenia. Each of the parental couple needs approval. Each bolsters his or her own standing by withholding approval from others. These two unpromising parents share a reluctance to admit either their mutual influence or the rules of their system. "Each member perceives open declaration as extremely dangerous. Therefore, everyone cooperates in keeping it hidden."

The contrast is with other couples, in which each parent still wants their own view of the relationship to prevail but also accepts that it might not. The claim is that parents of schizophrenic children cannot accept this. So, although each wants to control the relationship, the only solution is not to define it. "Thus the great game begins and its secret rules are formed." The parents "become expert in the use of paradox, taking advantage of that possibility, specific to man, to communicate simultaneously on the verbal and the non-verbal level, jumping from one logical class to a member of that class, as if they were the same thing, thus becoming acrobats in the world of the Russellian paradox."[14] "At the beginning of our work with these families, it often happened that we were taken in by the family's game to the point that our resulting frustration and anger became transferred to the relationship between ourselves."[15]

This account contains a large ratio of assertion to support. What is the evidence that parents of children with schizophrenia are those who, to an exceptional degree, both need and withhold approval? Or that they are unusually reluctant to admit their mutual influence or the existence of family rules? Why should we believe in the great game and its secret rules? Or that the parents are such good acrobats with Russellian paradox?

Some of the systems approach is overconfident speculation. But one thought about systems is important. Families *are* "systems" in the sense that their members interact and interpret each other. Changes in one person are likely to have reverberations on others, whose responses may in turn feed back. Therapists need to take account of these complications.

Families Across Generations

Some therapists add an extra dimension to this, seeing families as systems stretched across time. Patterns in families may have part of their origin in parents' own past family problems, particularly with their own parents. The first line of Philip Larkin's "This Be the Verse" is often remembered: "They fuck you up, your mum and dad." Less remembered is the start of the second verse: "But they were fucked up in their turn / By fools in old-style hats and coats." And no doubt *those* fools in their turn . . . the patterns may go back generations.

Sophocles, blaming the gods, noticed how disasters can cascade down the generations:

> When high gods shake a house
> That family is going to feel the blow
> Generation after generation.
> It starts like an undulation underwater,
> A surge that hauls black sand up off the bottom,
> Then turns itself into a tidal current
> Lashing the shingle and shaking promontories.
>
> I see the sorrows of this ancient house
> Break on the inmates and keep breaking on them
> Like foaming wave on wave across a strand.
> They stagger to their feet and struggle on
> But the gods do not relent, the living fall
> Where the dead fell in their day
> Generation after generation.[16]

Larkin and Sophocles meet here, but so do systems theorists and Freudians. It is not surprising that the tidal current across generations is strong if the father or grandfather is Oedipus.

How a family's past is preserved in stories can be important. John Byng-Hall thought about how his own family's stories affected him. In 1756 his ancestor, Admiral Byng, was sent to defend Minorca from a French attack. Finding his fleet heavily outnumbered, he fired token shots and avoided disaster by sailing away. He was found guilty of cowardice and was executed on the quarterdeck.

The story was passed down. Throughout his own youth, John Byng-Hall was preoccupied with worries about whether he would be a coward. In colonial Kenya there was danger from the Mau Mau and from wild animals. Would he run from a charging lion? Because he wanted to join the Navy, at the age of 12 he spent time on a naval cruiser. He remembers being terrified when standing at attention on the quarterdeck, trying to hide his fear from the ship's second in command. He links these anxieties and fears to memories of the Admiral Byng story. He later spent time researching evidence suggesting that Admiral Byng may have been made a scapegoat for the failings of others.[17]

Not every family history has an Admiral Byng, so the way the remote past reached into John Byng-Hall's own life may be very unusual. But as a therapist he reflected more generally on the effects of other families' memories of their—usually closer—history. He suggests two false beliefs that may be harmful. One is the belief that family history has no relevance. The other is that the family members now have no choice but to repeat the patterns of the past. He suggests that these opposed beliefs are similar. Families who think they cannot avoid it, reenact the past consciously. And those who deny the relevance of the past do so unwittingly.[18]

What Should Be the Aims of Family Therapy?

In the literature on families as systems, the interesting points are independent of the abstract theories. Little work is done by thoughts about "systems" seen as homeostatic mechanisms. What comes over as valuable is the intuitive feel for particular people, how they see and react to each other, and how they do or do not get on. Where people are in danger of being trapped into reliving the family past, what matters is again independent of "systems." It is the rejection of fatalism: knowing the past may be relevant but seeing the possibility of breaking free.

Families with different problems generate different aims: helping them cope with the needy and demanding grandparent now living with them;

helping homophobic parents listen to their son who has come out as gay; helping the teenager to talk about previously hidden childhood traumas and helping the parents to listen.

Therapy may take the form of helping families live with conflicts or disagreements that cannot be eliminated. "Our religion tells us that homosexuality is sinful, but we do see you have to decide about your own life." It might even help the teenager say, "I can't give way on having to be myself, but I do see this hurts you and I wish it didn't." It may take the form of helping family members listen to each other and see that no single person's narrative has the whole truth. It may involve helping people escape from bad cycles of mutual blame and see the possibility of better ways of getting on with each other.

Put so generally, these aims inevitably sound platitudinous. The controversial questions are about how to realize them. What strategies should family therapists adopt? This is discussed in some reflective papers by family therapists.[19]

One discussed blaming a person's illness on an unhealthy allocation of responsibility: "Putting all the problems in some sort of externalized thing like dad's depression or mum's anxiety. It seems a very helpful thing for them." Perhaps. But equally a family's difficulties may really stem from one of them developing Alzheimer's, schizophrenia, or depression. Obviously families will sometimes deceive themselves, using mistaken causal accounts to rationalize their problems. But there is a troubling hint of "therapist knows best" in these comments.

Katja Kurri and Jarl Wahlstrom used a couple's therapy session to illustrate help in escaping cycles of mutual misunderstanding and blame. The account also brings out some linked problems.

One therapist invites the husband to consider whether his thoughts about his wife's "emotionality" play a role in his agitated shouting, and asks him to consider why *she* reacts as she does. This implies that the husband might accept some responsibility for the situation. But later the therapist is said to emphasize the good intentions of both husband and wife: "The therapist's statement emphasizes the reformulation of the transactional pattern as expressing good intentions on both sides. The therapist appears here to deconstruct blame . . . If the intentions are good but the outcome undesired, then it appears as if something like bad luck or fate is in operation. In that case none of the participants could be held responsible for the course of events. The responsibility is given to the transactional pattern, so to speak."

As with the Milan school's view of schizophrenia, it invites skepticism to ascribe responsibility for the relationship's going wrong not to human agency but to fate, bad luck, or "the transactional pattern." Yet there are cases of mutual misunderstanding despite good intentions on both sides. In such cases, exposing the good intentions may help the couple escape from mutual recrimination. But intentions are not always good. What should happen when only one of the couple is open to reasonable criticism for being selfish or insensitive?

Kurri and Wahlstrom rightly see a problem for the moral neutrality of therapists. There may be no neutral way of formulating a critical comment about only one of a couple. They ask whether therapists can be neutral between two "discourses." The "discourse of autonomy" emphasizes a person's right to make choices and to pursue his or her own interests. The "discourse of relationality" emphasizes emotional responsiveness to others. If, in a couple, he is strong on autonomy and she feels he is emotionally insensitive to her, what should the therapist do? Kerri and Wahlstrom say, approvingly, that the conflict was resolved by the "principle of relational autonomy," which "indicates that identity and autonomy are generated from a matrix of relations." The therapists' interventions "produced a situation where the partners' autonomy was necessarily understood as relational."

The principle of relational autonomy seems too platitudinous and too vague to be much of a success in changing behavior. ("Yes, I agree my identity evolved in the context of relationships, but I still don't see why in this case I should put my autonomy second to what I see as my wife's unreasonable feelings.") And is it really true that therapists have to decide between "reinforcing" one or other of the values or else both? Is it really for the therapist to decide on priorities for the couple, guided by some principle that somehow combines the two values? What would be wrong with asking questions designed to make the conflict of values explicit and asking whether the couple are willing to explore compromises?

The Therapist as Freud or as Socrates?

> Searching through and talking about my emotions was no more than the psychiatrists wanted to do, of course, but I couldn't, and didn't want to, tell them. At that time, they would have started telling me my own story back; they would

> have made me into this character in their own version of events.
>
> —Grace Bowman, *A Shape of My Own: A Memoir of Anorexia and Recovery*

Why *not* ask questions to make the conflict of values between husband and wife explicit? Here there is a clash between two models of therapy. With some caricature, these can be seen as the therapist as Freud and the therapist as Socrates. The therapist as Freud says, "I have special psychological knowledge—in this case knowledge of how identity is generated from a matrix of relations—and my interventions will be designed to help you understand yourselves as I do." The therapist as Socrates says, "I don't know the answers, but I will ask questions to help make your values explicit. If you turn out to have different values, I will ask questions designed to find out whether you can still get on with each other. Everything will depend on the answers you decide to give."

An obvious limitation of the model of Socrates is that his questions explored only beliefs and not emotions. For therapists, Freud's approach was a clear advance. But another of Freud's ideas is more debatable: belief in special psychological knowledge, possessed only by initiates, giving the therapist a privileged interpretation. The Milan school's belief that systems theory gives greater insight than the family has into "the family's game" is in this sense thoroughly "Freudian." This belief in the therapist's privileged interpretation is still influential, even if the esoteric knowledge less often comes from psychoanalysis.

A deep ethical issue concerns the role of truth. Here the Freudian and Socratic models may pull in different directions. Does it matter in family therapy how far each of the different narratives is true? The therapist as Socrates may think this is worth exploring. If one of the family has paranoid fantasies about the rest, the others may want to "put the record straight," to whatever extent that is possible. The therapist as Socrates may be willing to discuss the evidence. The therapist as Freud, who perhaps "knows" that the real problems are about systems and boundaries, might try to exclude the issue as unhelpful. Paradoxically, the Socratic approach may sometimes be more helpful, because of the importance people attach to their true history being recognized.

There are parallels to political peacemaking, as between Israelis and Palestinians. Is it better to forget the disputed past and start afresh? Or do both sides need acknowledgment of the truths in their respective narratives? It might not be enough to say, "We accept that your version is true for you, just as theirs is true for them." This may elicit the response that this account is not just "true for us": "We want some recognition that these events actually happened."

In the case of the mutually blaming couple, when the therapist suggests that they both had good intentions, is this said because it is true or because it is helpful? Of course, if true, it is likely to be helpful. But supposing it is not true? Should it still be suggested, because believing it may help the couple escape the bad cycle? The therapist as Freud might say yes, claiming to understand their problem better than they do. The therapist as Socrates, not claiming a privileged view, lacks this reason for deception.

Moving the family toward a shared view, allowing escape from mutual blame, is often assumed to require the therapist's neutrality between the rival versions. Empathy with one can be seen as siding against others. John Stancombe and Sue White report that this leads to therapists changing the subject, or changing the blame-laden account into a nonblaming version. As they point out, either response may leave the person who expressed blame feeling that the core of his or her version has gone unheard and so saying it again. Neutrality may reinforce blame.

This problem arises only because of some disingenuousness in the therapist as Freud. She *has* heard the expression of blame. Fearing the consequences of indicating this, she gives the impression of not having heard. Hence the evasive or off-the-point responses that give the family an irritating sense of being manipulated. The therapist as Socrates may feel that all points are worth taking seriously, and doing so might not send a message about taking sides. ("Sarah, I understand that you are blaming Henry for causing the problem by getting so angry. Henry, I know you have a different view, and we will come to that in a moment. But first let's explore Sarah's view.") This may lead to a shared account that does some justice to both views. That more complex account, created by acknowledging rather than evading the partisan points, could even be both helpful and true.

According to Stancombe and White, some such account, based on different bits of the partisan versions, is what therapists construct for themselves. They are said to do this "in the backstage" as part of creating a neutral version to be "performed frontstage without compromising the therapist's 'neutrality.'"

The therapist as Freud is clearly visible in this contrast between the backstage account and the frontstage one offered to the family. Why all this make-believe? Why not go for the Socratic version, using sympathetic questioning to coax the family into themselves constructing the complex account? Perhaps this is what, at their best, therapists already do. Modest therapists understand how small is their knowledge of a family compared to what the family themselves know. They will expect the family's own constructed complex account to be richer than anything concocted "backstage." Good family therapists, instead of being in the grip of a theory, have the human sensitivity that goes with being a good listener. Then, with Socratic openness to what they hear, they will help the family dig themselves out of whatever trap they are in. Using gentle questioning, not to move families but to help them *move themselves,* is a wonderful thing for a therapist to do.

I argued this in the *Journal of Family Therapy,* commenting on the articles cited above. The editor, Dr. Ivan Eisler, made good criticisms in an editorial. He expressed sympathy for the Socratic over the Freudian approach. But "Glover's discussion of the *Freudian* and *Socratic* positions did not always fit my own preconceptions of what they might mean and kept switching like the corners of the Necker cube from inside to outside." He supported using gentle questions to help families move themselves. But was this a liking for the Socratic position per se? "Or is it based on our conceptualization of the process of change (clearly a *Freudian* position in Glover's terms)?" Therapists who ask questions aimed at eliciting new narratives conducive to change are clearly Socratic, "but the intention is, in Glover's terms, that of therapist as *Freud.*" This rightly complicates the account I gave. Freudian intention can motivate Socratic method. (I am happy for Ivan Eisler's acute point to be the last word here. He is a therapist and I am a philosophy professor. In each role, as we both know, leaving things open can be more fruitful than seeking a decisive verdict.)

Self-Discovery and Self-Creation

> And so it was, in term one of my third and last year at Oxford, that I met with Louise. She calls herself a *humanistic therapist* and talks to you without looking down at you . . .

> Louise taught me to take care of myself. She allowed me to see that the best part of growing up is acknowledging a part of us that always remains a child, and to cherish that child always. I discovered feelings I had not admitted, not even recognised, in the past. Fear. I was so afraid. Afraid of uncertainty. Afraid of not being good enough. Afraid of disappointing my parents, other people. Afraid that I was not, could not be, perfect.
>
> —Emily Halban, *Perfect: Anorexia and Me*

Emily Halban brings out some help a psychotherapist can give. Talking to the person seeking help without looking down is essential for creating the atmosphere for a shared enterprise of assisted self-exploration and self-interpretation. Most of us now know that people are sometimes partly unaware of their own motives and emotions. Any therapist must have the hope, and with luck the satisfaction, of helping the growth of self-understanding.

This self-discovery is one kind of (possibly unintended) self-creation. At the minimum, the person changes from being less aware to being someone more aware. Sometimes the self-knowledge may be enough. But the second, conscious layer of self-creation can be more important. Reclaiming feelings not admitted or recognized may help a person deal with problems through conscious change. It helps to control, or perhaps even eliminate, the emotions and motives from the dark that were once so influential. As in much psychiatry, a core aim must be the move from passivity to actively taking control. The rejection of fatalism is again essential: It is essential to see that it is possible to take some control of your own life.

Part of this therapy is helping people to think through their own deepest values. Alasdair MacIntyre has denied that therapists do this. A therapist "treats ends as given, as outside his scope; his concern also is with technique, with effectiveness," so therapists cannot engage in moral debate.[20] If MacIntyre's view of therapists is correct, it should not remain so. One aim of therapy is to promote self-understanding, which can feed into self-creation. And self-understanding includes the articulation of a person's values.

MacIntyre chides therapists for not engaging in moral debate. A lot depends on what that is taken to be. A woman seeking an abortion while in therapy is not going to be helped by a pro-life therapist attacking her moral outlook. That would be Therapist as Freud with a vengeance. But Therapist as Socrates will probe values. Asking questions to elicit hidden values is central to helping self-understanding. "Treating ends as given, as outside his scope," would be crippling. Part of the Socratic aim is to help people create themselves by seeing what they most deeply want to be.

Horse and Rider

> One thing is needful—to "give style" to one's character—a great and rare art! It is practiced by those who survey all the strengths and weaknesses of their nature and then fit them into an artistic plan until every one of them appears as art and reason and even weaknesses delight the eye. Here a large mass of second nature has been added; there a piece of original nature has been removed—both times through long practice and daily work at it. Here the ugly that could not be removed is concealed; there it has been reinterpreted and made sublime . . . In the end, when the work is finished, it becomes evident how the constraints of a single taste governed everything large and small. Whether this taste was good or bad is less important than one might suppose—if only it was a single taste!
>
> —Friedrich Nietzsche, *The Gay Science*

Few of us spend our lives, in the spirit of Nietzsche, as full-time landscape gardeners of the self. But many of us have some rough idea of the sort of person we want to be. And we often have a very clear idea of what we do *not* want to be. This sense of moral identity is part of the story. As well as caring about being one kind of person rather than another, people also value how they get there. They want to have some control. We cannot just choose our own characteristics. But it matters that, at least to some extent, we can shape the kind of person we are.

Not all self-creation is conscious. Through major decisions about our life, we influence unintentionally the sort of person we become. We are molded by choosing the person we marry or live with, by the friends we

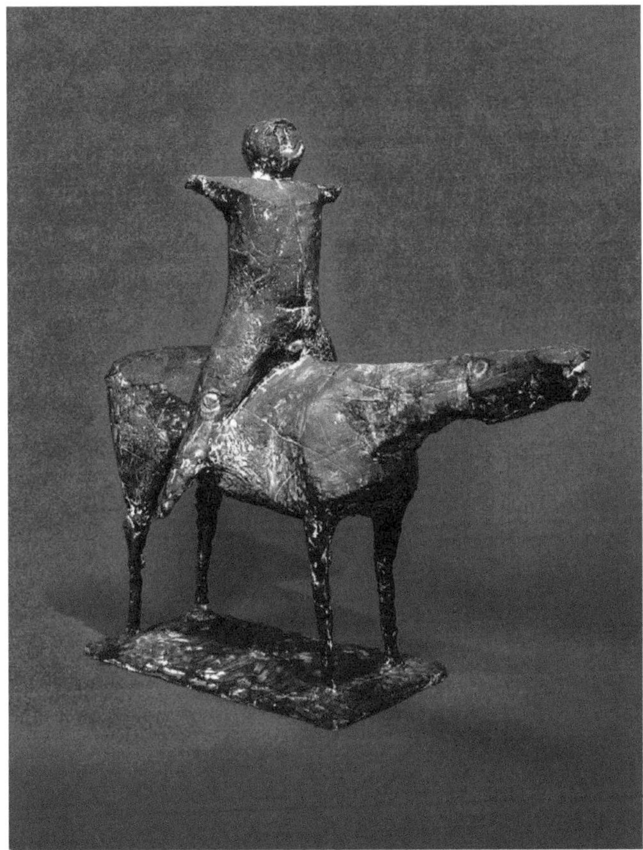

Figure 28.1: Marino Marini (1901–1980), *Horseman. Bronze,* Private collection. Copyright © 2012. Photo Art Resource/ Scala, Florence.

choose, the job we take and the place where we live. And there is Aristotle's path: from actions to habits to character.

Then there is the minimally conscious kind of self-creation described by Sigmund Freud. The I (*das Ich,* often translated as "the Ego") tries to bring the blind and conflicting unconscious impulses of the It (*das Es,* often translated as "the Id") under some kind of coherent conscious control. But Freud insists that the unconscious desires can be strong enough to limit this: "Often a rider, if he is not to be parted from his horse, is obliged to guide it where it wants to go."[21] Marino Marini's rather Freudian sculpture in Figure 28.1 captures this.

In Freud's view, psychoanalysis helps us control the unconscious desires through understanding them. He thought of this as a work of reclamation like the draining of the Zuyder Zee.

"How do I feel about his success?" Answering such a question may be only partly discovery. If, on asking the question, what floats to the surface feels a bit like jealousy, this initial feeling can be questioned. "Am I really so mean-spirited?" Reflection can, sometimes, lead to rejecting the attitude. The mixture of discovery and decision can be microlevel self-creation.[22]

There are limits to self-creation. To make a sculpture out of wood requires respecting the natural constraints of shape and grain. Self-creation is bound up with self-discovery: finding our own shape and grain. We cannot just choose what will prompt the thought about the real me. This is a reminder of another limit to Aristotle's thought about being responsible for our own character. What we are like depends partly on physical and chemical states of the brain, on experiences in childhood and even in the womb, and on the culture we live in. At most we only partly create ourselves. Some starting positions might make a particular self-creative project unattainable.

There are two different ways in which our self-creation is not fully ours. One is that how we are makes some transformations too difficult: we can only guide the horse where it is willing to go. The other is that the desires and values guiding our self-creation are not simply chosen by us. They too depend partly on things outside our control. We are horse and rider. Genetic inheritance, parents, early experiences, and chance encounters influence both the kind of horse *and* the kind of rider we are.

29

Entrapment in Eating Disorders

> I believe people become anorexic for two main reasons. First, they gain something from being ill—the control and focus they need. Then there is the addictive side, followed by the mental turmoil that is so difficult to break out of no matter how desperately you want to.
>
> —Sara, "Starving out of Shame," in *Anorexics on Anorexia*

Eating disorders are a case study in the interface between the scientific and the human sides of psychiatry. As suggested throughout this book, these "sides" are not warring but complementary.

Accounts from Outside and Inside

In trying to bring out the role of human interpretation of anorexia nervosa and bulimia nervosa (here shortened to anorexia and bulimia), I will contrast such interpretation with two brief and clear scientific accounts by respected leading researchers.

The first is the textbook account given by Janet Treasure and Ulrike Schmidt.[1] They point out that the classification of eating disorders has "a degree of fluidity" and that many guidelines for managing them are not firmly evidence-based. They report that evidence about causes of anorexia is often poor—the evidence is better for bulimia—and that genetic mechanisms account for more than 50 percent of the variance in the risk of developing an eating disorder. Parental problems such as alcoholism, depression, and drug abuse are more strongly linked to bulimia than to anorexia. Cognitive and behavioral therapy for bulimia is at least moderately effective in about 70 percent of cases.

The second account, by Christopher G. Fairburn, discusses the therapeutic techniques and the theoretical approach behind this degree of success.[2] He says the core pathology of these disorders is cognitive: "This psychopathology is the over-evaluation of shape and weight and their control . . . people with eating disorders judge their self-worth largely, or even exclusively, in terms of their shape and weight and their ability to control them." He discusses ways of reducing the importance attached to these things relative to other things in life.

It is hard to disagree that the self-evaluation of people with these disorders gives exaggerated emphasis to weight and to the ability to control it. In this way the "core pathology" is obviously *partly* cognitive. But perhaps the core could be extended to include the emotionally charged responses that bulk large in first-person accounts. For a deeper understanding of where the exaggerated emphasis on shape, weight, and control come from, we may need a better idea of how people with anorexia or bulimia feel about themselves and their lives.

Treasure and Schmidt also discuss "clinical conceptualizations" of anorexia: "Bruch developed a psychodynamic hypothesis centred on insecure attachment and the lack of attunement between the infant and the caretaker. Family models emphasise either causal or maintaining factors risk. The Maudsley model is a manualised form of family treatment evolving from the evidence implicating expressed emotion as a key factor in maintenance. Cognitive behavioural formulations for anorexia nervosa have also been described. Neurodevelopmental models have also been translated into treatment models including trait management."[3]

Treasure and Schmidt suggest thinking of bulimia in terms of this sequence:

> Early experiences (e.g., parenting, loss) → core beliefs → "hot" cognitions → intolerable emotional states → "escape"/blocking behaviors (binge eating, comfort eating).

They indicate that the "escape"/blocking behaviors feed back to influence both core beliefs and intolerable emotional states.[4]

Both the clinical conceptualizations of anorexia and the temporal or causal flow given for bulimia are at a striking level of abstraction. The sequential account gives no details about the particular "core beliefs," "hot cognitions," and "intolerable emotional states" found in bulimia.

The Waller and Kennerley article on which the Treasure and Schmidt account is based includes a flowchart, giving a typical illustration of its actual content.

It starts with a TRIGGER (Colleague says "You look really well.")
This leads to IMMEDIATE INTERPRETATION ("He thinks I look fat.")
This leads to SCHEMA ACTIVATED

Felt sense: ugliness.
Physiological responses: nausea, adrenaline.
Cognitive responses: negative images of self in past and future; confirmation to self that "I am unlovable."
Emotional responses: fear, self-repugnance.

This leads to PROBLEM REACTION (High levels of distress; drive to eat or exit.)

The example is helpful. "He thinks I look fat" is less abstract than "hot cognitions." But the flowchart stays very close to this immediate dubious or false interpretation of the colleague's comment, and how that in turn triggers and reinforces preexisting thoughts and feelings about being unlovable. Nothing is said about reaching behind the self-repugnance to how it arose. The sequence is still abstract compared to the felt pressures that are so vivid when people tell their own stories. In their own accounts, matters of identity are prominent. Once again the abstract clinical account flattens the contours of the person's inner landscape.

First-person accounts in turn have real weaknesses. They may contain mistakes, self-deception, or deliberate falsehoods. (Though I see no evidence of these in the passages to be quoted.) More interestingly, they may have distortions of selection and emphasis. And obviously it is worth investigating possible contributing factors (genetic, epigenetic, neurochemical, early environmental, or others), which the person is unlikely to know about. Equally obviously, the view from inside may also tell us a lot that the external perspective omits or sidelines. Probably no causal story fits everyone. But it is worth looking for recurring patterns even if they are not universal. The periodic table of the elements is not the best model for the messy human geography of psychiatry.

At the very least, the intuitive human interpretation of a few first-person accounts should throw up questions to be tested with larger numbers and control groups. With luck, this will get closer to the human reality behind the abstractions of "hot cognitions" or "intolerable emotional states."

Entrapment

> Although the illness made me extremely ill, I could not have coped with life without it.
>
> —Kate, "Anorexic Anger," in *Anorexics on Anorexia*

Many are drawn into eating disorders by problems and pressures. The diet regime offers some control over their lives. It replaces being overwhelmed with a needed feeling of achievement. But the sense of control can itself be addictive and the liberation a trap.

Accounts of experiences of anorexia or bulimia vary. People react differently to the same problems or similarly to different problems. One woman who had suffered terrible sexual abuse looked back on her anorexia as partly a strategy of escape: "I am certain that, to an extent, I was trying to get rid of my feminine characteristics. By reducing my body size I hoped I would no longer be seen as a sexual object that could be used and abused."[5] Another woman found that refusing to eat helped reduce her parents' arguing: "The longer I did not eat the more attention my parents gave me and the less time they spent arguing. I felt happier because they were not so angry with each other all the time but I was worried that if I ate they would stop looking after me and would start arguing again."[6]

One woman remembered family problems forced on her at 13. These included her father's drunkenness and her mother's affair and self-induced abortion. To support the family her mother had to go out to work: "I felt I had lost my innocence and childhood; I felt older but not wiser. I felt I had to be the mother figure. I did not want this. I think this was the start of my anorexia. I looked at myself and felt I wanted to be a child without these responsibilities." Having lost a lot of weight, she saw anorexia as a protective friend: "At the time I felt great—full of life and in control of everything . . . Anorexia was my friend and sheltered me from my father's coldness and drunkenness, away from my brother's delinquency and away from my mother's cosy confessions about the boss's husband."[7]

The idea of anorexia as a friend recurs. One woman had felt panic about exams and about leaving the security of school for the "real world" of looking for a job: "All I wanted to do was block out these new pressures, not to have to make any decisions and be able to concentrate on food, calories and exercising . . . Eventually I cut myself off from everyone; the only friend I had was Anorexia."[8] Another woman saw bulimia in a similar way: "I like to be alone and do my own thing, yet at the same time I get incredibly, uncomfortably lonely. An eating disorder became almost like a friend. As long as I have it, I don't need anyone else . . . I've always had this sort of 'something is missing' type of feeling. Two things thus far have ever served to fill that void—having an eating disorder and love."[9]

Like anorexia, bulimia can be seen as a solution to a problem. One woman grew up in a large extended family where life revolved round huge communal meals. Sharing food represented sharing love and affection, and she found the pressure to eat impossible to resist. "In those moments the debate in my head was usually whose feelings are first . . . Purging came as a way to please both. It was secretly rejecting what I didn't want, without letting those around me know I didn't want what they thought I should have."[10]

A third of people with anorexia develop bulimia within five years.[11] Sometimes they slide because it makes binge eating possible again. "Why drive myself insane trying to find something to eat that I won't feel guilty about when I could just eat whatever I wanted and then purge?"[12]

One frequent pattern of response starts with an eating disorder being welcomed as a way to block out pressures and stress: "I had needed to lose a little weight but it is obvious to me that I had problems and issues I needed to deal with and that dieting had provided me with something to focus on other than these problems."[13] Another woman said her bulimia "was clearer and safer to me than the chaos of my feelings and of relationships; or perhaps just clearer than trying to make sense of them."[14]

Then there is the "high" about losing weight, with the morale-boosting sense of taking control of part of their lives: "The feeling of lightness—of happiness—and a fuzzy, airy kind of an energy, which seemed to be irreplaceable. This is the high—every addiction has one—something that makes you feel good, something that is worth the low, or so it seems . . . With each new shape I made for myself, I was more optimistic, more alert, more euphoric and more in charge."[15] And this can give the hope of taking charge of themselves more generally: "I had such will-power that I knew I would make the end of my course and manage to survive in the safety of my anorexic world."[16]

The comforting feeling of being in control can make changes seem threatening: "I was just too ill mentally and I no longer wanted help. I was too deep into my Anorexia and the illness had completely taken me over. I felt in complete control and I did not want that taken away from me."[17] That fear of losing control is sometimes remembered as holding back efforts to escape: "Recovery took such a long time because by giving up my eating disorder I lost so much more as well—my 'safe' world of food and weight, the high I felt at being able to refuse food and the sense of power this gave me."[18]

In this way the liberating sense of control can itself become an addiction. Some compare their experiences to other addictions: "I would certainly class much of my behaviour now as compulsive and ritualistic . . . I know that a lot of my problems occur through habit in the same way as alcoholism or drug addiction."[19] In recovery there can be the same need for total abstinence to avoid sliding back: "It is like being an alcoholic. With alcoholism, if you have this problem you can no longer drink, even a mouthful. With Anorexia you have to keep away from the scales and one missed meal can lead to a never-ending downward spiral of weight loss."[20]

To experience fasting and weight loss as addictive brings awareness of being in a trap: "Anorexia can be addictive to an extent. You get addicted to the 'fasting high' and the regular weight loss but it is a horrible illness. I don't believe that people become seriously underweight in order to feel slim and look good . . . It feels to me as if there is much more to it than that, and in many ways anorexics become trapped in the illness . . . a disease that spreads until it completely consumes every part of you."[21]

Because one outcome of anorexia is death, the thought of being completely consumed can be the literal truth. One man used other powerful images for his entrapment and its possible outcome: "Anorexia for me was like being trapped in a prison where the prisoner is incarcerated in a deep pit and can see daylight above but has no way of reaching it. I was in a tunnel with no light at the end and a train travelling towards me."[22]

The Anorexic Lifestyle and Human Flourishing

Is anorexia compatible with a good human life? The rejection of any contrast between the two is sometimes found on "Pro Ana" websites. These reflect a range of opinions and purposes. Some aim simply to provide a space where people with anorexia can share and discuss problems with each other, when it is often hard to find others who will listen sympathetically. Other sites have a message. Some see eating disorders as terrible illness, urging (and advising about) escape and recovery. At the other end are some advocating anorexia as a lifestyle: "Volitional, proactive anorexia is not a disease or disorder . . . There are no victims here. It is a lifestyle that begins and ends with a particular faculty human beings seem in drastically short supply of today: the will . . . Contrary to popular misconception, anorexics possess the most iron-cored, indomitable wills of all. Our way is not that of the weak . . . If ever we completely tapped that potential in our midst . . . we could change the world. Maybe we could even rule it."[23]

One of Doris Lessing's books has the title *Prisons We Choose to Live Inside.* The Internet gives helpful access to supportive groups of like-minded people—which could also make it easier, almost without noticing, to live inside a self-built prison. Of course the quoted passage is very unusual. Neither the world-domination project nor the rhetoric of the iron will is likely to win many converts. Stripped of the heroics, though, it contains a thought worth pursuing: Is anorexia a lifestyle choice without victims?

No. The death rate, especially for anorexia, is high. One study puts the annual rate at 5.1 per 1,000 persons.[24] Another study, of people with anorexia being served by an eating disorders service, suggests that anorexics have a tenfold increase in risk of early death.[25] Those who die from anorexia are its victims. So are the devastated families of a daughter, sister, son, or brother either dead or still starving themselves. That there *are* victims is both true and central.

One possible reply to this is that anorexia is not a disorder but a lifestyle. People are not seen as psychiatrically disordered when they take up dangerous sports. There is one death for about every ten successful ascents of Mount Everest.[26] Those who die (and their families) can be seen as victims of mountaineering. But our society values the freedom to take the risk more than avoiding the deaths. Why should choosing an anorexic lifestyle be treated differently?

One difference comes from the "entrapment" side of anorexia. There is not the same pattern of people being driven to climb Mount Everest to escape intolerable pressures and stress.

The other main contrast comes from the features of a good life that anorexia takes away. Chapter 20 suggested that strands in a good human life include being at peace with yourself and being to some extent in control. The first-person accounts do not give the impression of inner peace: "Then there is the addictive side, followed by the mental turmoil that is so difficult to break out of no matter how desperately you want to."[27] They also suggest that the promise of control is an illusion: "Then control took control and I was left with no control."[28] Relationships are another strand of the good life. But accounts of eating disorders suggest that they have disastrous impacts on relationships with family and friends. Another strand, creativity, is engulfed by the anorexic lifestyle. "It's like a disease that spreads until it completely consumes every part of you."[29]

Narrowness is a feature of some kinds of religion. Jeanette Winterson describes the effect of her adopted mother's religion on her walk down the High Street. "We went past Woolworth's—'A den of vice.' Past Marks and Spencer's—'The Jews killed Christ.' Past the funeral parlour and the pie shop—'They share an oven.' Past the biscuit stall and its moonfaced owners—'Incest.' Past the pet parlour—'Bestiality.' Past the bank—'Usury.' Past the Citizens Advice Bureau—'Communists.' Past the day nursery—'Unmarried mothers.' Past the hairdresser's—'Vanity.'"[30]

The demanding narrowness of some versions of anorexia comes out in the rules advocated on some Pro Ana websites. One of them has "Ana's Laws":

> Thin is beauty; therefore I must be thin, and remain thin, if I wish to be loved. Food is my ultimate enemy. I may look, and I may smell, but I may not touch!
>
> I must think about food every second of every minute of every hour of every day . . . and ways to avoid eating it.
>
> I must weigh myself, first thing, every morning, and keep that number in mind throughout the remainder of that day. Should that number be greater than it was the day before, I must fast that entire day.
>
> I shall not be tempted by the enemy (food), and I shall not give in to temptation should it arise. Should I be in such a weakened state and I should cave, I will feel guilty and punish myself accordingly, for I have failed her.
>
> I will be thin, at all costs. It is the most important thing; nothing else matters.

> I will devote myself to Ana. She will be with me wherever I go, keeping me in line. No-one else matters; she is the only one who cares about me and who understands me. I will honor Her and make Her proud.[31]

It is easy to see other people's mind-forged manacles. In a therapist's response to the narrower versions of anorexia, one Socratic question might be: "How is your way of seeing things less stifling than Mrs. Winterson's?"

There is a shriveling of personality and risks to health and life—this is why families, friends, and psychiatrists want to intervene. But offers of professional help are often refused. There is a broad consensus in medical ethics that a person who has the capacity to make the decision to refuse treatment must be left to die if that is what the person has chosen. To justify imposing a lifesaving intervention that has been refused, the person's refusal must be shown to be the result of thinking so faulty or distorted as to show incapacity. Anorexic starvation can be linked to errors of judgment or reasoning, but these are usually too minor to undermine competence. The dilemma is stark. Must they really be left to die? Or are there other ways to question whether the decision to obey "Ana" is really theirs?

30
Authenticity and Identity in Eating Disorders

> Anorexia is not merely about body dysmorphia. There is a far deeper-reaching perversion of the mind that occurs when you are caught within the grips of this beast. You forget yourself.
>
> —Emily Halban, *Perfect: Anorexia and Me*

> I came to lose all understanding of my own centre and my own edges.
>
> —Grace Bowman, *A Shape of My Own: A Memoir of Anorexia and Recovery*

Ideas of identity and self-creation are central to the human interpretation of anorexia and bulimia. This will be supported by considering the decision to reject lifesaving treatment for anorexia. Does this reflect the person's authentic values? Or distorted anorexic values? This contrast has obvious intuitive appeal, but giving a clear and defensible account of it raises issues of identity.

Can There Be Distorted Values?

Are there such things as distorted values? If there are, the anorexic fanaticism about weight and body shape, and the intense obsession with being in control, seem good candidates. Jacinta Tan, Tony Hope, and their colleagues asked women questions about their experiences of anorexia. Among those who remembered their values at the time of the disorder, two gave these responses: "I wasn't really bothered about dying, as long as I died thin." "I remember getting some tests back saying how my liver was really damaged and all this, and I thought it was really rather good! I can't imagine that I thought it, it felt like really quite an accomplishment! . . . And you do feel like you might not have achieved anything else, but hey, I've done this, I'm cool!"[1]

How should we regard the values these comments express? They suggest dangerous priorities that are far from normal. But the history of imposing psychiatric "treatments" for homosexuality is a reminder: *mere* deviance from the norm is not enough justification. Much more is needed to prove distorted values or incompetent thinking.

On one approach the values are pathological—distortions totally bound up with anorexia or bulimia. They were not there before onset; they disappear with cure; the strength with which they are held varies according to the severity of the disorder. This strong linkage leaves it open whether the values are caused by the disorder, or cause the disorder, or are an intrinsic feature of the disorder. Any of these interpretations can seem to support stigmatizing the values as pathological.

But caution is needed. Tan and her colleagues rightly say, "It is insufficient, we believe, to base incompetence solely on the fact that a value that plays a key role in the decision is caused by, or part of, a mental disorder." They point out that all sorts of things cause people's values to change from one time to another, without discrediting either the earlier values or the later ones. It needs to be shown that the influence of the disorder is distorting rather than neutral.

This is clearly right. In psychology, "depressive realism" is the view that, because normal thinking tends to be overly optimistic, people with depression are in some ways more realistic than others. This has been challenged. But, even if it is false, the evidence could have gone the other way. It *could* have been true that depression improves some judgments. So "caused by or part of a mental disorder" is not enough to show distorted judgment. There has to be some independent support for the claim about distortion.

The depth and genuineness of these anorexic values can be doubted. Some evidence comes from what people say when cured. There are problems about hindsight, of course, but reports on anorexics' attitudes at the time also give grounds for doubt. The values seem to reflect not the person but the trap they have fallen into. (Hostages, captured in a crisis by some dictatorial regime, are sometimes filmed explaining to the world how reasonable their captors are.) The man who recalled that his anorexia had felt like being trapped at the bottom of a deep pit, or like facing an approaching train in a dark tunnel, probably never felt the anorexic values to be entirely his.

Ambiguous attitudes can be found in things said when still in the grip of anorexia:

> *What is the importance of your weight and body size to you?*
> I don't know, really, I think. I suppose if I were answering the question for anyone else I would probably say it was of no importance, because all my friends are of different sizes and it doesn't make any difference, but just for me it's different, I feel like I suppose because I got so caught up in it that it is really important, but I don't know why, but it is; I feel really guilty of myself, putting weight on . . . makes me feel really different.
> *Is it like there's a split, there's an intellectual part that knows it's not important, that the world doesn't revolve around your weight, but there's a feeling side that feels that its massively important.*
> Yeah, definitely.[2]

Values can be assessed for distortion in two different ways. One approach, as in Chapter 29, compares anorexic values with ideas of a good human life. Alternatively, values can be seen as distorted because they are not rooted in, or are opposed to, the person's authentic values.

Authentic and Inauthentic Values

What are someone's authentic values? They are what the person most deeply cares about. When people ask themselves what they deeply care about, the answer often comes from a mixture of decision and discovery.

Someone wonders about how much she cares about observing her ethnic or religious group's taboo on marrying a person outside the group. She does not find an answer just by asking how she feels about it. She decides what she cares about, perhaps thinking about the reasons for the taboo and judging they are not good.

Another person may ask himself whether he values having children, weighing it against the expense and the distraction from his work. He decides that he does not much value having children. His partner gets pregnant and the baby is born. Then he may discover that, despite his previous decision, this is something he cares deeply about.

Evidence about other people's authentic values takes different forms. Authenticity is supported by stability: when someone's patriotism has been consistent across a lifetime, it is hard to deny that it is really his. Intensity is relevant: it is hard to challenge the authenticity of the religious commitment of a person who has suffered persecution rather than deny her religion.

The dimension of depth and shallowness is important. In the Broadmoor interviews, some of the answers seemed shallow. Sometimes they followed conventional views about not swearing, or about letting a woman go through the door first. Sometimes the answers seemed more or less random, suggesting a lightness rather than the impact of experience or any serious thought about what matters. (This was visible in the shallowness of supporting capital punishment by the casual thought that the country is too crowded, contrasted with the impact witnessing an execution had on George Orwell's thinking.) Another indicator of depth is evidence of serious thought about moral identity: about who you are and what kind of person you want to be.

The "Thank You" Test

A possible support for the idea that a person's real values are temporarily eclipsed by psychiatric disorder comes from the "thank you" test. Suppose a young woman deep into anorexia is devoting herself to following "Ana's Laws." She waves away offers of help, saying she has no disorder or problems. Suppose that later, in a moment of weakness, she agrees to see a cognitive and behavioral therapist. The therapy works. Now she sees everything differently. She perhaps even thanks the therapist for curing her. The thanks are taken as evidence of a return to her values before the anorexia. This seems to bolster the view that the anorexic outlook was a temporary pathological deviation from her otherwise stable, and so authentic, values.

Even without the words "thank you," many people later do repudiate what they said when anorexic: "At home and at college, I was lonely and miserable but I didn't know what to do about it. I wasn't prepared to try something different. I had few friends, no boyfriends, rarely went out to socialize. If anyone had asked, I'd have said, 'I like my life just the way it is.' I can see how sad that is in retrospect but at the time I was so locked in to myself that I truly believed it."[3]

When her patient Gertrude later talked about having suffered when she starved herself, Hilde Bruch reminded her that she had always said it was not unpleasant. Gertrude replied, "I remember now how I felt at that time, and how I talked about it. It was not really lying because starving was what I wanted to do, but I remember feeling terribly uncomfortable. I remember what I *thought* and how I really *felt*. I thought it was just wonderful—that I was molding myself into that wonderful ascetic pure image, and I told myself I was not hungry; but what I felt was entirely different . . . I felt I had to do something I didn't want to do for a *higher purpose*. That took over my life . . . If you indulge in being a person who doesn't eat and who stays up all night, then you can't admit 'I feel miserable' or 'I feel hungry' . . . I violently defended it, but I was truly miserable. I am so terrified of it now that I think of it with almost physical horror. I have it definitely in my memory that I have experienced the pain of hunger; now I could never conceive of doing it again."[4]

Hilde Bruch, commenting on this, said that all her patients who came to accept their natural body size looked back on self-starvation with horror. Understandably, she drew the conclusion that "an anorexic patient cannot be considered outside the danger of relapse unless she has honestly reported on the terror of starvation and her inability to repeat it."[5]

It fits the "thank you" test when someone admits that her earlier claim "I like my life just the way it is" was wrong. But there is a worry about the test. Bruch's idea that sincerely recanting what you said before is the only way of showing you are cured can seem alarmingly like the view of the authorities in George Orwell's *1984*:

> "You are improving. Intellectually there is very little wrong with you. It is only emotionally that you have failed to make progress. Tell me, Winston—and remember, no lies: you know that I am always able to detect a lie—tell me, what are your true feelings towards Big Brother?"
>
> "I hate him."
>
> "You hate him. Good. Then the time has come for you to take the last step. You must love Big Brother. It is not enough to obey him: you must love him."

There are important differences between *1984* and the psychiatric "thank you" test. Winston Smith's recantation and his gratitude for coming to love Big Brother were coerced by close exposure of his face to rats. To preserve their own power, the authorities wanted him to change his attitude. They did not care about his own values and interests. Without coercion he would not have come to love Big Brother, so there is no reason to think it was an authentic value of his. A therapist may hope to save a client from starvation and death by appealing to things the client cared about before becoming anorexic. The contrast is obvious. In the absence of coercive manipulation in the interests of others, the "thank you" test can give support to authenticity.

Emma Baldock has argued that the causal origin of values is one important kind of evidence in assessing their authenticity. Value changes coming from the growth of a brain tumor are unlikely to be authentic. Those coming from reflection or the person's own responses to experiences are more likely to be. This is linked to self-creation. People's character and the things they do are more truly theirs when coming from their own thoughts and choices or from their own reactions to experiences (as in Orwell's reaction to the execution). They are less likely to be so when brought about by some disruption of this evolving self-creation, whether by external manipulation or by a brain tumor.[6]

The Sense of Self in Eating Disorders

Like anyone else, people who develop eating disorders have a sense of self, a view of the kind of person they are. Are there patterns in how this influences their disorder? Or in how the disorder in turn shapes their sense of self?

They often do not like what they see in the mirror—the body they hope to change by dieting. "When an anorexic looks in the mirror, her own form looks large, rounded and curved. Her eyes sharpen on the other bodies around her while her interpretation of her own image is skewed. Others see her as thin—skeletal—but she struggles to understand their perspective. Two sets of eyes see the size of the body completely differently. She fears her own shape—it becomes, like a monstrous creation, the seat of all discomfort, pain and anxiety, while the idea of an alternative, thinner shape provides comfort, stability and reassurance."[7]

Some accounts indicate that people with anorexia do not like the self they encounter when they turn from the kind of body they have to the kind of person they are. There is a mixture of guilt and self-hatred. "If I had a 'bad' day then I would blow it out of all proportion as if I did not deserve to be happy and deserved to be suffering like this. I felt guilty if I experienced any feelings of happiness, no matter how small."[8] Another said, "I hated my father, I hated my brother, but more than anything I hated myself."[9]

Eating disorders can express this self-dislike and perhaps can also be an appeal for recognition: "I wanted to be sickly skinny as a statement of being sad, angry and not a part of the world I hated, but more like a walking dead person. I felt dead and empty on the inside and I wanted a skeletal body to reflect that."[10]

The self-hatred can slide into self-punishment by means of the eating disorder. One person with anorexia said, "If I was hurt or upset about something I would take it out on myself and not eat. That was where I channelled my anger. Food had become a weapon to use against myself, and dieting had made me discover its powers."[11]

A woman with bulimia said, "The pain is crippling. Worse than any period pain ever . . . Laxatives just mess up your large intestine and carry a whole lot of other bad health side effects. Do I care? Not at all. The whole point of this is to harm ourselves, to get rid of the bad food and inflict pain on ourselves. We are bad, fat, ugly people, and we deserve to be punished."[12]

Bad Self-Evaluations and "Being Good"

Where do these dark self-evaluations come from? No story fits everyone. But one conjecture comes from the way some of them were "good" children. Sometimes they felt that "being good" was what their hard-pressed parents needed from them: "I tried to make things 'right' for my mother by being 'good.' So I took the role of the quiet, uncomplaining one of the family, never saying 'no' to anyone or anything, so at mealtimes I ate all I was given and if more was offered I accepted whether I was hungry or not."[13]

But often "being good" was an appeal for the recognition, approval, and unconditional acceptance they felt they had been denied.

> I felt that my Father, who had always ignored me because I was not a boy, would pay me attention if I achieved high marks.[14]

> I wanted to be good enough. I wanted my parents' approval. I wanted them to be proud of me. I could never get this from them, my personality was not what they wanted.[15]
>
> I also felt that I had to be a perfectionist in all that I did so that my father would be proud and notice me.[16]
>
> I never had a real friend apart from my Nan (Dad's Mum). She accepted me unconditionally. As for my parents, they were proud of my swimming trophies, my Guide's certificate, my academic prowess and my "good deeds" to the less fortunate. I was a good and obedient child.[17]

Some people's accounts note their perfectionism, linked to wanting to fulfill their parents' hopes. Responses of disappointment could trigger guilt, sometimes amounting to self-hatred. "I was also a perfectionist. I wanted to be the best, at everything and immediately . . . I felt there was pressure from home too. Every time my grades slipped just a little I felt extremely guilty and felt I had let them down terribly. I hated myself for that."[18] Later the disappointment and resulting guilt could come from not making progress toward escaping the disorder: "But above all it was always the disgrace of disappointing my parents who were pouring so much of themselves on to me, my recovery. I couldn't deal with disappointment, because along with disappointment there came guilt, and a deep sense of unworthiness—and both, in turn, were anorexia's favourite fodder."[19]

The obsessive perfectionism can go beyond wanting to please their parents. They may worry about how other people in general regard them. "I got my first job. Being the typical perfectionist I am I worked night and day to create a good impression . . . I completely wore myself out and gradually became more and more depressed. I reached the stage where I knew I needed help and so I visited my doctor . . . I was taken into hospital the day after the visit for an indefinite period. My first thought was for my job; I didn't want to lose it and I was also extremely concerned about what other people would think . . . Everything I did had total control. In my eating I *had* to control what I ate—I had to have the perfect image."[20]

Pressures, Other-Dependence, and the Sense of Self

Some people's evaluations of themselves, whether positive or negative, greatly reflect the opinions of others. Richard Keshen cites Virginia Woolf's diary entries after she read reviews of her novel *The Years.* One said it was quite good. Virginia Woolf wrote, "And so it is." When another called her a first-rate novelist, she wrote that "after all that agony, I'm free, round, can go full ahead." Three weeks later two other reviews called the book dead and disappointing: "So I'm found out and that odious rice pudding of a book is what I thought—a dank failure."[21]

Keshen stresses loss of autonomy in "other-dependence." Bending too much to others' opinions, and fearing negative reactions, the person may defer excessively to those whose responses have such power. Standing back and criticizing other people's evaluations can be the way to greater autonomy. (Keshen points out that Virginia Woolf herself illustrates the possible complexity of all this. She was in many ways highly autonomous, as well as being other-dependent in the way the quoted responses illustrate. She was also acutely aware of the "invisible presences": "public opinion; what other people say and think; all those magnets which attract us to be this way to be like that, or repel us the other and make us different from that . . . I see myself as a fish in a stream; deflected; held in place; but cannot describe the stream."[22])

In eating disorders the other-dependent distress can complicate family relationships. The young woman sliding into anorexia may take her family's disappointment to show they do not understand her. She in turn may feel disappointed by them, creating a circle of mutual blame. Simona Giordano suggests that she may think, "If I should feel bad about disappointing them, they should feel bad about disappointing me."[23] The pressures toward an identity reflecting the values of others can arouse resentment. One woman with bulimia described how she had felt herself shrinking into a shell of a person: "I didn't think I was truly the person people wanted me to be but I didn't want to show them who the true me was. So I pretended to be what other people wanted. However, the less I spoke up and the more of myself I hid, the deeper I got into the eating disorder and the more resentful I became of the family I was so desperately trying to please."[24]

Other-dependence, with its excessive desire to please, can create emptiness at the person's core: "I was sitting with these three people but I felt a terrible fragmentation of myself. There wasn't a person inside at all. I tried with whoever I was with to reflect the image they had of me, to do what they expected me to do. There were three different people, I had to be a different person to each; and I had to balance that. It was the same when I was a child and had friends. It was always in response to what they wanted."[25]

Inner Conflict: The Good and Bad Self

> Not only will he act upon different desires at different times, not only will action upon these different desires establish within him different habits, but at these different times the world will seem to him so different that it will not occur to him to will otherwise than he does. And at times the two centres can be so brought into conjunction that the world will seem to him these two different ways at one and the same time.
>
> —Richard Wollheim, *The Good Self and the Bad Self*

The question "What kind of person are you?" usually has no simple answer. One reason for this is inner conflict. People with eating disorders may dislike the person they are becoming. "My personality had also changed . . . the polite friendly Kate had gone . . . Anorexia turned me into a very nasty, dishonest, deceitful person. That was not the real me. I thought I was in control of my life when I was anorexic but in fact I was not in control at all. The illness was in control of me."[26]

The combination of self-dislike and not being in control recurs. "When I was anorexic I was obnoxious, saying what I felt in a way that was designed to cause hurt to others, but my father still visited me at the hospital each night. I did not know how to stop being awful although I really did want to."[27] The inner conflict is often in this way linked to the effect of the anorexia on the family. One woman knew that losing more weight would distress her family yet still hoped to lose more: "With every thrill I still got from losing another pound, I hurt people I loved so much and I died a little bit more inside."[28]

These conflicts sometimes give rise to the idea of being split into a "good self" and a "bad self." "Sometimes I feel that I am two different people, the person I am when I do not eat, who is good, kind, considerate, in control of her life, happy and full of energy . . . and the other person who has to lock herself away from the world and does not care about anything." And the worries about the responses of others may inhibit any self-creative project of combining elements from each "self." "The crazy thing, that is difficult to understand, is that I cannot let these two people merge into one; they have to remain separate from each other in the same way that my eating does, good and bad, black and white, separate . . . Yes, I know I'm not cured and that my thoughts are irrational, and yes, I do wish they were different, but I am not brave enough to join them together for fear that no-one will like the me that no-one meets."[29]

Obviously the thought about having a good self and a bad self is not confined to those who experience the conflicts of eating disorders. Perhaps everyone knows some kind of inner conflict. And many (most?) people think that some of their conflicts are between a good side and a bad side. In some of these accounts of eating disorders, however, the vehemence of the self-dislike suggests a self-image with a large and unusually intense bad side. When combined with dependence on the approval of others, this dark self-image can be a serious obstacle to becoming the person they themselves want to be. "I still have this intense and overwhelming need to be productive and to do the 'right thing.' I have an incredibly difficult time believing that anyone could care about me if I stopped being who they wanted and started being who I wanted. But I am learning."[30]

Reflection, Self-Creation, and Recovery

Why do people feel guilty when they do not meet others' expectations? Simona Giordano has argued that the expectations themselves are not the whole explanation. Guilt also depends on accepting that disappointing them is something to feel bad about.[31]

People made to feel guilty might not see alternatives. They might not notice their other-dependence. Or they might not have Richard Keshen's thought about critical reflection as the way out. The demands and expectations, when thought about, may seem unrealistic or unreasonable. Keshen advocates basing self-evaluation on autonomous reasons. This may sound unrealistic. Surely even those who come closest to autonomy must to some extent reflect the influence of other people's attitudes and responses? In Freud's image of the rider and the horse, even a dominant rider was once a child, subject to all the parental and other influences this implies. Keshen accepts this, saying that autonomous reasons do not have to meet the impossible standard of having no external causes. Instead, they are the reasons we make our own through critical thought about them, especially in dialogue with others.[32]

No self-creation is completely independent of others' evaluations. But one aim of therapy can be to help a person engage in dialogue that may help them decide which values to make their own. Of course, self-creation, with its links to critical reflection, need not come from psychiatric help: "A big part of my recovery came down to actually embracing change rather than opposing it . . . I was bored by the frustrating obsession with every inch of my body. I had had enough . . . In my early twenties, trying to forge a connection with myself as an independent adult and lose the remains of my teenage self was an important goal and I wanted to reach towards it."[33]

Many factors other than self-creation help recovery. But issues of identity are central to eating disorders. This is suggested by the way the process of recovery is often interwoven with turning from other-dependence toward self-creation. "Confidence in myself, in becoming the person I want to be and not the one anyone else wants me to be—this, I've discovered, is the underlying cause of my anorexic hell . . . Who am I? What is normal? What is right? How does food become a thing you need to live and not life itself? If only I knew. I am sure that I will find the answers once I develop into the person I am meant to be—the person that has never been able to develop. Everyone has their own character, personality and likes and dislikes over food. What does it matter if we cannot achieve ten out of ten all the time?"[34]

31

Dementia, Responsibility, and Identity

> In Alzheimer's disease there is the loss of the personality, a diminished sense of self-worth. A highly productive person has to wonder why he is still alive and what purpose the Lord has in keeping him on this earth. As I struggle with the indignities that accompany daily living, I am losing my sense of humanity and self-worth. Blessed is the person who can take the Alzheimer's patient back to that happier time when they were worthwhile and allow them to see the situation in which they were of some use.
>
> —Robert Davis, *My Journey into Alzheimer's Disease*

> For me now, any question of identity becomes profound and difficult. Without memory you lose the idea of who you are. I am struggling more than ever to find answers to questions of identity. I am flooded with early memories preserved in protected places in my brain where Alzheimer's does not reign supreme. These memories become the last remnants of my search for who I am.
>
> —Thomas Debaggio, *Losing My Mind: An Intimate Look at Life with Alzheimer's*

Some major psychiatric disorders can change the central core of a person. This raises acutely the problem of the boundary between the person and the illness. There are questions about where the boundary comes between medical treatment to cure an illness and interventions to change someone's character and personality. The boundary between the person and the illness is also important for decisions about responsibility. It seems unfair to blame people for things coming directly from illness.

Character Distortion and Responsibility: Frontotemporal Dementia

When a psychiatric or neurological disorder seems to take over and distort an individual's whole personality and character, how should we respond to what they do?

Frontotemporal dementia involves some major changes not typical of other dementias. At the mild end are breaches of etiquette and other social norms. More serious are emotional blunting, loss of empathy, and loss of the inhibitions that normally check bizarre or antisocial behavior. People with frontotemporal dementia tend not to feel remorse. In contrast to the standard account of antisocial personality disorder, though, they are rarely manipulative or given to deception.[1]

One man in his sixties had changed over four years. He showed less concern for others, intruded into people's offices, butted into their conversations, and would eat indiscriminately (including garbage). He stopped taking showers. He hoarded things and filled his pockets with restaurants' napkins and sugar. For the first time in his life he began stalking and trying to molest children. He was arrested for exposing himself to children. He could describe in detail what he had done and agreed it was wrong and harmful.

A man in his fifties had changed over two years. He started to laugh inappropriately. He became emotionally detached. He did not react to the death of his mother or visit his wife when she was in the hospital. He became disinhibited—without embarrassment blurting out distressing comments, belching, or being partly undressed in front of others. When driving he struck a van with passengers in it, but drove on. He could describe what he did, and knew hit-and-run driving was wrong, but said he did not feel a need to stop at the time.[2]

Such cases bring out the difficulty any legal system still using only the M'Naghten criteria for responsibility would have in responding adequately to crimes committed by people with frontotemporal dementia. Quite apart from the evidence of brain atrophy, clearly these two men have recently developed character-disrupting psychiatric problems. Treating them as fully responsible for their acts would be bizarre. But it is hard for a M'Naghten-based system to avoid doing so. Do they know the nature and quality of their acts? They can describe them clearly, together with their consequences. Do they know that molesting children or hit-and-run driving are wrong? They each admit the wrongness of what they did.

Under the M'Naghten rules, recognizing diminished responsibility would depend on stretching the word "know" to include an *emotional* awareness of the seriousness of the acts. It is not clear that M'Naghten-based systems would allow that stretching.

On the other hand, some might hold such people fully responsible. Accepting or rejecting an excuse is largely about how much an apparently bad action does or does not reflect the person's character. Excuses protect a person's character by disconnecting it from objectionable actions. So it seems strange to accept the excuse that psychiatric disorder has made someone's character worse. Does not this mean that the person's *present* character is open to precisely the criticism the objectionable action suggests?

People often change radically. They have religious conversions. They may change partners and jobs and emigrate. They take up drugs or enter convents. Any of these upheavals may change character sharply. But the immigrant or the nun are still praised or blamed for what they do. The new actions flow from the new character and personality. It is still appropriate to evaluate the person on the basis of what they do. Normally, with a kind of Aristotelian common sense, we do hold people responsible for their characters. Despite being newly acquired, the novice nun's piety and the immigrant's new patriotism still come into our picture of them. So why should a new willingness to molest children, shaped by dementia, be different?

Those who have to live with this behavior mainly do see it as different. Where a medical condition causes this kind of radical transformation, they see it in terms of the illness rather than the person. They may suggest (with varying degrees of literalness) that his very identity has been affected: "He isn't the man I married."[3] Blaming the person may show a lack of understanding.

It is not just that the original person has changed. We have seen some limits to Aristotle's view that character comes from habits, in turn coming from freely chosen actions. It does not do justice to the pressures often behind the slide into addiction. It fits dementia even less well. The nun's piety or the immigrant's patriotism come from upheavals they freely chose. But dementia is not the intended result of anyone's choices. So this disaster, although internal to the person's body, is seen as striking from "outside." The urge to blame is rightly checked.

Dementia and the Erosion of Identity

> Do you understand I am not dying, just disappearing before your eyes?
>
> —Thomas Debaggio, *Losing My Mind: An Intimate Look at Life with Alzheimer's*

To some extent others—family, friends, and caregivers—can support the person's identity. They often know what the person cares about. Dr. Catherine Oppenheimer describes a patient with dementia, lonely after losing her husband, and frightened. This patient called the emergency services a dozen times a day. She stubbornly fought attempts to persuade her to leave her home. Buying the house and making it a home had been a shared project with her husband: "To leave her home would have meant finally losing her husband and herself."[4]

Protection of identity can come from understanding, and from supporting attempts to communicate. Jennifer Radden cites the kind of undramatic everyday support that makes a difference. A man (J) with dementia was leaving his house. Where he was going his shabby, worn, and unmendable couch might put people off. But it was laden with memories: he had repaired it and had shared it with his dog. Should he take it with him? When he tried to decide, he "wavered and hesitated, forgot, remembered, and began over, entirely unable to keep in view all the factors and their respective weights." To help him with his decision, his two adult daughters held on to the different strands of the problem, giving him each strand as it was needed. Jennifer Radden says this recognition (of such things as his ability to repair furniture, his feeling for the dog, and his hopes for his new home) in turn supported these parts of his identity.[5]

When a medical condition brings about a radical transformation of someone's character, we are inclined to say, "It is not him but his illness." Whether or not this thought is accepted affects the relationship. Aggression that seems to reflect the person is resented. If it reflects only the illness, we may be more detached. But the boundary between the person and the illness is often elusive.

Even where someone with severe dementia acts most of the time in quite uncharacteristic ways, the question of how much of the original person is left may be complicated. People are more than their deliberate actions. Iris Murdoch wrote, "When we apprehend and assess other people we do not consider only their solutions to specifiable practical problems, we consider something more elusive . . . their total vision of life, as shown by their mode of speech or silence, their choice of words, their assessment of others, their conception of their own lives, what they think attractive or praiseworthy, what they think funny . . . what, making two points in the two metaphors, one may call the texture of a man's being or the nature of his personal vision."[6]

Toward the end of her life, Murdoch herself developed Alzheimer's disease. Her husband, John Bayley, described its severity: "The power of concentration has gone, along with the ability to form coherent sentences, and to remember where she is or has been. She does not know she has written twenty-seven remarkable novels, as well as her books on philosophy; received honorary doctorates from the major universities; become a Dame of the British Empire."[7] She started to ask many anxious, repetitive questions that faded out in midsentence. Bayley found her questions often hard to interpret: "At such times I feel my own mind and memory faltering, as if required to perform a function too far outside their own beat and practice."

The Person Still Glimpsed

> It is humiliating to give up our areas of responsibility. There is a distinct feeling of the loss of self and all that we have been. Yet all is not gone.
>
> —Robert Davis: *My Journey into Alzheimer's Disease*

> In interpreting dementia, it is important to avoid the tempting metaphors that describe someone as a shell, a husk, or being gone, by which we remove people from moral significance.
>
> —Stephen G. Post, *The Moral Challenge of Alzheimer Disease*

The thought that someone is quite gone can be mistaken. Sometimes Iris Murdoch was able to say something grimly appropriate, as that she was "sailing into the darkness." Even under these adverse conditions, John Bayley found that they still had a kind of communication: "like underwater sonar, each bouncing pulsations off the other, and listening for an echo." And he noted the need "to feel the unique individuality of one's spouse has not been lost in the common symptoms of a clinical condition."

Bayley was able to say, "Iris remains her old self in many ways." His account suggests that those ways had to do with the "something more elusive" about which she herself had written: the texture of her being, and especially what she thought funny. Speaking of times when he could not understand what she tried to convey, Bayley said, "The continuity of joking can very often rescue such moments. Humour seems to survive anything. A burst of laughter, snatches of doggerel, song, teasing nonsense rituals once lovingly exchanged, awake an abruptly happy response, and a sudden beaming smile . . . Only a joke survives, the last thing that finds its way into consciousness when the brain is atrophied."

Sans Everything

Even in quite severe dementia, there is often something of the original person. But the blankness can grow. At a late stage of her illness, Iris Murdoch would pick up from the street old candy wrappings, matchsticks, and cigarette ends. Indoors, she made and rearranged piles of clothes, books, stones, cups, and shoes. Sometimes she was "silently scouring the house, or on the rampage downstairs, drumming on the front door and shouting to the outside world *'Help me—help!'*"[8]

Before the illness, the Iris Murdoch who wrote so well about the texture of a person's being or the nature of a personal vision would not have thought any of this hoarding and turmoil was hers. None of it comes from any conscious self-creation. It did not even come about in the less conscious Aristotelian way, through the ossifying of freely chosen actions into habits and then character. It came from atrophy of the brain. The lack of any element of self-creation is the main reason why the behavior reflects the illness and not the person. Through self-creation the person we become reflects our own values. We do not do things intended to bring on dementia. This disaster comes "from outside" in that it is not under our present or past control. The piles of stones, cups, and shoes reflected the illness, not the real Iris Murdoch.

32

Schizophrenia: The Person or the Illness?

Was't Hamlet wronged Laertes? Never Hamlet.
If Hamlet from himself be ta'en away,
And when he's not himself does wrong Laertes,
Then Hamlet does it not, Hamlet denies it.
Who does it then? His madness. If't be so,
Hamlet is of the faction that is wronged;
His madness is poor Hamlet's enemy.

—William Shakespeare, *Hamlet*

The boundary between the person and the illness is harder to draw in schizophrenia. Dementia mainly (but not always) comes on late in life. This makes it easier to see the demented period as a coda: something after the main part of someone's life. But the radical personality changes of schizophrenia usually come on relatively young.

Here I will put aside such issues as whether schizophrenia is a unitary condition or should be divided into subgroups, or whether it is a properly empirically based scientific concept.[1] At the start of this book I expressed my hopes that we might eventually achieve finer-grained, and possibly more biologically based, diagnostic categories. The objects of those hopes include schizophrenia. But to talk about common features shared by many people with the diagnosis, the word has to be used—with an appropriate tinge of skepticism.

The question of the boundary between the person and the illness hardly arises in acute schizophrenic crisis. Little coherent personality may show through the torrent of words, the delusions, the suspicious hostility, or the menacing stare. Most of this has all too clearly more to do with the illness than with a person's own characteristics.

In the periods of relative stability the boundary question is real. Even in stable periods, the person may still hear voices and behave strangely. The conjectures put forward in the discussion of delusions included a disruption of emotional intuition. This, if correct, could be linked to the weak grasp of the small change of everyday life that is part of the strangeness. When someone has been changed profoundly by psychiatric illness, it matters that the person underneath the changes is still recognized. There is something like this in Tove Jansson's magical book *Finn Family Moomintroll.* In a children's game of hide-and-seek, Moomintroll hides under the Hobgoblin's hat. He comes out radically changed.

> "You aren't Moomintroll," said the Snork Maiden scornfully. "He has beautiful little ears, but yours look like kettle-holders!"
>
> Moomintroll felt quite confused and took hold of a pair of enormous crinkly ears. "But I am Moomintroll," he burst out in despair. Don't you believe me?"
>
> "Moomintroll has a nice little tail, just about the right size, but yours is like a chimney sweep's brush," said the Snork.
>
> And, oh dear, it was true! Moomintroll felt behind him with a trembling paw.
>
> "Your eyes are like soup plates," said Sniff. "Moomintroll's are small and kind."
>
> "Yes exactly," Snufkin agreed.
>
> "You are an impostor!" decided the Hemulen.
>
> "Isn't there anyone who believes me?" Moomintroll pleaded. "Look carefully at me, Mother. You must know your own Moomintroll."
>
> Moominmama looked carefully. She looked into his frightened eyes for a very long time, and then she said quietly, "Yes, you are my Moomintroll."
>
> And at the same moment he began to change. His ears, eyes, and tail began to shrink, and his nose and tummy grew, until at last he was his own self again.
>
> "It's all right now, my dear," said Moominmama. "You see, I shall always know you whatever happens."[2]

It would be wonderful if such recognition could dispel psychiatric changes in this way. It cannot, of course. But the recognition can still be a lifeline.

Schizophrenia and Identity

Sometimes the person may seem much as before the illness. But often there is a deep transformation.[3] Someone friendly and humorous, lively and alert, may have become strangely unreachable: taciturn, sullen, uninterested in others, perhaps aggressive, and doing little beyond half-watching television. This new burnt-out personality may last a lifetime, either uninterrupted or alternating with acute episodes. Friends and family may have conflicting responses to the aggression the person they have known sometimes shows toward them. Should they react with exasperation or detachment? Does the aggression reflect the person or the illness?

Jay Neugeboren discusses this in his account of Robert, his younger brother with schizophrenia. Neugeboren would sometimes break down after painful visits to his brother in the hospital. For a time he got through the visits by thinking there were two Roberts. There was one he grew up with, and one now in the hospital: "It was as if, I would say, the brother I grew up with had died." This made things easier because it reduced blame or disappointment: "I could spend time with him without making him feel that he had, by becoming a mental patient, somehow failed me, or himself, or life."[4]

To see the original person as having died is extreme. But there is a strong case for the thought that the schizophrenic personality expresses the illness rather than the person's real self. The reasons are partly conceptual and partly moral.

The conceptual case starts by accepting that the strangeness and narrowing passivity are caused by the illness. As a thought experiment, imagine a treatment that, without other side effects, restored people from this negative state to how they were before the illness. This would be a cure for schizophrenia. It would then be natural to see the second personality as a temporary product of the illness. The hostility and aggression displayed during the illness would be put aside as not reflecting the person's real self. But if that would be the approach if there were a cure, why should the status of the schizophrenic personality be so different now?

Should not what counts as a feature of an illness be independent of whether a cure is available?

The moral case for seeing the schizophrenic personality as reflecting the illness rather than the person is linked to the desire not to give up on the possibility of a cure, a kind of keeping faith with the original person. There is the hope that the original version of the person might not be lost. On the analogy of a television screen where the picture has been replaced by visual chaos, there is the hope that, if only we could get the neurological or neurochemical tuning right, the original picture might be restored.

As with dementia, the new personality is the product of the illness rather than of any self-creative process. It does not reflect the choices or values of the person before the onset. It seems unfair that people's personalities have been so distorted by factors outside their control. Refusal to see the new personality as really reflecting them is a recognition of this. And blaming the person for things that reflect the new personality seems particularly unfair.

But there is also a strong case for saying that the schizophrenic personality is now the person's real self. Perhaps the personality of the 18-year-old before the onset of the illness is irretrievably lost. At least it may have been hidden for years. Refusal to recognize the new personality leaves the person as he is now in limbo, perhaps for the rest of his life. Jay Neugeboren recognizes this: "The sad truth is that who he is—his identity as Robert Neugeboren and nobody else, a human being forever in process, forever growing, changing and evolving—is made up, to this moment in time, largely of what most of us have come to call his illness. And if he gives that up . . . and does not hold on to his illness and its history as a legitimate, real, and unique, part of his ongoing self—what of him, at fifty-two years old, will be left?"[5]

The dilemma is acute. Is the schizophrenic personality an authentic expression of the person? To say yes seems to ignore how it was forced on the person by the illness. To say no seems to locate the authentic person in a distant past and to deny recognition to the only person actually here.

How should those close to a person with schizophrenia react to bursts of unprovoked hostility and aggression? Are reactive attitudes such as anger and resentment appropriate? Of course these attitudes are not entirely under our control. But to the extent that we can choose, either alternative is troubling. To have these responses seems unfair, for all the reasons that make it doubtful that the behavior reflects the person rather than the illness. But to inhibit the reactive attitudes, especially where the actions that trigger them are typical of the new personality, may be to exclude the person from the deeper emotional relationships.

Versions of Authentication

The question "Is he really like that or is it just his illness?" reflects a contrast between an aberration and something central or deep in a person. But the words "central" and "deep" are vague. What kinds of psychological changes support the view that something reflects not the person but the illness? What kinds of continuity support the alternative view? What makes up someone's individuality and uniqueness? The question "Is this the real person?" is not like the question whether a banknote is genuine. In the psychiatric case the tests of authenticity are multiple and conflicting. Deciding between them might be, not a matter of discovering some deep metaphysical truth, but of deciding which one, or which combination, best captures the things that matter most.

There are at least three different tests for authenticating a person's present character or personality as "really them." The first two are:

1. The original person test
2. The predominant person test.

These two names are self-explanatory. Take the person greatly changed by schizophrenia, but whose new character and personality have been stable for many years. Does the new personality reflect the real person? The original person test gives the answer no. The predominant person test gives the answer yes. This pair of tests can be called "external." It is largely possible to apply them from outside, without calling on the person's own view.

By contrast, the third, an internal test, appeals to the person's own perspective:

3. The self-creation test: Deep endorsement and active autobiography

Two things are relevant: the person's own reflective endorsement, and his or her active autobiographical story.

First, endorsement. In an approach to identity that takes the person's values seriously, people's own feelings about what they are really like are central. Taken off Prozac, Peter Kramer's patient Tess said, "I'm not myself." Her own endorsement of how she was on Prozac rather than her other state has to be taken seriously.

Not any endorsement is enough. People with mood disorders sometimes seesaw backward and forward between two states, giving different accounts of what their "myself" is in the different phases. What is needed is what can be called "deep endorsement": a relatively stable endorsement that reflects the person's deeper values, rather than the shallow, breathless endorsement given only in a manic phase. Deep endorsement can be hard to be sure about. The problem is like that raised by a person's mood swings when one is trying to evaluate the authenticity of that person's expressed wish not to be kept alive.

Also relevant is autobiography. The present character or personality is authenticated to the extent that there is a coherent autobiographical story of how it emerged. How I am now need not be the same as how I was. But there has to be an evolution of one out of the other. The demand for an autobiographical story may seem to exclude nothing. Surely any change in character can be recounted as a first-person story? ("He forced me to undergo surgery to remove bits of my brain, and since then he has given me daily injections of this drug. Now I do nothing at all except look forward to the next injection.") A merely passive story does not authenticate the new personality. Authentication needs an active, self-creative autobiographical story, at least in the minimal Aristotelian sense in which my new character or personality grows out of actions that I chose.

Some unself-conscious Aristotelian self-creation is the minimum required by the autobiographical test. Stronger authentication comes from more substantial forms of self-creation. Perhaps I set out to become the kind of person I am now. If the project reflects my deepest values, this support from the endorsement test greatly strengthens the authentication. Some suggest, plausibly, that our deepest values are decisive in settling such questions of identity. Viktor Frankl, reflecting on his experience of how even in the Nazi concentration camps people sometimes gave meaning to their lives, said promptings of conscience came from interpreting the situation in the light of a set of values: "These values, however, cannot be espoused and adopted by us on a conscious level—they are something that we *are*."[6]

All three tests are relevant. But there is a case for giving priority to the self-creative test. This comes from the point of asking the question about "the real me." A large part of its point comes from the way people value the more substantial kind of self-creation: being shaped by what they care about. Psychiatry, in its concern with the good life, should be shaped by the value people place on this.

33

Self-Creation, Values, and Psychiatric Disorder

> An indication of the power of medicine to reshape a person's identity is contained in the sentence Tess used when, eight months after first stopping Prozac, she telephoned me to ask whether she might resume the medication. She said, "I am not myself."
>
> —Peter Kramer, *Listening to Prozac*

How far does the idea of self-creation help draw the boundary between the person and the illness in mood disorders and in schizophrenia?

Depression and Recreating the Self: Landscape as Metaphor

Anthropologists report that in some cultures depression is seen as "loss of soul," expressed in metaphors of emptiness.[1] Metaphors are part of how people interpret and shape themselves.

Jennifer Radden has asked why we think a bleak landscape is melancholy. Part of her answer cites the way traditional descriptions have linked melancholy with coldness, darkness, and isolation. In the ancient accounts of opposite humors, "melancholy was always placed with coldness (and dryness). As the seasons came to be added to such schemas, melancholy was associated with things autumnal. The link with darkness is similarly ancient: as a disease of the black bile, melancholy was described as common in those of dark hair and complexion . . . The emphasis upon out-of-the-way, unpeopled landscapes seems to hearken to the isolation and (self-imposed) loneliness of misanthropy, which from the earliest descriptions has been noted as an aspect of melancholy."[2] She makes it clear that the metaphors linking mind and landscape run both ways, with the two directions interacting with each other.

Richard Mabey, the distinguished nature writer, has described how a mixture of self-interpretation and landscape helped his progress away from severe depression. His move from the Chiltern Hills to the flat Norfolk landscape became an internalized metaphor.[3]

He fell in love with Poppy. Walking through the harvest fields, she told him about sadness in her life, and he told her about his depression, and his mother's illness and her death. Depression had stopped him from writing for two years. Poppy told him to keep a diary for her while she was away. Under the beech tree he wrote about his garden, the birds, the wood, and his past.

> And the more I wrote the less my life seemed to resemble that of the marginalised voyeur I'd cast myself as. I'd been places, made friends, and made, I began to remember, a mark. Writing again was not just a relief in itself, the regaining of an identity, but a key that began to unlock pieces of me that had been dormant for years . . . At the end of Poppy's holiday I realised I'd written what was virtually a short book, and that I had my life back again. My friends, the sea, the hard work, that symbolically comforting beech, and above all Poppy's care, had broken the grip of my illness. But it was regaining that imaginative relationship with the world beyond that was my "nature cure."[4]

Richard Mabey knows the idea of nature cure goes back at least as far as the Romans. The thought has been that the landscapes of the country should "take you out of yourself." "But that was not how it happened with me. I'd tried repeatedly to exorcise my depression by this kind of exposure, but I was too disconnected by then, and all I felt was a kind of rebuke, a clear statement that I was no longer part of that world . . . What healed me, I think, was almost the exact opposite process, a sense of being taken not out of myself but back in, of nature entering me, firing up the wild bits of my imagination." He saw that if there was a moment when he was cured, it was when Poppy made him write: "It was those first stumbling imaginative acts that reconnected me, more than the autumn breeze through the trees. The physical rejoining came later, and my translation from the depths of forest country to the bright and shifting landscape of the fens was a huge metaphorical support."[5]

Our Landscape: Depression and Temperament

Some geologists use levels of the mind as an image for different layers of landscape. Richard Fortey does this in *The Hidden Landscape:* "Lying beneath the thin skin of recorded history in our islands, geology has the same role in landscape as does the unconscious mind in psychology: ubiquitous but concealed."[6] It is worth borrowing back the comparison and, running it the other way, letting the geological layer of landscape stand for the more permanent aspects of a person's psychology, not for mood but for temperament.

Rainer Maria Rilke's *Tenth Elegy* starts with thoughts of jubilation on emerging from an emotionally dark time. But the jubilation includes celebrating the dark times themselves:

> How dear you will be to me then, you nights of anguish.
> Inconsolable sisters, why didn't I kneel to you, submissive,
> And lose myself in your dishevelled hair?
>
> By looking through our bitter times towards their end
> We squander our sorrows. But they are a season of us,
> Yes, our winter foliage, our dark evergreen. Not only a
>   season,
> But also our landscape, settlement and fortress,
> Our depths and our home.[7]

People prone to depression may want to recognize their "dark evergreen," to accept times of depression as a "season of us." A season could be a passing mood. But something more permanent—temperament—is Rilke's "landscape," where the metaphor moves away from trees to geology.

In a humane psychiatry, not only short-lived mood but even more permanent temperament may be open to modification. Someone might want to escape a temperament found devastatingly life-wrecking. (Of course there are huge ethical questions here about the genuine autonomy of the choice and about what counts as "life-wrecking.") The effect of Prozac on Peter Kramer's patient Tess may be a case in point. But some are skeptical about how radically Prozac transforms personality. Lauren Slater, in her account of Prozac in her own life, wonders how far the idea of radical change would survive long-term study of the patients.[8] At first Prozac did transform her, but then its powers faded, "the stilts shrinking to fine high heels on my best days, on my worst days to stunted flats."

Lauren Slater also asks whether the transformed self might have been present within the original self. People's reports about their previous personality may be colored by their present depression. Before Prozac, Slater would have described her early years in terms of the roots of her depression. But Prozac brought back many more positive memories that give a quite different color to her past. "In altering my present sense of who I am, Prozac has demanded a revisioning of my history, and this revisioning is perhaps the most stunning side-effect of all."[9] She finds it hard to choose between two ways of seeing what Prozac does: either as transforming the self or as restoring the original self.

It is striking that Lauren Slater's account from the inside, like Richard Mabey's account of depression, centers on changes in her conception of herself. If the "revisioning" of her history leads her to decide that Prozac has restored her, the original person test will authenticate her present self. Even if she settles for the "transformation" account, her present self can still be authenticated by the autobiographical test. Her active autobiographical story and her endorsement are what count. For either kind of authentication, her self-interpretation is crucial. The landscape, settlement, and fortress are ours only if *we* feel they are our depths and our home.

Our Home? Manic Depression

But how we feel about them is not always stable. In manic depression (sometimes called bipolar disorder), people's oscillations of mood may affect their view of where their depths and their home are to be found.

Manic depression often includes nightmare psychotic episodes as well as the bouts of depression that sometimes prompt suicide. But its seriousness can be expressed equally in the mania. Felicity Bryan describes her mother's manic phases:

> The sufferer, when manic, feels capable of anything. Their mind is in overdrive . . . My thoughtful mother who took such generous interest in other people was now a horribly intrusive busybody. I remember, aged 17, receiving a 25-page letter

> telling me, all too coherently, what a tart I was. Stopping my mother's letters before they reached the recipient was a full-time job . . . Old friends would get long, apparently well-argued letters saying they must not be ashamed of the fact that they were unattractive, fat, that their husbands were unfaithful to them, that they were Jewish. Stopping her spending sprees was also a nightmare. A pantechnicon would arrive from the local nursery stuffed with unwanted trees and shrubs . . . She could not be left alone. She was a danger to herself. For a daughter, the worst thing was the complete change in her personality. I loathed this arrogant person who was turning our family life upside down . . . Then the depression would come. Betty would look back on her manic behaviour, not recognising herself, and be filled with remorse.[10]

For Betty, the manic states were obviously no kind of home.

Lithium and other treatments can often restrain the severity of the mood swings, allowing some escape from the oscillation between despair and an out-of-control wildness. But the price of the escape can present poignant choices.

Dr. Kay Redfield Jamison is a psychologist who has co-authored a standard textbook on manic-depressive illness. She knows it as a scientist and has experienced it from inside. Her autobiography gives a striking personal account of this condition and its dilemmas. For Kay Jamison, the medication (lithium) is essential. There are terrible costs of leaving the illness uncontrolled. There would be intoxicating experiences, but "when the black tiredness inevitably followed, I would be subdued back into the recognition that I had a bad disease, one that could destroy all pleasure and hope and competence." She saw "how draining and preoccupying it had become just to keep my mind bobbing above water."[11] The choice was not about whether to have medication but about the dose.

Long-term use of lithium can be seen as changing temperament. To the extent that the effects of a particular dose are stable, choosing a dose for the long term can be to choose a temperament. Such a choice needs reflection in the light of having experienced the alternatives. The question is what you most deeply care about.

Kay Jamison reflects on her different states on different doses of lithium. Higher doses make episodes of mania and depression less likely, but at a cost. She had found some of her manias exhilarating. In one psychotic episode, she had the experience of flying through space, past the ravishingly colored rings of Saturn. Long afterward, she missed that experience. (As Felicity Bryan's account of her mother shows, not everyone finds the manic phases so exhilarating. They can be as troubling as the depressions.) But Jamison found it hard to adapt to normality. "The intensity, glory, and absolute assuredness of my mind's flight made it very difficult to believe, once I was better, that the illness was one that I should willingly give up."

The higher dose controlled her moods rigidly. But a lower dose, like the structural supports in buildings designed for earthquakes, "allowed my mind and emotions to sway a bit." Her emotions were more even and predictable, through being more resilient to stress. The lower dose also gave greater clarity of thinking and intensity of experience: "It was as though I had taken bandages off my eyes after many years of partial blindness . . . I realized that my steps were literally bouncier than they had been and that I was taking in sights and sounds that previously had been filtered through thick layers of gauze."

The greater flexibility of the way the lower dose controlled her moods, together with the clarity of thinking and intensity of experience, suggests that it is in the lower-dose temperament that she has found her depths and her home. She says that the clarity and intensity now recovered "had once formed the core of my normal temperament."

The question is complex. Jamison uses the metaphor of home—but to express a reaction against both illness and medication. Soon after starting on lithium, she was reading Kenneth Grahame's *Wind in the Willows.* She got to where Mole, smelling his old home after a long time away, is desperate to find it again. Having found it, Mole sits before the fire, seeing how much he had missed the warmth and security of the "friendly things which had long been unconsciously a part of him." Reading this, Kay Jamison broke down: "I missed my home, my mind, my life of books and 'friendly things,' my world where most things were in their place, and where nothing awful could come in to wreck havoc . . . I longed for the days that I had known before madness and medication had insinuated their way into every aspect of my existence."

This pull of the world before madness and medication must weigh against identifying with having the illness, even on lower medication. But this too is not the whole story. Given the choice, would she choose to have manic depression? Without lithium, she would simply say no: the depressions are just too awful. But with lithium? She says she has felt more deeply, experienced things more intensely, thought on a different level, loved more and laughed more, through the intensity coming from her illness. In a phrase Rilke would have liked, she has "appreciated more the springs, for all the winters." So perhaps she does see the controlled version of the illness as her home. In the end she says, "Strangely enough I think I would choose to have it."

Schizophrenia and Self-Creation

In schizophrenia, the relation between the person and the illness can seem very different from the inside. Simon Champ has described something of his changing conceptions of himself, his illness, and the relations between them.[12] At first his energies were consumed by the fight against his symptoms. He accepted the label "schizophrenic": "My illness was central to my identity." Later he came to see schizophrenia as something more positive, while still identifying with it. He would challenge people about it: "Hi, I'm Simon and I'm schizophrenic." But over time he gained more control over his symptoms: "I was recovering my personhood and saw the illness as influencing rather than defining me."

Simon Champ started to campaign on behalf of people like himself. And he reacted against the passivity of "suffering" from schizophrenia: "I had only really made progress in my own recovery when I stopped seeing myself as a 'victim' and relinquished more passive roles in my treatment." But he still had to overcome a negative self-image absorbed from society: "Many places inside me were still darkened by my internalization of society's treatment and attitudes to people who had experienced a mental illness . . . As I worked through the anger I felt at the treatment I had received, I felt a renewed sense of hope for my own life."

He reflected on his sense of his own identity, which previously had been linked to ideas about employment and about masculinity. His decided that his sense of worth need not depend on paid work: he could make other contributions. He also changed his ideas about manhood, coming to see that "real men do indeed cry."

Simon Champ's escape from passivity was based on self-interpretation and self-creation. Coming to terms with his illness, he says, has involved a deep communication with himself: "a communication that has given me the most precious thread, a thread that has linked my evolving sense of self, a thread of self-reclamation, a thread of movement toward a whole and integrated sense of self, away from the early fragmentation and confusion I felt as I first experienced schizophrenia."

Untreated schizophrenia can be the shipwreck of a person's life, at times a madness in which it is hard to see how people in its throes could be at peace with themselves. The success of biological psychiatry so far is measured by the degree of relief it can bring to the terrible symptoms of such illnesses: the medications that eliminate or contain the paranoia, the incoherent thought, the paralyzing passivity, the threatening "voices." Understandably this relief is often given priority over more elusive aims about preserving identity or about self-creation.

But Simon Champ's account lends support to a psychiatry that goes beyond a purely biological approach. The support is in showing what is sometimes possible, not in showing how many other cases are the same. Not everyone has Simon Champ's self-reflective capacities. In some people the grip of the illness may be too strong for them to escape from passivity. Obviously any general extrapolation from a single case would be flimsy.

Simon Champ's use of the word "self-reclamation" has echoes of Freud's metaphor of reclaiming the Zuyder Zee. Psychiatric help can be thought of as having two goals: the traditional medical goal of containing or eliminating the symptoms of illness, and the humanist goal of restoring autonomy, including the capacity for self-reclamation.

Restoring the person's autonomy will often require the removal, or at least the containment, of the symptoms of the illness. It is not easy to be autonomous when passive and withdrawn or when being shouted at by menacing "voices." Attacking the symptoms often has to start without the person's own active involvement. He or she may be too deluded or too indifferent to make self-creative decisions. But if the symptoms can be driven back far enough to make personal involvement possible, there can be the further aim of restoring autonomy and self-creation. And then, as in Simon Champ's case, the self-reclamation may contribute to dealing with the symptoms. The medical and the humanist goals are interwoven.

Medication of the symptoms may still be needed. But the restoration of autonomy may need other kinds of help too. These include encouraging the person to talk and a willingness to listen. (The aim is not any old talk, but the long, recurring Socratic conversation that goes deep inside the person. Though to start with, any old talk may be better than nothing.) Other help may include encouraging campaigning, as Simon Champ did for people like himself.

Autonomy cannot be organized by other people. There can only be encouragement and the giving of opportunities. Perhaps no one kind of encouragement works for everyone. But for autonomy to be restored, the person has to move away from the purely passive role, as Simon Champ did. Powers of autonomy and self-creation grow through being used.

Simon Champ's account shows how the self-creative, autobiographical approach can make other ways of posing the question about the real self seem too crude. From outside, the question may seem to be "Is the person's real self what he was before the illness, or what he is now?" But from the inside, Simon Champ's self-creative project has complex links with himself at different stages: "You do not simply patch up the self you were before developing schizophrenia . . . you have to actually recreate a concept of who you are that integrates the experience of schizophrenia." Although the new created self is not just a reproduction of the original self, there is a kind of continuity with it. He describes the peace of mind he now has—"as if I've come home to myself, a self changed, a self I last felt at 17, and yet now I'm 40. All those years of experiences separate me from the teenager I was, but somewhere inside I'm complete again, as I used to be then."

EPILOGUE

Psychiatry and Our Depths

"Our depths and our home." A few words about the other metaphor taken from Rilke: the metaphor of depth.

(Here I am conscious of cheating slightly. The word Rilke uses is *Boden*. Literally, this means "ground" or "bottom," as in "the bottom of the sea." To use the word "bottom" when talking of people has irrelevant associations. The translation could have read "our ground and our home." I preferred to exploit the associations with the bottom of the sea, and chose "depths." The idea of our bitter times as being part of the depths of a person seemed true to Rilke's intentions. But now I am starting from this English word rather than from what Rilke actually said.)

While writing this book, I did not notice how often I drew on the contrast between depth and shallowness. Looking back, it needs some clarification.

The first contrast here between shallowness and depth was in the discussion of the Broadmoor interviews. The suggestion was that seeing morality in terms of opening doors for women, or thinking that swearing is as bad as bullying, is shallow because of the stress on the conventional and the trivial. The contrast was with what gives moral depth: either personal reflection on why things matter or an intuitive feel for other people and what they care about. Command moralities are shallow because unreflective obedience cannot draw on these things.

Depth and Self-Understanding

"Deep versus shallow" is a contrast not of one dimension but of several. "What is deep in a person" can refer simply to what is inaccessible to consciousness. Psychoanalysis in its early days was sometimes called "depth psychology" because of its efforts to delve below what is conscious. The same use of "deep" was found in the account David Hicks gave of the "psychiatry" in Guantanamo: "They probed and tinkered in recesses so deep, parts of ourselves we are not conscious of or in touch with in our daily lives and may not even connect with and discover in our lifetimes."

Another version of depth is found in what was called earlier the deep sense of self: a secure and untroubled awareness of the distinct person you are. In some of the Broadmoor interviewees its absence may have created a hunger for recognition, with attempts to impress other people that they were "really someone."

Another use of the deep/shallow contrast has to do with moral identity: the sort of person you hope to be and the values shaping that hope. Thinking about choices made by addicts raises the contrast between two ways of settling inner conflicts. Some are settled by brute strength of desire. The other approach involves asking questions about what you happen to want. These other decisions go deeper because in them people discover or express more of themselves. In turn, the kind of person someone wants to be can reflect shallowness or depth. Some of the interviewees hoped mainly to be someone with the skills of a chef or the talents of Bruce Forsyth. Others, by contrast, were aware that their previous life of earning money and getting drunk at pubs and clubs was "lived basically on one level" and saw there could be more than this. "I need the experiences outside, you know, to develop."

People can be deepened through experiences that matter to them, as some were by the Shakespeare productions in Broadmoor. One in the audience felt a sense of peace and wholeness at the deaths at the end of *King Lear.* Another said Hamlet could have been his mother or brother: "So it did have a lot of meaning. I hope you understand this." These experiences can leave a lasting imprint: one patient spoke of "something I'll take with me for the rest of my life." They may deepen people by enlarging their understanding: "It also brought home to me how we compound our miseries through our own destructive feelings of bitterness and vengeance . . . If only we could learn not to act on impulsive urges of revenge."

Depth and authenticity are interwoven with each other in the question of whether an action—perhaps something strange done by a person with schizophrenia, or the refusal to eat by someone with anorexia—is an expression of the illness or of the person. The question reflects a contrast between an aberration and what is central or deep in a person. As Viktor Frankl pointed out, someone's identity is partly *constituted* by the values that go deepest: values that "cannot be espoused and adopted by us on a conscious level—they are something that we *are*." But this needs supplementing with Martha Nussbaum's thought that it is no simple matter to find out what the deepest parts of ourselves are. Helping people find their depths may call on many Socratic conversations.

Depth and Attitudes toward Others

One of the great costs of ruthlessly self-interested amoralism is that it rules out the deepest relationships. Love and friendship are incompatible with pure self-interested calculation. The depth of relationships also varies with the extent to which attitude spirals evolve (attitudes toward attitudes, and so on, spiraling upward). The strength of the case against trying to medicate away the low psychological states involved in grief varies in different people. It depends on how far the grief is part of the seriousness and depth of the relationship that person had with the person whose loss they are grieving.

The Broadmoor interviews brought out some contrasts between shallow and deep respect for other people. The deep attitude of respect goes beyond the conventional politeness of opening doors for women, and beyond respecting people's legal or moral rights. It is a way of seeing people, caught in Rainsborough's thought that "the poorest he that is in England hath a life to lead as the greatest he." (We would now of course explicitly include the poorest she.) The key is not just abstract assent to a platitude, but emotional awareness that other people as much as ourselves have a life to lead that is as desperately important to them as mine is to me.

This awareness goes with trying to understand another person's interpretation of the world—and sometimes how it may have been disrupted. The depth here is going beneath the visible surface of a person. As George Herbert wrote, "A man that looks on glass, / On it may stay his eye; / Or if he pleaseth, through it passe, / And then the heav'n espie." Though in the depths beneath the surface, it is not always heaven that comes into view. Sometimes it is the vulnerable child Ted Hughes noticed, peering through the slits in the defensive armor of adulthood. In postcombat stress it may be the dark side of what human beings can do. But understanding this darkness can give more depth than looking away from it.

Binocular Vision in Psychiatry

People are deep or shallow in different ways. Some are reflective but have little human intuition. Others are the reverse. And so on. People come in different places on the continuum in different contexts. Depth and shallowness are relevant to psychiatric interpretation. Judging how to help a person may require trying to look into their depths.

The metaphor of visual depth perception is useful. To see the physical world in depth, we use our two eyes. The brain decodes the slightly discrepant pictures they give to get information about the relative distance of things. Knowledge of physical depth is extracted from the incompatibilities of binocular vision.

This is a metaphor for psychiatry, a field where there are truths that at first look incompatible. People are not transparent, yet often they can be interpreted. To some extent we create ourselves. Yet what we are like is quite severely constrained by factors outside our control. Psychiatric disorder can have such strange features that "domesticated" accounts often falsify it. Yet, *humani nihil a me alienum puto:* it is essential not to forget the extent of the shared human condition on both sides of the boundary. A major psychiatric disorder is a tragedy to be prevented if possible. Yet it may be something the person who has it would not change, "our winter foliage, our evergreen."

On each of these issues there is a tension between what comes before the word "yet" and what comes after it. But there are no deeply incompatible truths: paradoxes exist to be resolved. Each side of the opposition may be part of the truth. Psychiatric disorder can make people in some ways radically strange without obliterating all the human psychology they share with others.

The philosophical interest is greater when the tension goes deeper. How far is self-creation compatible with the constraints of temperament and of environment? How can we take with sufficient seriousness the testimony of someone who is not sorry to have schizophrenia without falling into the shallowness of belittling how terrible it is? These are foundational questions for a philosophical account of psychiatry and of the conditions it treats. In trying to answer each question, we have to start from the two perspectives. It is only by combining whatever is ultimately defensible in each that we go deeper.

Seeing things from apparently incompatible standpoints gives a metaphor for psychiatry as a whole. We will never understand mental disorder unless we see it, as modern psychiatry does, in the clear light of scientific empiricism. But there is also the subjective perspective, which tells us so much that is not visible from the outside. To see to the depths of people with psychiatric disorder, the two perspectives have to be combined in binocular vision. We need the external scientific story. And the view from inside, interpreted with empathy but also with searching questions.

NOTES

ACKNOWLEDGMENTS

INDEX

NOTES

Prologue

1. Karl Jaspers, *Allgemeine Psychopathologie,* translated by J. Hoenig and Marian W. Hamilton as *General Psychopathology* (Baltimore: Johns Hopkins University Press, 1997).

1. Socratic Questions in Broadmoor

1. T. Millon, E. Simonsen, and M. Birket-Smith, "Historical Conceptions of Psychopathy in the United States and Europe," in *Psychopathy: Antisocial, Criminal and Violent Behavior,* ed. T. Millon, E. Simonsen, M. Birket-Smith, and R. D. Davis (New York: Guilford Press, 1998), 3–31.
2. Hervey Cleckley, *The Mask of Sanity: An Attempt to Clarify Some Issues about the So-Called Psychopathic Personality,* first published 1941, with revisions until the posthumous 5th ed., edited by Emily S. Cleckley (Augusta, Ga., 1988).
3. Ibid., 403.
4. Ibid., 7.
5. Ibid., 361.
6. Ibid., pp. 369–370, and 383.
7. Ibid., 161.
8. Robert D. Hare, *The Hare Psychopathy Checklist–Revised* (Toronto: Multi-Health Systems, 1991).
9. Robert D. Hare, "Psychopathy and Antisocial Personality Disorder: A Case of Diagnostic Confusion," *Psychiatric Times* 13, no. 2 (1996).

3. Childhood and After

1. Stephen Darwall, "Two Kinds of Respect," *Ethics* 88 (1987): 36–49.

4. Interpreting This Landscape

1. Christopher Reid, ed., *Letters of Ted Hughes* (London: Faber and Faber, 2007), 513–514.

5. Shakespeare Comes to Broadmoor

1. Peter Brook, *The Empty Space* (London: Penguin Books, 1972), 149–150.
2. Clark Baim, Sally Brooks, and Alan Mountford, *The Geese Theatre Handbook* (Hook: Waterside Press, 2002), 20, 43, 182–185; Andy Watson, "Lift Your Mask," in *The Applied Theatre Reader,* ed. Tim Prentki and Sheila Preston (London: Routledge, 2009), 47–54.
3. Murray Cox, ed., *Shakespeare Comes to Broadmoor* (London: Jessica Kingsley, 1994); Murray Cox and Alice Theilgaard, *Shakespeare as Prompter: The Amending Imagination and the Therapeutic Process* (London: Jessica Kingsley, 1994).
4. Antony Sher, *Beside Myself* (London: Arrow Books, 2002), 336–339.
5. Erving Goffman, *Asylums: Essays on the Social Situation of Mental Patients and Other Inmates* (London: Penguin, 1968), 280.

6. Hopes for the Future of Psychiatry

1. There are sobering accounts of the efforts of the pharmaceutical industry to influence psychiatric thinking. See Marcia Angell, *The Truth about the Drug Companies: How They Deceive Us and What to Do About It* (New York: Random House, 2004), chap. 8, "Marketing Masquerading as Education," 135–155; David Healy, *Let Them Eat Prozac: The Unhealthy Relationship between the Pharmaceutical Industry and Depression* (New York: NYU Press, 2004); Charles Medawar and Anita Hardon, *Medicines Out of Control? Antidepressants and the Conspiracy of Goodwill* (The Netherlands: Aksant Academic, 2004).
2. Thomas G. O'Connor, Yoav Ben Shlomo, Jon Heron, Jean Golding, Diana Adams, and Vivette Glover, "Prenatal Anxiety Predicts Individual Differences in Cortisol in Pre-Adolescent Children," *Biological Psychiatry* 56, no. 3 (2005): 211–217; K. M. Radtke, M. Ruf, H. M. Gunter, K. Dohrmann, M. Schauer, A. Meyer, and T. Elbert, "Transgenerational Impact of Intimate Partner Violence on Methylation in the Promoter of the Glucocorticoid Receptor," *Translational Psychiatry* 1 (2011), published online.
3. Bruce N. Cuthbert and Thomas R. Insel, "Toward New Approaches to Psychotic Disorders: The NIMH Research Domain Criteria Project," *Schizophrenia Bulletin* 36, no. 6 (2010).
4. Sarah E. Morris and Bruce N. Cuthbert, "Research Domain Criteria: Cognitive Systems, Neural Circuits, and Dimensions of Behavior," *Dialogues in Clinical Neuroscience* 14, no. 1 (2012): 29–37.
5. Gary Kasparov, "The Chess Master and the Computer," *New York Review of Books*, February, 11, 2010.
6. Diego Rasskin-Gutman, *Chess Metaphors: Artificial Intelligence and the Human Mind* (Cambridge, Mass.: MIT Press, 2009), chap. 5.
7. Gail Silver, "Coming to Terms, Making Changes, Moving On," in *Voices beyond the Border: Living with Borderline Personality Disorder*, ed. Lucy Robinson and Vicky Cox (Brentwood, Essex: Chipmunkapublishing, 2006), 154.

7. "A Skill So Deeply Hidden in the Human Soul"

1. Ernst Gombrich, *Art and Illusion*, 2nd ed. (London: Phaidon Press, 1961), 251.
2. Martin Gayford, *A Bigger Message: Conversations with David Hockney* (London: Thames and Hudson, 2011), 47–53.
3. Rosaleen A. McCarthy and Elizabeth A. Warrington, *Cognitive Neuropsychology: A Clinical Introduction* (San Diego: Academic Press, 1990), 23–55.
4. Glyn W. Humphreys and M. Jane Riddoch, *To See but Not to See: A Case Study of Visual Agnosia* (London: Erlbaum Associates, 1987).
5. Ibid., 32–33.
6. A. B. Rubens and D. F. Benson, "Associative Visual Agnosia," *Archives of Neurology* 24 (1971): 305–316.
7. Norman Geschwind, "Disconnexion Syndromes in Animals and Man," in *Selected Papers on Language and the Brain* (Boston: Reidel, 1974), 165–186.
8. Humphreys and Riddoch, *To See but Not to See*, 62.
9. Geschwind, "Disconnexion Syndromes," 167.

10. D. E. Lyons, L. R. Santos, and F. C. Keil, "Reflections of Other Minds: How Primate Social Cognition Can Inform the Function of Mirror Neurons," *Current Opinion in Neurobiology* 16, no. 6 (2006): 230–234.
11. Gregory Hickock, "Eight Problems for the Mirror Neuron Theory of Action Understanding in Monkeys," *Journal of Cognitive Neuroscience* 21, no. 7 (2009): 1229–1243.
12. Marco Iacoboni, *Mirroring People: The New Science of How We Connect with Others* (New York: Farrar, Straus and Giroux, 2008).
13. Hickock, "Eight Problems."
14. Gilbert Ryle, *The Concept of Mind* (London: Hutchinson, 1949), 172.
15. Marcel Proust, *Remembrance of Things Past,* trans. C. K. Scott Moncrieff and Terence Kilmartin (London: Chatto and Windus, 1981), 2:63–65.
16. Janet Malcolm, *The Journalist and the Murderer* (London: Granta Books, 2004), 128.

8. Intuitive Interpretation

1. Ted Hughes, *Poetry in the Making* (London: Faber and Faber, 1967), 121.
2. M. H. Johnson et al., "Newborns' Preferential Tracking of Face-Like Stimuli and Its Subsequent Decline," *Cognition* 40 (1991): 1–19.
3. A. W. Young, "To Find the Mind's Construction in the Face," in *Face and Mind* (Oxford: Oxford University Press, 1998), 1–66.
4. Marcel Proust, *Remembrance of Things Past,* trans. C. K. Scott Moncrieff and Terence Kilmartin (London: Chatto and Windus, 1981), 1:20.
5. David Sylvester, *Interviews with Francis Bacon* (London: Thames and Hudson, 1975), 58.

9. Reflective Interpretation

1. Nicholas Humphrey, *The Inner Eye* (London: Faber and Faber, 1986), 36–40.
2. Nicholas Humphrey, *Consciousness Regained: Chapters in the Development of Mind* (Oxford: Oxford University Press, 1984), 21.
3. Simon Baron-Cohen, *Mindblindness: An Essay on Autism and Theory of Mind* (Cambridge, Mass.: MIT Press, 1995), 31–58. See also Peter Carruthers and Peter K. Smith, eds., *Theories of Theories of Mind* (Cambridge: Cambridge University Press, 1998); Simon Baron-Cohen, Helen Tager-Flusberg, and Donald J. Cohen, eds., *Understanding Other Minds: Perspectives from Developmental Cognitive Neuroscience,* 2nd ed. (Oxford: Oxford University Press, 2000).
4. Martin Davies and Tony Stone, eds., *Mental Simulation: Evaluations and Applications* (Oxford: Blackwell, 1995); Alvin I. Goldman, *Simulating Minds: The Philosophy, Psychology and Neuroscience of Mindreading* (Oxford: Oxford University Press, 2006).
5. W. V. O. Quine, "Two Dogmas of Empiricism," in *From a Logical Point of View* (Cambridge, Mass.: Harvard University Press, 1953), 42.
6. Jerry Fodor, *The Modularity of Mind* (Cambridge, Mass.: MIT Press, 1983), 107.
7. Virginia Woolf, "A Sketch of the Past," in *Moments of Being,* 2nd ed. (San Diego: Harcourt Brace, 1985), 135.

8. Leo Tolstoy, *Anna Karenina,* trans. Richard Pevear and Larissa Volokhonsky (London: Penguin, 2001), 564–565.

10. "A Gulf Which Defies Description"

1. George Walter, ed., *Everyman's Poetry* (London: J. M. Dent, 1996), 41.
2. Karl Jaspers, *General Psychopathology,* tran. Paul R. McHugh (Baltimore: Johns Hopkins University Press, 1997), 447.
3. P. O. Svanberg et al., "Promoting a Secure Attachment: A Primary Prevention Practice Model," *Developmental Psychology* 42, no. 4 (2006): 627–642; M. G. Groeneveld et al., "Enhancing Home-Based Child Care Quality through Video-Feedback Intervention: A Randomized Controlled Trial," *Clinical Child Psychology and Psychiatry* 15, no. 3 (2010): 363–378.
4. Jaspers, *General Psychopathology,* 581.

11. Autism and Interpretation

1. Lorna Wing, *The Autistic Spectrum: A Guide for Parents and Professionals,* new ed. (London: Robinson, 1996), 92–102.
2. Clare Sainsbury, *Martian in the Playground: Understanding the Schoolchild with Asperger's Syndrome* (London: Book Factory, 2000), 18.
3. Naoki Higashida, *The Reason I Jump,* translated from the Japanese by K. A. Yoshida and David Mitchell (London: Sceptre, 2013), 71.
4. Francesca Happé, Angelica Ronald, and Robert Plomin, "Time to Give Up on a Single Explanation for Autism," *Nature Neuroscience* 9 (2006): 1218–1220.
5. Jim Sinclair, "Don't Mourn for Us," *Our Voice,* newsletter of the Autism Network International, 1993.
6. Temple Grandin, *Thinking in Pictures and Other Reports from My Life with Autism* (London: Bloomsbury Press, 2006), 21.
7. Donna Williams, *Nobody Nowhere: The Remarkable Autobiography of an Autistic Girl* (London: Jessica Kingsley, 1999).
8. Ibid., 21.
9. Ibid., 44.
10. Ibid., 27.
11. Ibid., 38.
12. Ibid., 45.
13. Ibid., 46.
14. Grandin, *Thinking in Pictures,* 5.
15. Gunilla Gerland, *A Real Person: Life on the Outside,* trans. Joan Tate (London: Souvenir Press, 1996), 203.
16. Higashida, *The Reason I Jump,* 55–56.
17. Williams, *Nobody Nowhere,* 20.
18. Ibid., 55.
19. Ibid., 52.
20. Ibid., 17.
21. Ibid., 20.

22. Ibid., 185–188.
23. Ibid., 59–60.
24. Ian Hacking, "Autistic Autobiography," *Philosophical Transactions of the Royal Society* B, 364 (2009): 1467–1473.
25. Oliver Sacks, *An Anthropologist on Mars* (New York: Knopf, 1995).

12. Interpreting Delusions

1. Joan Didion, *The Year of Magical Thinking* (London: Harper Perennial, 2006), 32, 37.
2. Anonymous, "An Autobiography of a Schizophrenic Experience," *Journal of Abnormal and Social Psychology* 51 (1955): 677–690.
3. Gerd Gigerenzer and Reinhard Selten, eds., *Bounded Rationality: The Adaptive Toolbox* (Cambridge, Mass.: MIT Press, 2002).
4. David C. Boyles, *My Punished Mind* (New York: Universe, 2004), 11–12.
5. Ibid., 14, 22.
6. E. F. Torrey, *Surviving Schizophrenia,* 3rd ed. (New York: Harper Collins, 1995), quoted in Ian Gold and Ian Hohwy, "Rationality and Schizophrenic Delusion," in *Pathologies of Belief,* ed. Max Coltheart and Martin Davies (Oxford: Blackwell, 2000), 161.
7. Albert Einstein, "Autobiographical Notes," trans. Paul A. Schilpp, in *Albert Einstein: Philosopher-Scientist,* ed. Paul A. Schilpp, 3rd ed., Library of Living Philosophers (La Salle, Ill.: Open Court, 1970), 49.
8. Susan A. Clancy, *Abducted: How People Come to Believe They Were Kidnapped by Aliens* (Cambridge, Mass.: Harvard University Press, 2005), 8.
9. B. A. Maher, "Anomalous Experience and Delusional Thinking: The Logic of Explanations," in T. F. Oltmans and B. A. Maher, *Delusional Beliefs* (New York: Wiley, 1988), 15–33.
10. Christopher D. Frith, *The Cognitive Neuropsychology of Schizophrenia* (Hove, UK: Taylor and Francis, 1992).
11. Christopher Peacocke, *Truly Understood* (Oxford: Oxford University Press, 2008), 275–279.
12. John Campbell, "Schizophrenia: The Space of Reasons and Thinking as a Motor Process," *Monist* 82 (1999): 609–625. The view of delusions as disorders of self-monitoring has been presented here very schematically. For one developed version, see G. Lynn Stephens and George Graham, *When Self-Consciousness Breaks: Alien Voices and Inserted Thoughts* (Cambridge, Mass.: MIT Press, 2000).
13. John Custance, *Wisdom, Madness and Folly: The Philosophy of a Lunatic* (London: Gollancz, 1951), 31, 52.
14. H. D. Ellis and A. W. Young, "Accounting for Delusional Misidentifications," *British Journal of Psychiatry* 157 (1990): 239–248; A. W. Young, "The Neuropsychology of Abnormal Beliefs," in *Pathologies of Belief,* ed. Max Coltheart and Martin Davies (Oxford: Blackwell, 2000).
15. Fyodor Dostoyevsky, *The Idiot,* trans. Alan Myers (Oxford: Oxford University Press, 1992), 237.

16. Gerard Manley Hopkins, "Comments on the Spiritual Exercises of Saint Ignatius Loyola," in *Poems and Prose of Gerard Manley Hopkins,* ed. W. H. Gardner (Harmondsworth: Penguin, 1953), 147–148.
17. Amos Tversky and Daniel Kahneman, "Judgement under Uncertainty: Heuristics and Biases," in Daniel Kahneman, Paul Slovik, and Amos Tversky, *Judgements under Uncertainty: Heuristics and Biases* (Cambridge: Cambridge University Press, 1962), 3–20.
18. Amos Tversky and Daniel Kahneman, "Causal Schemas," in Kahneman, Slovik, and Tversky, *Judgements under Uncertainty.*
19. Philippa A. Garety and David R. Hemsley, *Delusions: Investigations into the Psychology of Delusional Reasoning,* Maudsley Monographs 36 (Hove, UK: Psychology Press, 1997), 86–106.
20. Anonymous, "Autobiography."
21. John Campbell, "Rationality, Meaning and the Analysis of Delusion," *Philosophy, Psychiatry and Psychology* 8 (2001): 89–100.
22. Francis King and George Matthews, eds., *About Turn: The British Communist Party and the Second World War—The Verbatim Record of the Central Committee Meetings of 23 September and 2–3 October 1939* (London: Communist Party of Great Britain, 1990).
23. Nicholas Tomalin and Ron Hall, *The Strange Last Voyage of Donald Crowhurst* (Camden, Maine.: International Marine/McGraw Hill, 1970), 207–212.
24. Custance, *Wisdom, Madness and Folly,* 73.
25. Louis Sass, *The Paradoxes of Delusion: Wittgenstein, Schreber and the Schizophrenic Mind* (Ithaca, N.Y.: Cornell University Press, 1994).
26. Daniel Paul Schreber, *Memoirs of My Nervous Illness,* trans. and ed. Ida MacAlpine and Richard A. Hunter (New York: New York Review of Books, 2000).
27. Ibid., 115.
28. Ludwig Wittgenstein, *Philosophical Investigations,* trans. G. E. M. Anscombe (Oxford: Blackwell, 1953), pt. 1, sec. 8.
29. Jerry Fodor, *The Modularity of Mind* (Cambridge, Mass.: MIT Press, 1983).
30. Dostoyevsky, *The Idiot,* 477.
31. Daniel Dennett, "Cognitive Wheels: The Frame Problem of AI," in *Brainchildren: Essays in Designing Minds* (Cambridge, Mass.: MIT Press, 1998), 181–205.
32. Antonio Damasio, *Descartes' Error* (London: MacMillan, 1996), 34–51.
33. K. W. M. Fulford, "Value, Illness and Failure of Action," in *Philosophical Psychopathology,* ed. George Graham and G. Lynn Stephens (Cambridge, Mass.: MIT Press, 1994), 212–213.

13. Waking Dreams

1. Hans Prinzhorn, *Artistry of the Mentally Ill,* trans. Eric von Brock (New York: Springer, 1972). See also Susan Ferleger Brades, Martin Caiger-Smith, and Andrew Patrizio, *Beyond Reason, Art and Psychosis, Works from the Prinzhorn Collection* (London: South Bank Centre, 1996).
2. Mohr, quoted in Christopher Turner, "The Influencing Machine," *Cabinet Magazine,* 2004.

3. Prinzhorn, *Artistry of the Mentally Ill,* 66–68.
4. William Blake, "A Descriptive Catalogue of Pictures, Poetical and Historical Inventions, Painted by William Blake" in *William Blake: Seen in My Visions,* ed. Martin Myrone (London: Tate, 2009), 45–46.
5. Henry Crabb Robinson, "Diary Account of Blake," 1–2, in *Blake, Coleridge, Wordsworth, Lamb, etc., Being Selections from the Remains of Henry Crabb Robinson,* ed. Edith J. Morley (Manchester: Manchester University Press, 1922), quoted in Peter Ackroyd, *Blake* (London: Vintage, 1969), 361–362.
6. Ibid.
7. Marius Romme and Sandra Escher, *Accepting Voices,* translated and expanded from the Dutch edition (London: Mind, 1994).
8. Karl Jaspers, *Strindberg and Van Gogh,* trans. Oskar Grunow and David Woloshin (Tucson: University of Arizona Press, 1977), 187.
9. Kay Redfield Jamison, *Touched with Fire: Manic Depressive Illness and the Artistic Temperament* (New York: Free Press Paperbacks, 1993), 233.
10. Letter to Theo van Gogh, August 22, 1880. All letters quoted here are to his brother Theo.
11. Letter, January 4, 1890.
12. Letter, February 12, 1890.
13. Letter, May 11, 1890.
14. Letter, August 21 or 22, 1888.
15. Letter, October 8, 1899.
16. Letter, September 3, 1888.
17. John Custance, *Wisdom, Madness and Folly: The Philosophy of a Lunatic* (London: Gollancz, 1951), 31.
18. Aldous Huxley, *The Doors of Perception and Heaven and Hell* (Harmondsworth: Penguin, 1959), 20–26.
19. Letter, December 31, 1889, or January 1, 1890.
20. Letter, September 26, 1888.
21. Jaspers, *Strindberg and van Gogh,* 176.
22. Letter, July 1880.

14. The Need for Boundaries

1. Michael Burleigh, *Death and Deliverance: "Euthanasia" in Germany, 1900–1945* (Cambridge: Cambridge University Press, 1994), 115–119.
2. Anatoly Koryagin, "Compulsion in Psychiatry: Blessing or Curse?," *Psychiatric Bulletin* 14 (1990): 84.
3. Sidney Bloch and Peter Reddaway, *Russia's Political Hospitals* (London: Gollancz, 1977), 84.
4. Ibid., 94–96.
5. Solomon Volkov, *Conversations with Joseph Brodsky: A Poet's Journey through the Twentieth Century,* trans. Marian Schwartz (New York: Free Press, 1998), 67–68.
6. *The Guardian,* September 29, 1973, quoted in Sidney Bloch, "Psychiatry: An Impossible Profession?," *Australian and New Zealand Journal of Psychiatry* 31 (1997): 172–183.

7. Human Rights Watch and the Geneva Initiative on Psychiatry, *Dangerous Minds: Political Psychiatry in China Today and Its Origins in the Mao Era* (New York: Human Rights Watch, 2002), a report mainly written by Robin Munro.
8. Chenzou District Mental Hospital, Hunan Province, Medical Group of the Mental Clinic of PLA Hospital, no. 165, "Analysis of a Survey of 250 Cases of Mental Illness," in Human Rights Watch et al., *Dangerous Minds,* 191–204.
9. Jia Rubao, "More on the Essential Nature of Mental Illness" (1977), in Human Rights Watch et al., *Dangerous Minds,* 218.
10. "China Encyclopedia of Public Security" (1990), in Human Rights Watch et al., *Dangerous Minds,* p. 121.
11. Human Rights Watch et al., *Dangerous Minds,* p. 61.
12. Handwritten account, ibid., 123–125.
13. Shen Jun and Gong Yantao, "A First Look at the Forensic Psychiatric Evaluation of Falun Gong Cases," in Human Rights Watch et al., *Dangerous Minds,* p. 282.
14. Lynette A. Jackson, *Surfacing Up: Psychiatry and Social Order in Colonial Zimbabwe, 1908–1968* (Ithaca, N.Y.: Cornell University Press, 2005), 4–6.
15. *Reports on the Public Health, 1938,* quoted in ibid., 140.
16. Ibid., 147–149.
17. David Anderson, *Histories of the Hanged: Britain's Dirty War in Kenya and the End of Empire* (London: Orion Books, 2006).
18. Dr. J. C. Carothers, *The Psychology of Mau Mau* (Nairobi: Government Printer, 1954).
19. Mwangi Mweru, quoted in Anderson, *Histories of the Hanged,* 296.
20. M. Gregg Bloche and Jonathan H. Marks, "Doctors and Interrogators at Guantanamo Bay," *New England Journal of Medicine* 353, no. 1 (2005): 6–8.
21. Jason Leopold, "An Interview with Former Guantanamo Detainee David Hicks," *Truthout,* February 2011.
22. Jock McCulloch, *Colonial Psychiatry and "the African Mind"* (Cambridge: Cambridge University Press, 1995), 67–71.
23. Ibid., 71–72.
24. Cited in Peter Tatchell, "Aversion Therapy Exposed," *THUD,* August 2, 1996, www.petertatchell.net ; "Go Ahead Caller, I'm Listening," *Daily Telegraph,* February 13, 2004.
25. Peter Tatchell, obituary of Hans Eysenck, *The Guardian,* September 13, 1997.
26. Sigmund Freud, letter, April 9, 1935, quoted in Ernest Jones, *The Life and Work of Sigmund Freud,* edited and abridged by Lionel Trilling and Steven Marcus (Harmondsworth: Penguin, 1964), 624.
27. Anna Freud, quoted in Elisabeth Young-Bruehl, *Anna Freud: A Biography,* 2nd ed. (New Haven, Conn.: Yale University Press, 2008), 327.
28. Peter Strudwick, "The Ex-Gay Files: The Bizarre World of Gay-to-Straight Conversion," *The Independent,* February 1, 2010.
29. Patrick Devlin, "Mill on Liberty in Morals," in *The Enforcement of Morals* (Oxford: Oxford University Press, 1970), 107, 116.
30. Ibid., v.

15. Personality and Sexuality

1. Anonymous, quoted by Dakota, August 7, 2007, http://recoveryourlife.com/forum.
2. **The Solution.**

> Finally they got the Singles problem under control, they made it scientific. They opened huge Sex Centres—you could simply go and state what you want and they would find you someone who wanted that too. You would stand under a sign saying *I Like to Be Touched and Held* and when someone came and stood under the sign saying *I Like to Touch and Hold* they would send the two of you off together.
>
> At first it went great. A steady stream of people under the sign *I Like to Give Pain* paired up with the steady stream of people from under *I Like to Receive Pain. Foreplay Only—No Orgasm* found its adherents, and *Orgasm Only—No Foreplay* matched up its believers. A loyal Berkeley, California, policeman stood under the sign *Married Adults, Lights Out, Face to Face, Under a Sheet,* because that's the only way it was legal in Berkeley—but he stood there a long time in his lonely blue law coat. And the man under *I Like to Be Sung to While Bread Is Kneaded on My Stomach* had been there weeks without a reply.
>
> Things began to get strange. The *Love Only—No Sex* was doing fine; the *Sex Only—No Love* was doing really well, pair after pair walking out together like wooden animals off a child's ark, but the line for *38D or Bigger* was getting unruly, shouting insults at the line for *8 Inches or Longer,* and odd isolated signs were springing up everywhere, *Retired Schoolteacher and Parakeet—No Leather; One Rm/No Bath/View of Sausage Factory.*
>
> The din rose in the vast room. The line under *I Want to Be Fucked Senseless* was so long that portable toilets had to be added and a minister brought in for deaths, births and marriages on the line. Over under *I Want to Fuck Senseless*—no-one, a pile of guns. A hollow roaring filled the enormous gym. More and more people began to move over to *Want to Be Fucked Senseless.* The line snaked around the gym, the stadium, the whole town, out into the fields. More and more people joined it, until *Fucked Senseless* stretched across the nation in a huge wide belt under the Milky Way, and since they had to name it they named it, they called it the American Way.

In Sharon Olds, *The Gold Cell* (New York: Knopf, 1987).

16. Dysfunction?

1. Allen V. Horwitz and Jerome C. Wakefield, *The Loss of Sadness: How Psychiatry Transformed Normal Sorrow into Depressive Disorder* (Oxford: Oxford University Press, 2007), 17.
2. Tim Crow, "Schizophrenia as the Price That *Homo sapiens* Pay for Language: A Resolution of the Central Paradox in the Origin of the Species," *Brain Research Reviews* 31 (2000): 118–129.
3. Jonathan Burns, "From 'Evolved Interpersonal Relatedness' to 'Costly Social Alienation": An Evolutionary Neurophilosophy of Schizophrenia," in *Maladapting Minds: Philosophy, Psychiatry and Evolutionary Theory,* ed. Pieter R. Adriaens and Andreas de Block (Oxford: Oxford University Press, 2011), 289–307.

4. Randolph M. Nesse and Eric D. Jackson, "Evolutionary Foundations for Psychiatric Diagnosis: Making *DSM-V* Valid," in Adriaens and Block, *Maladapting Minds,* 173–197.
5. Isaac Marks and Randolph Nesse, "Fear and Fitness: An Evolutionary Analysis of Anxiety Disorders," in *The Maladapted Mind: Classic Readings in Evolutionary Psychopathology,* ed. Simon Baron-Cohen (Hove, UK: Psychology Press, 1997).
6. Chris Stringer, *The Origin of Our Species* (London: Allen Lane, 2011).
7. Tracy Thompson, *The Beast: A Journey through Depression* (New York: Penguin, 1996), 53.
8. Alan Hollinghurst, review of Richard Wollheim, *Germs: A Memoir of Childhood, The Guardian,* September 18, 2004.
9. Richard Wollheim, *Germs: A Memoir of Childhood* (London: Waywiser Press, 2004), 248.
10. Ibid., 248–250.
11. R. L. Gregory and Jean G. Wallace, "Recovery from Early Blindness: A Case Study," in *Concepts and Mechanisms of Perception* (London: Duckworth, 1974), 65–229.

17. Harm

1. Jerome C. Wakefield et al., "Extending the Bereavement Exclusion for Major Depression to Other Losses," *Archives of General Psychiatry* 64 (2007): 433–439.
2. George W. Brown and Tirril Harris, *Social Origins of Depression: A Study of Psychiatric Disorder in Women* (London: Tavistock, 1979).
3. Jonathan Shay, *Achilles in Vietnam: Combat Trauma and the Undoing of Character* (New York: Scribner, 1994), 198–199.
4. Julian Barnes, *Levels of Life* (London: Jonathan Cape, 2013), 73.
5. Ibid., 71, 113.
6. Bennett Foddy and Julian Savulescu, "A Liberal Account of Addiction," *Philosophy, Psychiatry & Psychology* 17, no. 1 (2010): 1–22.
7. Daniel Gavron, *The Kibbutz: Awakening from Utopia* (Lanham, Md.: Rowman and Littlefield, 2000), 187.
8. Shmual Gollan, in ibid., 165.
9. Arnon Columbus, in ibid., 131.
10. Carmela, in Nurit Leshem, "Shirat Hadeshe," quoted in ibid., 168.
11. Nikolai Bukharin, *The Economics of the Transformation Period* (London: Pluto Press, 1971).
12. For qualifications of this, see Steven Pinker, *The Better Angels of Our Nature* (London: Allen Lane, 2011).
13. Robert Nozick, *Anarchy, State and Utopia* (New York: Basic Books, 1974), 42–45.

18. What Is Autism?

1. Jim Sinclair, "Don't Mourn for Us," *Our Voice* 1, no. 3 (1993).
2. "ME": sharon.theawfultruth.blogspot.co.uk, January 6, 2012.

3. Naoki Higashida, *The Reaon I Jump*, trans. K. A. Yoshida and David Mitchell (London: Hodder and Stoughton, 2013), 72–73.
4. Sandy Starr, “Is Autism Just Another Identity?,” paper presented at the Centre of Medical Law and Ethics/Institute of Psychiatry, King’s College London conference, “Autism, Ethics and the Good Life,” April 2012. Transcript at www.spiked-online.com.
5. Clare Sainsbury, *The Martian in the Playground* (Bristol: Lucky Duck, 2000), 33.

19. Crossing the Medical Boundary?

1. Peter Kramer, *Listening to Prozac* (New York: Penguin, 1993), 1–21.
2. David Fryer, “Insecurity: The Restructuring of Unemployment and Mental Health,” Claudia Dalbert, “Justice Concerns and Mental Health during Unemployment,” and Bjorgulf Claussen, “Suicidal Ideation in the Long-Term Unemployed: A Five-Year Longitudinal Study,” all in *Unemployment and Health, Intergenerational and Interdisciplinary Perspectives*, ed. Thomas Kieselbach, Anthony H. Winefield, Carolyn Boyd, and Sarah Anderson (Bowen Hills: Australian Academic Press, 2006); Vijaya Murali and Femi Oyebode, “Poverty, Social Inequality and Mental Health,” *Advances in Psychiatric Treatment* 19 (2013): 4.
3. Eric Newhouse, “Half of Vets Returning from Iraq and Afghanistan Need Medical Attention,” *Truthout*, November 16, 2011.
4. Timothy Williams, “Suicides Outpacing War Deaths for Troops,” *New York Times News Service*, June 8, 2012; Murtaza Haider, “Losing War: One Veteran Every 80 Minutes,” *Dawn.com* (blog), March 28, 2012, http://www.dawn.com/news/706062/losing-war-one-veteran-every-80-seconds.
5. Marcia Angell, *The Truth about the Drug Companies: How They Deceive Us and What to Do about It* (New York: Random House, 2004), 119. See also Charles Medawar and Anita Hardon, *Medicines Out of Control? Antidepressants and the Conspiracy of Goodwill* (Amsterdam: Aksant Academic, 2004), www.aksant.nl; and David Healy, *Let Them Eat Prozac: The Unhealthy Relationship between the Pharmaceutical Industry and Depression* (New York: New York University Press, 2004).
6. Yair Ettinger, “Rabbi’s Little Helper,” *Haaretz.com*, April 6, 2012. I know of this case through this report. *Haaretz* has the reputation of being a reliable newspaper, and I know no reason to doubt the report. If it turns out to be misleading, the account given here should be treated as a thought experiment. My concern is not with the activities of a particular religious community, but with the issues raised by the kind of case described.

20. Strands in a Good Human Life

1. Council of Civil Service Unions and Cabinet Office, *Work, Stress and Health: The Whitehall II Study* (London: Authors, 2004).
2. Viktor Frankl, *Man’s Search for Meaning*, rev. ed. (New York: Washington Square Press, 1984), 83–115.
3. Ibid., 90.

4. Galen Strawson, "Against Narrativity," in *The Self?*, ed. Galen Strawson (Oxford: Blackwell, 2005), 73.
5. Virginia Woolf, "A Sketch of the Past," in *Moments of Being*, 2nd ed. (San Diego: Harcourt Brace, 1985), 70–71.

21. Brain, Mind, and Agency

1. Thomas Nagel, "What Is It Like to Be a Bat?," in *Mortal Questions* (Cambridge: Cambridge University Press, 1979), 165–180.
2. David Chalmers, *The Conscious Mind: In Search of a Fundamental Theory*, 2nd ed. (Oxford: Oxford University Press, 1998), 93–111.
3. Robert Kirk, *Zombies and Consciousness* (Oxford: Clarendon Press, 2005).
4. Oliver Sacks, *Awakenings*, rev. ed. (Harmondsworth: Penguin Books, 1976), 317–318.
5. Josef Breuer and Sigmund Freud, *Studies in Hysteria*, trans. Nicola Luckhurst (London: Penguin, 2004).
6. Richard Kanaan, David Armstrong, Philip Barnes, and Simon Wessely, "In the Psychiatrist's Chair: How Neurologists Understand Conversion Disorder," *Brain* (2009): 1–8. http://brain,oxfordjournals.org/.
7. J. Grafman, "Conceptualizing Functional Neuroplasticity," *Journal of Community Disorders* , 33, no. 4 (2000): 345–355.
8. Eleanor A. Maguire, David G. Gadian, Ingrid S. Johnsrude, Catriona D. Good, John Ashburner, Richard S. J. Frakowiak, and Christopher D. Frith, "Navigation-Related Structural Change in the Hippocampi of Taxi Drivers," *Proceedings of the National Academy of Sciences of the United States of America* 27 (2000): 4398–4403.
9. Karl R. Popper and John C. Eccles, *The Self and Its Brain: An Argument for Interactionism* (Berlin: Springer, 1977).
10. Ibid., 120.
11. Ibid., 355.
12. Ibid., 366.
13. Michael Lockwood, *Mind, Brain and the Quantum: The Compound I* (Oxford: Blackwell, 1989), 8.
14. David Deutsch, *The Beginning of Infinity: Explanations That Transform the World* (London: Allen Lane, 2011), 295–296.
15. Lockwood, *Mind, Brain*, 251–259.
16. Ibid., 159, 176.
17. Kenneth S. Kendler, "Towards a Philosophical Structure for Psychiatry," *American Journal of Psychiatry*, 162, no. 3 (2005): 433.
18. Dylan Evans, *Placebo: The Belief Effect* (London: HarperCollins, 2003), chap. 4, 70–95.
19. B. Libet, C. A. Gleason, E. W. Wright, and D. K. Pearl, "Time of Conscious Intention to Act in Relation to Onset of Cerebral Activity (Readiness Potential): The Unconscious Initiation of a Freely Voluntary Act," *Brain* 106 (1983): 623–642.
20. B. Libet, "Do We Have Free Will?," *Journal of Consciousness Studies* 6, nos. 8–9 (1999): 47–57.

21. Daniel M. Wegner, *The Illusion of Conscious Will* (Cambridge, Mass.: MIT Press, 2002).

22. Psychiatric Conditions and the Framework of Responsibility

1. Aristotle, *Nicomachean Ethics,* trans. Sir David Ross (London: Oxford University Press, 1925), bk. 3.
2. Nigel Walker, *Crime and Insanity in England.* I: *The Historical Perspective* (Edinburgh: Edinburgh University Press, 1968), 91. From here to the end of this section of this chapter, I draw on this excellent historical account.
3. James Fitzjames Stephen, paper presented to the Juridical Society, quoted in ibid., 105; Barbara Wootton, *Social Science and Social Pathology* (London: Allen and Unwin, 1959), 233.
4. Margaret G. Spinelli, "Maternal Infanticide Associated with Mental Illness: Prevention and the Promise of Saved Lives," *American Journal of Psychiatry* 161 (2004): 1548–1557.
5. "Postpartum Psychosis," *PregnancyInfo.net,* www.pregnancy.info.net/postpartum_psychosis.html.
6. Duncan Campbell, *A Stranger and Afraid: The Story of Caroline Beale* (London: Macmillan, 1997), 28–29. I have drawn heavily on this account.
7. Ibid., 36.
8. Ibid., 124–125.
9. Ibid., 185–186.
10. Ibid., 167, 260.
11. Spinelli, "Maternal Infanticide."
12. P. F. Strawson, "Freedom and Resentment," in *Freedom and Resentment and Other Essays* (London: Methuen, 1976), 1–25. For a subtle and sympathetic critical discussion of Strawson, see R. Jay Wallace, *Responsibility and the Moral Sentiments* (Cambridge, Mass.: Harvard University Press, 1996).

23. What Is Addiction?

1. Bennett Foddy and Julian Savulescu, "A Liberal Account of Addiction," *Philosophy, Psychiatry & Psychology* 17, no. 1 (2010): 1–22.
2. W. Schultz, P. Apicella, and T. Ljungberg, "Responses of Monkey Dopamine Neurons to Reward and Conditioned Stimuli during Successive Steps of Learning a Delayed Response Task," *Journal of Neuroscience* 13 (1993): 900–913.
3. William James, *The Principles of Psychology* (New York: Dover, 1950), 2:541.
4. Kent C. Berridge and Terry E. Robinson, "Drug Addiction as Incentive Sensitization," in *Addiction and Responsibility,* ed. Jeffrey Poland and George Graham (Cambridge, Mass.: MIT Press, 2011), 21–53.
5. Steven E. Hyman, "Addiction: A Disease of Learning and Memory," *American Journal of Psychiatry* 162 (2005): 1414–1422.
6. Foddy and Savulescu, "Liberal Account," 3–7.
7. Ibid., 6.
8. Mark Griffiths, "Does Internet and Computer 'Addiction' Exist? Some Case Study Evidence," *Cyberpsychology and Behavior* 5, no. 2 (2000): 211–218.

9. Quoted in Alexander Nehamas, *Only a Promise of Happiness: The Place of Beauty in a World of Art* (Princeton: Princeton University Press, 2007), 129.
10. Dostoyevsky's letter to his brother Michael, quoted in Jessie Coulson's Introduction to her translation of *The Gambler* (Harmondsworth: Penguin Books, 1966), from which the quoted passage is taken.
11. Mark D. Griffiths, "Is 'Loss of Control' Always a Consequence of Addiction?," *Frontiers in Psychiatry* 4, no. 36 (2013).
12. Mark Griffiths, *Gambling and Gaming Addictions in Adolescence* (Leicester: British Psychological Society / Blackwell, 2002).
13. Foddy and Savulescu, "Liberal Account," 10.
14. J. M. Fischer and M. Ravizza, *Responsibility and Control: A Theory of Moral Responsibility* (New York: Cambridge University Press, 1998).

24. Unwilling Addiction as Diminished Control

1. Plato, *Republic*, 425e, 426a.
2. Samuel Taylor Coleridge, letter to Joseph Cottle, April 26, 1814.
3. *Nicomachean Ethics,* bk. 7.
4. Here I sidestep a number of complications. See, for instance, David Wiggins, "Weakness of Will, Commensurability, and the Object of Deliberation and Desire," in *Needs, Values, Truth: Essays in the Philosophy of Value* (Oxford: Basil Blackwell, 1987), 239–267.
5. Lee N. Robins, Darlene H. Davis, and David N. Nurco, "How Permanent Was Vietnam Drug Addiction?," *American Journal of Public Health* 64, no. 12 (1974): 38–43; Lee N. Robins, "Vietnam Veterans' Rapid Recovery from Heroin Addiction: A Fluke or Normal Expectation?," *Addiction* 88 (1993): 1041–1054.
6. Nigel Walker, "Liberty, Liability, Culpability," in *Psychopathic Disorders,* ed. Michael Craft (London: Mass Market Paperback, 1966).
7. Richard J. Herrnstein and Drazen Prelec, "A Theory of Addiction," in *Choice over Time,* ed. George Loewenstein and Jon Elster (New York: Russell Sage Foundation, 1992), 331–360.
8. Sunny S. J. Lin and Chin-Chung Tsai, "Sensation Seeking and Internet Dependence of Taiwanese High School Adolescents," *Computers in Human Behavior* 18, no. 4 (2002): 412–426; Mehwash Mehroof and Mark D. Griffiths, "Online Gaming Addiction: The Role of Sensation Seeking, Self-Control, Neuroticism, Aggression, State Anxiety, and Trait Anxiety," *Cyberpsychology, Behavior, and Social Networking* 13, no. 3(2010): 313–316.
9. Jaime Derringer et al., "Predicting Sensation Seeking from Dopamine Genes," *Psychological Science* 21, no. 9 (2010): 1282–1290.
10. J. Coid, M. Yang, P. Tyrer, A. Roberts, and S. Ulrich, "Prevalence and Correlates of Personality Disorder in Great Britain," *British Journal of Psychiatry* 188 (2006): 423–431.
11. C. A. J. Dejong, W. van den Brink, F. M. Harteveld, and E. G. van der Wielen, "Personality Disorders in Alcoholics and Drug Addicts," *Comprehensive Psychiatry* 34, no. 2 (2003): 87–94.

12. Owen Flanagan, "What Is It Like to Be an Addict?," in *Addiction and Responsibility,* ed. Jeffrey Poland and George Graham (Cambridge, Mass.: MIT Press, 2011), 275, 278.
13. Caroline Knapp, *Drinking: A Love Story* (London: Quartet Books, 1996), 17.
14. B. Hurwitz, C. Tapping, and N. Vickers, "Life Histories and Narratives of Addiction," State-of-Science Review, Foresight Brain Science, Addiction and Drugs Project, Office of Science and Technology, London, 2005.
15. Keith E. Stanovich and Richard F. West, "Individual Differences in Reasoning: Implications for the Rationality Debate," *Behavioral and Brain Sciences* 23 (2000): 645–665; Daniel Kahneman, *Thinking Fast and Slow* (London: Allen Lane/Penguin, 2011).
16. A. David Redish, Steve Jensen, and Adam Johnson, "A Unified Framework for Addiction: Vulnerabilities in the Decision Process," *Behavioral and Brain Sciences* 31 (2006): 415–487; David Redish, *The Mind within the Brain: How We Make Decisions and How Those Decisions Go Wrong* (New York: Oxford University Press, 2013), 171–192.
17. R. Holton, "Rational Resolve," *Philosophical Review* 113 (2004): 507–535.
18. Roy F. Baumeister, Mark Muraven, and Dianne M. Tice, "Ego Depletion: A Resource Model of Volition, Self-Regulation and Controlled Processing," *Social Cognition* 18, no. 2 (2000): 130–150.
19. Kathleen D. Vohs and Todd F. Heatherton, "Self-Regulatory Failure: A Resource-Depletion Approach," *Psychological Science* 11, no. 3 (2000): 249–254.
20. Neil Levy, "Addiction, Responsibility and Ego-Depletion," in *Addiction and Responsibility,* ed. Jeffrey Poland and George Graham (Cambridge, Mass.: MIT Press, 2011), 89–111.
21. Janet Treasure, "Motivational Interviewing," *Advances in Psychiatric Treatment* 10 (2004): 321–337.
22. Mark Muraven, "Autonomous Self-Control Is Less Depleting," *Journal of Research in Personality* 42 (2008): 763–770.
23. Mark Muraven and Roy F. Baumeister, "Self-Regulation and Depletion of Limited Resources: Does Self-Control Resemble a Muscle?," *Psychological Bulletin* 126 (2000): 247–259.
24. Hanna Pickard and Steve Pearce, "Addiction in Context: Philosophical Lessons from a Personality Disorder Clinic," in *Addiction and Self-Control: Perspectives from Philosophy, Psychology and Neuroscience,* ed. Neil Levy (Oxford: Oxford University Press, 2013).
25. R. Jay Wallace, "Addiction as Defect of the Will: Some Philosophical Reflections," *Law and Philosophy* 18 (1999): 621–654.
26. Pickard and Pearce, "Addiction in Context," 2013.
27. Steve Pearce and Hanna Pickard, "Finding the Will to Recover: Perspectives on Agency and the Sick Role," *Journal of Medical Ethics,* doi: 10.1136/jme.2010.035865.
28. George Ainslie, *Breakdown of Will* (Cambridge: Cambridge University Press, 2001), chaps. 5 and 6; Ainslie, "Free Will as Recursive Self-Prediction: Does a Deterministic Mechanism Reduce Responsibility?," in *Addiction and*

Responsibility, ed. Jeffrey Poland and George Graham (Cambridge, Mass.: MIT Press, 2011), 55–87.

25. Character, Personality Disorder, and Responsibility

1. I have taken the account of his childhood and personal life from Robert G. L. Waite, *The Psychopathic God: Adolf Hitler* (New York: Basic Books, 1977), republished by Da Capo Press, (New York, 1993). Waite gives sources for the claims made here. There are obvious reasons for caution about psychohistory, especially about retrospective diagnosis. (A good survey of the many conflicting "diagnoses" of Hitler by psychiatrists and others is William Carr, *Hitler: A Study in Personality and Politics* (London: Edward Arnold, 1978), chap. 5.) On the personal details and the childhood, it is hard to be confident about all the particular claims, but Waite's sources are sufficiently varied to make the general picture plausible.

   In the major English-language biography of Hitler, Ian Kershaw cites a skeptical review of Waite by Rudolph Binion (*Journal of Psychohistory* [1977]: 295–300) and says that "attempts to find in the youngster "the warped person within the murderous dictator" [Waite's words] have proved unpersuasive" (Ian Kershaw, *Hitler, 1889–1936: Hubris* [London: Penguin, 2001], 13, 607 n. 64.) With proper skepticism, Kershaw says the impact of Hitler's childhood on his character is "a matter of speculation" and that "assumptions have to remain guesswork." But he also says that "it takes little to imagine that his later patronizing contempt for the submissiveness of women, the thirst for dominance (and the imagery of the Leader as a stern, authoritarian father-figure), the inability to form deep personal relationships, the corresponding cold brutality towards humankind, and—not least—the capacity for hatred so profound that it must have reflected an immeasurable undercurrent of self-hatred concealed in the extreme narcissism that was its counterpoint must surely have had roots in the subliminal influences of the young Adolf's family circumstances" (Kershaw, *Hitler*, 13.)
2. A. Caspi, J. McClay, T. E. Moffitt, J. Mill, J. Martin, I. Craig, A. Taylor, and R. Poulton, "Role of Genotype in the Cycle of Violence in Maltreated Children," *Science* 297 (2002): 851–854; T. E. Moffitt and A. Caspi, "Evidence from Behavioural Genetics for Environmental Contributions to Antisocial Conduct," in *The Explanation of Crime, Context, Mechanisms and Development*, ed. P. O. Wikstrom and R. J. Sampson (Cambridge: Cambridge University Press, 2006), 108–152.
3. T. E. Moffitt, "Genetic and Environmental Influences on Antisocial Behaviors: Evidence from Behavioral-Genetic Research," *Advances in Genetics* (Elsevier) (2005).
4. D. Foley, B. Wormley, J. Silberg, H. Maes, J. Hewitt, L. Eaves, and B. Riley, "Childhood Adversity, MAOA Genotype, and Risk for Conduct Disorder," *Archives of General Psychiatry* 61 (2004): 738–744.
5. David Hume, *A Treatise of Human Nature* (1739), bk. 2, pt. 3, sec. 1.

26. The Sense of Self

1. Jan Morris, *Conundrum* (New York: Harcourt Brace Jovanovich, 1974), 38.
2. Michael B. First, "Desire for Amputation of a Limb: Paraphilias, Psychosis or a New Type of Identity Disorder," *Psychological Medicine* 34 (2004): 1–10.
3. P. D. McGeoch, D. Brang, T. Song, R. Lee, M. Huang, and V. S. Ramachandran, "Xenomelia: A New Right Parietal Syndrome," *Journal of Neurology, Neurosurgery and Psychiatry* 82 (2011): 1314–1319.
4. Sean O'Connor, reply to a disabled person whose own legs do not work and who was shocked by someone wanting to cast away functioning legs, Treadmarkz: Leaving Treadmarkz Across the Universe, poster, July 17, 2008.
5. Gunilla Gerland, *A Real Person: Life on the Outside,* trans. Joan Tate (London: Souvenir Press, 1997), 208–209, 220–221.

27. Moral Identity and Moral Injury

1. "Falklands Veterans Claim Suicide Toll," BBC website, January 13, 2002.
2. Diane Silver, "Beyond PTSD: Soldiers Have Injured Souls," *Miller-McCune,* reproduced on *Truthout,* September 3, 2011.
3. Eric Newhouse, "Half of Vets Returning from Iraq and Afghanistan Need Medical Attention," *Truthout,* November 16, 2011.
4. Tony McNally, *Watching Men Burn: A Soldier's Story* (London: Monday Books, 2007),121–122.
5. Ibid., 125–126.
6. Ibid., 157–158.
7. Ibid., 201.
8. Bernard Williams, "Moral Luck," in *Moral Luck and Other Essays* (Cambridge: Cambridge University Press, 1981), 27–39.
9. Nancy Sherman, *The Untold War: Inside the Hearts, Minds and Souls of Our Soldiers,* (New York: W. W. Norton, 2010), 99.
10. Karl Marlantes, *What It Is Like to Go to War* (London: Corvus, 2012), 27.
11. Bill Moyers interview with Karl Marlantes, *Moyers and Company,* reproduced on *Truthout,* August 1, 2012.
12. Marlantes, *What It Is Like,* 50.
13. Jonathan Shay, *Achilles in Vietnam: Combat Trauma and the Undoing of Character* (New York: Scribner, 1994), 78–79.
14. McNally, *Watching Men Burn,* p. 140.
15. Sherman, *The Untold War,* 90.
16. Bill Moyers interview with Karl Marlantes.
17. Jonathan Shay, *Achilles in Vietnam: Combat Trauma and the Undoing of Character* (New York: Scribner, 1994); Jonathan Shay, *Odysseus in America: Combat Trauma and the Trials of Homecoming* (New York: Scribner, 2002). This chapter owes a lot to these books, and borrows heavily from Shay's rethinking of post-traumatic stress disorder as moral injury.
18. Bill Moyers interview with Karl Marlantes.
19. Shay, *Achilles in Vietnam,* xxii.
20. Ibid., 31 and 33.

21. Joshua E. S. Phillips, *None of Us Were Like This Before* (London: Verso, 2010), 186.
22. Edward Tick, *War and the Soul* (Wheaton, Ill.: Quest Books, 2005), 100.
23. Rachel Yehuda, in *Psychological Trauma,* ed. Rachel Yehuda (Washington D.C.: American Psychiatric Press, 1998), xiv.
24. Paul Carey, David J. Castle, and Dan J. Stein "Anxiety Disorders," in *Essential Psychiatry,* 4th ed., ed. Robin M. Murray (Cambridge: Cambridge University Press, 2008), 160–162.
25. Bill Moyers interview with Karl Marlantes.
26. McNally, *Watching Men Burn,* 226, 238, 241.
27. Marlantes, *What It Is Like,* 32.
28. Shay, *Achilles in Vietnam,* 185–187.
29. Bernard J. Verkamp, *The Moral Treatment of Returning Warriors in Early Medieval and Modern Times* (Scranton, Pa.: University of Scranton Press, 2006), 2–8.
30. Shay, *Achilles in Vietnam,* 188–194.
31. Tick, *War and the Soul,* 190–194.
32. Marlantes, *What It Is Like,* 32.
33. Larry Dewey, *War and Redemption: Treatment and Recovery in Combat-Related Posttraumatic Stress Disorder* (Burlington, Vt.: Ashgate, 2004), 199–200.

28. Psychotherapy, Autonomy, and Self-Creation

1. Paul Biegler: *The Ethical Treatment of Depression: Autonomy through Psychotherapy* (Cambridge, Mass.: MIT Press, 2011).
2. *Treatment Choice in Psychological Therapies and Counselling,* Department of Health, London 2001; Graeme Whitfield and Chris Williams, "The Evidence Base for Cognitive-Behavioural Therapy in Depression: Delivery in Busy Clinical Settings," *Advances in Psychiatric Treatment* 9 (2003): 21–30.
3. Ludwig von Bertalanffy, *General Systems Theory: Foundations, Development, Applications,* rev. ed. (New York: George Braziller, 2003); Gregory Bateson *Steps to an Ecology of Mind,* 2nd ed. (Chicago: University of Chicago Press, 2000); Mara Selvini Palazzoli, *Paradox and Counter-Paradox: A New Model of the Therapy of the Family in Schizophrenic Transaction,* trans. Elisabeth V. Burt (Northvale, N.J.: Jason Aronson, 1978).
4. Bertalanffy, *General Systems Theory,* 32, 55–56.
5. Ibid., 215, 219.
6. Bateson, *Ecology of Mind,* 190.
7. Ibid., 186–193.
8. Robin M. Murray and Kimberlie Dean, "Schizophrenia and Related Disorders," in *Essential Psychiatry,* 4th ed., ed. Robin M. Murray, Kenneth S. Kendler, Peter McGuffin, Simon Wessely, and David J. Castle (Cambridge: Cambridge University Press, 2008), 284–319.
9. Palazzoli, *Paradox and Counter-Paradox,* 8.
10. John Byng-Hall, *Rewriting Family Scripts: Improvisation and Systems Change* (New York: Guilford Press, 1995).
11. Palazzoli, *Paradox and Counter-Paradox,* 3–4.

12. Ibid., 3–4.
13. Murray and Dean, "Schizophrenia and Related Disorders."
14. Palazzoli, *Paradox and Counter-Paradox,* 21–25.
15. Ibid., 16–17.
16. *The Burial at Thebes:* Sophocles' *Antigone,* trans. Seamus Heaney (London: Faber and Faber, 2004), 28.
17. John Byng-Hall, "Family Legends: Their Significance for the Family Therapist," in *Family Therapy: Complementary Frameworks of Theory and Practice,* ed. Arnon Bentovim, Gill Gorrell Barnes, and Alan Cooklin (London: Academic Press, 1987), 177–192.
18. John Byng-Hall, "Dysfunction of Feeling: Experiential Life of the Family," in Bentovim, Gorrell Barnes and Cooklin, *Family Therapy,* 75–93.
19. Ceri Bowen, Peter Stratton, and Anna Madiff, "Psychological Functioning in Families That Blame: From Blaming Events to Theory Integration," John Stancombe and Sue White, "Cause and Responsibility: Towards an Interactional Understanding of Blaming and 'Neutrality' in Family Therapy," Katja Kurri and Jarl Wahlstrom, "Placement of Responsibility and Moral Reasoning in Couple Therapy," and Michelle O'Reilly, "The Complaining Client and the Troubled Therapist: A Discursive Investigation of Family Therapy," all in *Journal of Family Therapy* 17, no. 4 (2005).
20. Alasdair MacIntyre, *After Virtue* (London: Duckworth, 1977), 30.
21. Sigmund Freud, *The Ego and the Id,* trans. Joan Riviere, revised by James Strachey (New York: W. W. Norton, 1989), chap. 2.
22. Stuart Hampshire and H. L. A. Hart, "Decision, Intention and Certainty," *Mind* 67 (1958); Richard Moran, *Authority and Estrangement: An Essay on Self-Knowledge* (Princeton: Princeton University Press, 2001), 55–60.

29. Entrapment in Eating Disorders

1. Janet Treasure and Ulrike Schmidt, "Eating Disorders," in *Essential Psychiatry,* 4th ed., ed. Robin M. Murray, Kenneth S. Kendler, Peter McGuffin, Simon Wessely, and David J. Castle (Cambridge: Cambridge University Press, 2008), chap. 9.
2. Christopher G. Fairburn, *Cognitive Behaviour Therapy and Eating Disorders* (New York: Guilford Press, 2008), chaps. 2 and 8.
3. Treasure and Schmidt, "Eating Disorders," 184–185. Citations have been omitted.
4. The sequence is "adapted" from Waller and Kennerley, "Cognitive-Behavioural Treatments," in *Handbook of Eating Disorders,* 2nd ed., ed. Janet Treasure et al. (Chichester: John Wiley, 2003).
5. Helen, in Rosemary Shelley, ed., *Anorexics on Anorexia* (London: Jessica Kingsley, 1997), 102.
6. Carla, in ibid., 30–31.
7. Alison, in ibid., 76–77.
8. Kirsty, in ibid., 126–127.
9. "There Goes Alice Down the Hole," in *Bulimics on Bulimia,* ed. Maria Stavrou (London: Jessica Kingsley, 2009), 25–26.

10. "Surrounded by People but Completely Alone," in Stavrou, *Bulimics on Bulimia,* 42–43.
11. Treasure and Schmidt, "Eating Disorders," 182.
12. "Binging and Purging to Stay Alive," in Stavrou, *Bulimics on Bulimia,* 20.
13. Sara, in Shelley, *Anorexics on Anorexia,* 63–64.
14. "Running Away but Going Nowhere," in Stavrou, *Bulimics on Bulimia,* 49.
15. Grace Bowman, *A Shape of My Own: A Memoir of Anorexia and Recovery* (London: Viking, 2006), 66.
16. Fiona, in Shelley, *Anorexics on Anorexia,* 21.
17. Kate, in ibid., 14.
18. Simon, in ibid., 58.
19. Anne, in ibid., 68.
20. Alison, in ibid., 79.
21. Sara, in ibid., 64.
22. Callum, in ibid., 139.
23. Quoted in Mim Udovitch, "A Secret Society of the Starving," *New York Times Magazine,* September 8, 2002.
24. J. Arcelus et al., "Mortality Rates in Patients with Anorexia Nervosa and Other Eating Disorders: A Meta-Analysis of 36 Studies," *Archives of General Psychiatry* 68, no. 7 (July 2011): 724–731.
25. E. J. Button et al., "Mortality and Predictors of Death in a Cohort of Patients Presenting to an Eating Disorders Service," *International Journal of Eating Disorders* 43, no. 5 (July 2010): 387–392.
26. Andrew Sutherland, "Why Are So Many People Dying on Everest?," *BMJ* 333.7565 (2006): 452.
27. Sara, "Starving out of Shame," in Shelley, *Anorexics on Anorexia.*
28. Emily Halban, *Perfect: Anorexia and Me* (London: Ebury Publishing, 2008), 7.
29. Sara, in Shelley, *Anorexics on Anorexia,* 64.
30. Jeanette Winterson, *Why Be Happy When You Could Be Normal?* (London: Jonathan Cape, 2011), 86–87.
31. proanalifestyle.blogspot.com, July 23, 2007.

30. Authenticity and Identity in Eating Disorders

1. Jacinta Tan, Tony Hope, Anne Stewart, and Raymond Fitzpatrick, "Competence to Make Treatment Decisions in Anorexia Nervosa: Thinking Processes and Values," *Philosophy, Psychiatry & Psychology* 13, no. 4 (2006): 267–282. See also J. Tan, R. A. Hope, and A. Stewart, "Competence to Refuse Treatment in Anorexia Nervosa," *International Journal of Law and Psychiatry* 26, no. 6 (2003): 697–707; Tan, Hope, and Stewart, "Anorexia Nervosa and Personal Identity: The Accounts of Patients and Their Parents," *International Journal of Law and Psychiatry* 26, no. 6 (2003): 533–548.
2. Quoted in Tan, Hope, and Stewart, "Competence to Refuse."
3. "An Addictive Personality, Food and Alcohol," in *Bulimics on Bulimia,* ed. Maria Stavrou (London: Jessica Kingsley, 2009), 112.
4. Hilde Bruch, *The Golden Cage* (Cambridge, Mass.: Harvard University Press, 2001), 16–18.

5. Ibid., 18.
6. Emma Baldock, "A Test of Authenticity for the Liberty to Make High Cost Treatment Decisions with Special Application to Anorexia Nervosa," PhD thesis, King's College London, 2009.
7. Grace Bowman, *A Shape of My Own: A Memoir of Anorexia and Recovery* (London: Viking, 2006), 118.
8. Simon, in Rosemary Shelley, ed., *Anorexics on Anorexia* (London: Jessica Kingsley, 1997) 55–56.
9. Helen, in ibid., 105.
10. "The Hardest Part Is Wanting to Recover," in Stavrou, *Bulimics on Bulimia,* 62.
11. Sara, in Shelley, *Anorexics on Anorexia,* 62.
12. "I Want to be Like You," in Stavrou, *Bulimics on Bulimia,* 128.
13. Joanne, in Shelley, *Anorexics on Anorexia,* 49.
14. Alison, in ibid., 76.
15. "Not Good Enough," in Stavrou, *Bulimics on Bulimia,* 98.
16. Joanne, in Shelley, *Anorexics on Anorexia,* 49.
17. Cherry, in ibid., 87.
18. Kate, in ibid., 12.
19. Emily Halban, *Perfect: Anorexia and Me* (London: Ebury Publishing, 2008), 77–78.
20. Fiona, in Shelley, *Anorexics on Anorexia,* 22, 25.
21. Richard Keshen, *Reasonable Self-Esteem* (Montreal: McGill-Queen's University Press, 1996), 20–34.
22. Virginia Woolf, "A Sketch of the Past," in *Moments of Being,* 2nd ed. (San Diego: Harcourt Brace, 1985), 80.
23. Simona Giordano, *Understanding Eating Disorders: Conceptual and Ethical Issues in the Treatment of Anorexia and Bulimia Nervosa* (Oxford: Clarendon Press, 2005).
24. "Surrounded by People but Completely Alone," in Stavrou, *Bulimics on Bulimia,* 43.
25. A patient, quoted in Hilde Bruch, *The Golden Cage: The Enigma of Anorexia Nervosa* (Cambridge Mass.: Harvard University Press, 1978), 49, reprinted 2001.
26. Kate, in Shelley, *Anorexics on Anorexia,* 14, 18.
27. Cherry, in ibid., 88–91.
28. Lisa, in ibid., 136.
29. Cherry, in ibid., 92–93.
30. "Surrounded by People," 47.
31. Giordano, *Understanding Eating Disorders,* 159–163.
32. Keshen, *Reasonable Self-Esteem,* 28–33.
33. Bowman, *Shape of My Own,* 243.
34. Joanne, in Shelley, *Anorexics on Anorexia,* 49, 51.

31. Dementia, Responsibility, and Identity

1. Julie F. Snowden, David Neary, and David M. A. Mann, "Frontotemporal Dementia, Old Age Psychiatry Papers," *British Journal of Psychiatry* 180 (2002): 140–143; Mario F. Mendez, Jill S. Shapira, and Ronald E. Saul, "The Spectrum

of Sociopathy in Dementia," *Journal of Neuropsychiatry and Clinical Neurosciences* 23 (2011): 132–140.

2. These two accounts come from Mario F. Mendez, "The Unique Predisposition to Criminal Violations in Frontotemporal Dementia," *Journal of the American Academy of Psychiatry and Law* 38, no. 3 (2010): 318–323.
3. Tony Hope, "Personal Identity and Psychiatric Illness," in *Philosophy, Psychology and Psychiatry,* ed. A. Phillips Griffiths (Cambridge: Cambridge University Press, 1996), 131–143.
4. Catherine Oppenheimer, "I Am, Thou Art: Personal Identity in Dementia," in *Dementia: Mind, Meaning and the Person,* ed. Julian C. Hughes, Stephen J. Louw, and Steven R. Sabat (Oxford: Clarendon Press, 2006), 202.
5. Jennifer Radden, "Into the Darkness: Losing Identity with Dementia," in Hughes, Louw, and Sabat, *Dementia,* 83.
6. Iris Murdoch, "Vision and Choice in Morality," in *Existentialists and Mystics: Writings on Philosophy and Literature,* ed. Peter Conradi (London: Penguin, 1999), 80–81.
7. John Bayley, *Iris: A Memoir* (London: Duckworth, 1998), 34–45. The following quotations are also from this source.
8. John Bayley, *Iris and the Friends* (London: Duckworth, 1999), 232.

32. Schizophrenia

1. Richard Bentall, ed., *Reconstructing Schizophrenia* (London: Routledge, 1990); Man Cheung Chung, K. W. M. (Bill) Fulford, and George Graham, eds., *Reconceiving Schizophrenia* (Oxford: Oxford University Press, 2007).
2. Tove Jansson, *Finn Family Moomintroll,* trans. Elizabeth Portch (London: Puffin Books, 1961).
3. There is an interesting discussion of some different versions of the new schizophrenia-related personality in Paul Lysaker and John Lysaker, *Schizophrenia and the Fate of the Self* (Oxford: Oxford University Press, 2008), chap. 4.
4. Jay Neugeboren, *Imagining Robert: My Brother, Madness and Survival* (New York: Henry Holt, 1997), 252–253.
5. Ibid., 303.
6. Viktor Frankl, *Man's Search for Meaning* (New York: Rider, 1959), 169.

33. Self-Creation, Values, and Psychiatric Disorder

1. Richard A. Schweder, "Menstrual Pollution, Soul Loss, and the Comparative Study of Emotions," in *Culture and Depression: Studies in the Anthropology and Cross-Cultural Psychiatry of Affect and Disorder,* ed. Arthur Kleinman and Byron Good (Berkeley: University of California Press, 1985), 182–215.
2. "Melancholy, Mood and Landscape," in Jennifer Radden, *Moody Minds Distempered* (New York: Oxford University Press, 2009), 180–187.
3. Richard Mabey, *Nature Cure* (London: Chatto and Windus, 2005).
4. Ibid., 62–64.
5. Ibid., 223–224.
6. Richard Fortey, *The Hidden Landscape: A Journey into the Geological Past* (London: The Bodley Head, 2010).

7. O wie werdet ihr dann, Nächte, mir lieb sein,
gehärmte. Das ich euch knieender nicht, untröstliche
        Schwestern,
hinnahm, nicht in euer gelöstes
Haar mich gelöster ergab. Wir, Vergeuder der Schmerzen.
Wie wir sie absehn voraus, in die traurige Dauer,
ob sie nicht enden vielleicht. Sie aber sind ja
unser winterwähriges Laub, unser dunkeles Sinngrün,
einer der Zeiten des heimlichen Jares-, nicht nur
Zeit-, sind Stelle, Siedelung, Lager, Boden, Wohnort.
8. Lauren Slater, *Prozac Diary* (London: Penguin, 1998), 186–200.
9. Ibid., 191.
10. Felicity Bryan, "Once We Had a Daughter," *The Guardian,* April 22, 2006.
11. Kay Redfield Jamison, *An Unquiet Mind: A Memoir of Mood and Madness* (London: Picador 1996), 161–169. The following quotations in the text are from this source, pages 91–97 and 217–18.
12. Simon Champ, "A Most Precious Thread," in *From the Ashes of Experience: Madness, Survival, Growth,* ed. Phil Barker, Peter Campbell, and Ben Davidson (London: Whurr, 1999), 113–126.

ACKNOWLEDGMENTS

Central to this book are the interviews with men in Broadmoor Hospital who have a diagnosis of antisocial personality disorder. They were carried out in conjunction with parallel interviews by the Broadmoor psychiatrist Dr. Gwen Adshead, with the support of her able research assistants Sarah Nicholson and Chris Brown. Gwen was a delight to work with, and I learned an enormous amount from her. I am grateful to Val Pancucci for transcribing the interviews. I also want to thank those who were interviewed. They were often willing to tell me very personal things. I thank them for agreeing to be interviewed and agreeing to their (anonymized) comments being used in writing up the project.

The Wellcome Trust funded the project. They have had to wait a long time for any published results from my part of it. I thank them for their support and patience.

Part of the Wellcome project was a parallel set of interviews with people with a diagnosis of frontotemporal dementia, a condition that also can lead to antisocial behavior. This came from a generous invitation from Professor Martin Rossor of the National Hospital for Neurology and Neurosurgery. I will never forget sitting in the corner of his office for a morning, while at regular intervals patients came in to be told that their diagnosis was this form of dementia. Martin was the ideal doctor: sharply focused on the results of the imaging, and also honest, clear, and calmly supportive. My interviews were much less good. Some patients were at an early stage of dementia. Asked about ethics, they gave fine answers belied by their reported behavior. Most of the others were too far gone to understand the questions. I was not creative enough to find ways of dealing with this. I gave up on this part of the project. I wish I had managed a better response to Martin's imaginative idea.

As well as quoting from the Broadmoor interviews, I have quoted a lot in the book from the growing number of first-person accounts of psychiatric disorder. One of the main themes of the book is the way accounts from the inside should help in redrawing the psychiatric map. I thank all the people whose published accounts I have quoted.

Art is also a way into the inside of these conditions. I have been particularly struck by the art of Laura Freeman, as it appears on her website. I thank her for permission to use several of her powerful pictures.

This book also grew out of "Towards Humanism in Psychiatry," my 2003 Tanner Lectures on Human Values at Princeton. I am grateful to the Trustees of the Tanner Lectures on Human Values, and to Princeton's Center for Human Values, for the invitation to give the lectures, and for permission to use material from the lectures in this book. I thank Princeton University and the Center for Human Values for generous hospitality, and for inviting the very distinguished team of Peter Brooks, Antonio Damasio, Jonathan Lear, and Jennifer Radden to be the respondents to the lectures. I learned a lot and enjoyed the discussions enormously.

I have been writing this book on and off for a number of years, mainly while I was director of the Centre of Medical Law and Ethics, in the Law School at King's College London. From that time I have many warm memories of the generosity and friendship of colleagues and students alike.

This book has been influenced by colleagues in the Centre, either by their general support or by their own thoughts or research on psychiatry. These include Jennifer Bostock, Jill Craigie, Sue Eckstein, Bobbie Farsides, Don Hill, Penney Lewis, David Lloyd, Genevra Richardson, Rosamund Scott, Suzanne Shale, and Leslie Sherratt. Pat Walsh ran a group on ethical issues in autism, culminating in an outstanding conference run by Pat herself with Virginia Bovell and Francesca Happé. I have been influenced by them and by other speakers at the conference.

I am grateful to my successor as director, Leif Wenar, and to four successive heads of the Law School—John Phillips, Raymond Plant, Tim Macklem, and David Caron—for keeping me on to do some teaching after the standard retirement age. This has postponed what will be a great loss in my life. My students have no idea how much they have given me.

When I arrived at King's, a great stimulus was the warm welcome by the Institute of Psychiatry, especially by Channi Kumar, Robin Murray, George Szmukler, and Simon Wessely. I have learned from all of them.

My Tanner Lectures grew out of the 2002 Aubrey Lewis Lecture I gave at the IoP at the invitation of George Szmukler. Another stimulus was the invitation to help colleagues at the IoP and in the Philosophy Department in setting up and teaching the MSc course in Philosophy of Mental Disorder. Among those I learned from are Derek Bolton, Bill Fulford, David Papineau, Mark Sainsbury, and Richard Samuels. I also introduced and taught a psychiatric module in the MA in Medical Ethics and Law run by the Centre of Medical Law and Ethics. I am grateful to those (too many to name) in the courses for the special kind of stimulus that bright, responsive, and argumentative students give to their lucky teachers.

Among those whose thoughts, criticisms, experiences, or suggestions have influenced this book are Natalie Acton, Richard Ashcroft, Emma Baldock, Simone Bateman, Linda Begbie, Walter Bilderback, Felicity Bryan, Virginia Bovell, John Burbidge, John Campbell, Patrick Casement, Ann Davis, Heather Dyke, Ivan Eisler, Rai Gaita, Simona Giordano, Anita Grandy, Jim Hopkins, Monique Jonas, Richard Kanaan, Lucien Karhausen, Elleke Landeweer, Ruth Macklin, Dan Moros, Thomas Nagel, Gunilla Oberg, Christopher Peacocke, Liz Pellicano, Priscilla Roth, Alan Ryan, Thomas Schramme, James Stewart, Jim Strain, Jacinta Tan, Nadia Whittaker, Guy Widdershoven, and Charlotte Wilson.

My thanks to Clare Sainsbury, once an undergraduate I taught as part of her Philosophy, Politics and Economics course at New College, Oxford. More recently she has been a friend who in turn has taught me a huge amount about Asperger's syndrome in particular and about psychiatry more generally. My thanks to Tony Hope, who, much earlier, I once taught as part of his Philosophy, Psychology and Physiology course at New College. For many years he has been both a friend and the sort of psychiatrist and then ethics teacher his patients and students must have been really lucky to have.

Bill Ruddick has read much of this book and has commented on it with generosity and perceptiveness, in many subtle ways influencing it for the better.

Hanna Pickard has read the book and made valuable suggestions, especially about addiction, that I have followed up. At a point when I felt low about the book, her support for it was a lifeline.

Richard Keshen has read and commented on the book. He has done this with most of what I have written since I was his graduate supervisor in Oxford many years ago. Some of my best students end up teaching me.

He has influenced me over the years more than he can realize. While I was writing the section about William Blake, one of the pleasures was going with Richard and Mary Keshen to look at places in London with Blake associations. (At that time I thought of writing also about Virginia Woolf's psychiatric illness, an idea I gave up when I saw that I would not be able to do it nearly as well as Hermione Lee in her Virginia Woolf biography. But it was still a great pleasure to go with Vivette and with Richard and Mary to the Woolfs' home at Monk's House.)

Ian Malcolm, at Harvard University Press, has been an ideal editor. He has improved the book a lot through constructive critical comments. He has been wonderfully supportive of the book, to an extent only its grateful author knows.

Finally, my family. It is now impossible to disentangle the different strands of their contribution: intellectual, emotional, critical, and supportive, as well as through shared experience. Vivette, Daniel, David, and Ruth all have different angles on the questions discussed in this book and have influenced me enormously. In different ways Daniel and David have greatly influenced my thoughts about what to say and about how to say it. In recent years Vivette's research has been in biological psychiatry. Ruth is a child psychotherapist. I have been inspired by the work they each do. Their ways of seeing these matters are overlapping but different. To some extent I have internalized both perspectives. Have I really got good evidence for this claim? Is that comment a bit crude and unperceptive about the person discussed? The combination of the skeptical questions and the inspiration has improved the book a lot.

I dedicate the book to my grandson, Sam, in gratitude for many interesting conversations lit up by his lively, humorous, and questioning approach to life.

INDEX